The
Complete
Book of
Running
for Women

The
Complete
Book of
Running
for Women

**Everything You Need to Know About Training,
Nutrition, Injury Prevention, Motivation,
Racing and Much, Much More**

CLAIRE KOWALCHIK

POCKET BOOKS

NEW YORK LONDON TORONTO SYDNEY

The author of this book is not a physician, and the ideas, procedures, and suggestions in this book are not intended as a substitute for the medical advice of a trained health professional. All matters regarding your health require medical supervision. Consult your physician before adopting the suggestions in this book, as well as about any condition that may require diagnosis or medical attention. The author and publisher disclaim any liability arising directly or indirectly from the use of this book.

An *Original* Publication of POCKET BOOKS

POCKET BOOKS, a division of Simon & Schuster Inc.
1230 Avenue of the Americas, New York, NY 10020

Library of Congress Cataloging-in-Publication Data

Kowalchik, Claire.
    The complete book of running for women : everything you need to know about training, nutrition, injury prevention, motivation, racing and much, much more / Claire Kowalchik.
        p.   cm.
Includes bibliographical references and index.
ISBN 0-671-01703-9
1. Running for women.   2. Physical fitness for women.   I. Title.
GV1061.18.266 K68 1999
613.7'172'082—dc21   98-50318

First Pocket Books trade paperback printing March 1999

30 29 28 27 26

Cover design by Lisa Litwack, front cover photo © Jim Cummins/FPG
Book design by Alma Orenstein
Illustrations by Joann Owen Coy

Printed in the U.S.A.

In memory of my parents,
Hazel and Michael Kowalchik

Acknowledgments

MANY MINDS HAVE HELPED CREATE THIS BOOK. MY SINCERE thanks to the women of Making Strides, my Tuesday night running group, and the women runners everywhere who have shared their thoughts and experiences with me. To the staff of *Runner's World* magazine, especially executive editor Amby Burfoot, from whom I learned so much. To sports nutritionist Nancy Clark, M.S., R.D., and Judy Mahle Lutter, president of the Melpomene Institute for Women's Health Research, who reviewed many of the chapters of this book for accuracy.

And special thanks to my friend, mentor, and "coach," Budd Coates, for his help editorially as well as athletically: I wouldn't be the runner I am today without him.

Of course none of this would have happened without editor Greer Kessel Hendricks, who came to me with the idea for this book and shared my vision. Her support, enthusiasm, and editing have been invaluable to me.

And finally to my partner, Porter Shimer, for his love and unwavering confidence in my ability to get this book done on time.

Contents

Introduction

TO BE A RUNNER

MY FIRST EXPERIENCE RUNNING—OTHER THAN CHASING THE dog around the house—was when I was about 8 years old and my sister Kathy, the jock in the family, would challenge me to a race in the backyard. The distance couldn't have been much greater than 25 yards. I always accepted her challenge. I always lost.

Kathy could run and swim and bike, and she could play a mean game of basketball, tennis, and softball. Me? I remember once in fifth grade, the gym instructor stood behind me and helped me swing the bat just so I could hit the ball. How humiliating. I was 11 years old before I learned to ride a bike, and even then it was one with extra-fat tires. High-school P.E. class? You can imagine.

I felt totally inadequate over my physical ineptness. I envied my sister's multifaceted athleticism. I longed for some small show of athletic prowess, but none was to come for a long time.

I came to running again at age 27—not for the sport of it, but rather as a means to an end. I found that running relieved stress and made me fit. It soon replaced aerobics as my athletic activity of choice. I must admit that first year, I did *not* experience runner's high on too many occasions, but I stuck with it anyway for the great fitness gains, and gradually running changed for me. It offered more and more days of physical exhilaration—days when my body seemed to move effortlessly over the ground.

Eventually friends convinced me to enter races—a few 5-Ks, a couple of 10-Ks. Well . . . my late twenties didn't prove to be my athletic period either. My times were slow. I shuffled along in ungainly form, and racing just plain hurt. My fast-running friends told me I simply needed to train harder and longer every day. I did . . . I got slower. Racing hurt even more.

I was on the verge of giving up racing altogether but decided to give it one more shot. I suppose it was that childhood longing still smoldering. I sought training advice from Budd Coates, the head of my company's fitness center, a 2:13 marathoner and coach. Slowly but surely, I got faster. When I finally broke 50 minutes for a 10-K, I was thrilled. I continued to train diligently—each week, a speed workout, a long run, a hill effort—and I lowered all my race times. In my 13 years as a runner thus far, I've completed eight marathons, qualified for and run the Boston Marathon twice, and raced a mile in 5 minutes and 58 seconds. I have become an athlete.

Oh, I'll never be as fast a runner as many of my friends or certainly the many world-class athletes I met in my 8 years as the managing editor of *Runner's World* magazine, but I know the thrill of victory. It doesn't come simply with running my best races. I feel it when I can keep up with faster runners during a speed workout, when I'm running strong over a hilly course, or simply when I've conquered motivation deficit and run an invigorating 5-miler on a rainy day.

Through running, I found athleticism, but I've realized that, more important, I found strength. My body is lean, toned, and healthy. I can feel the power in my muscles, heart, and lungs. I have more energy and endurance for all things, and this is true mentally as well. Running penetrates. It drives beneath muscle and bone to our core strength. Running is an act of will. It requires mental as well as physical toughness. The more we do it, the stronger we become, the easier running is. Still, no matter how far or how fast I run on a given day, I know I have accomplished something that is difficult. This strength permeates the rest of my life. I feel good about myself, and I take that to my job and my relationships. I feel more capable, more independent. I take more risks because I believe that I can accomplish things I once thought impossible.

Running isn't only about performance and improvement and accomplishment, however. This I have learned also. Running is not simply a means to an end. It is an end in itself. When we become too caught in caretaking, which seems to be our wont as wives and mothers and daughters, or when we are too full with the pressures of meeting the demands of our supervisors and the needs of those we supervise, we can find a time and place in running that is our own.

Or running can be sharing—a time to talk deeply with a friend, a child, a spouse. My running partners are among my best friends.

Running can be play—on the beach, in the rain (yes, in the rain), in a new snow, among a group of friends on a trail run with a picnic afterward. Running can be contemplation, creativity, a working out of some pestering problem—or a birthing of new ideas for a work project, new lines for a poem, new measures for a song. And through running, we find a connection to nature.

Running has been all of these things for me, depending on my needs and desires. These days, I run most often simply because it feels good. And that is finally what running is all about—it feels good while you're doing it, and it leaves you with new energy when you're done.

Running offers us renewal each time we head out the door. It strips us down to our centers. It is sun, sweat, rain, breeze against our skin. It is blood pumping through our arteries, air filling our lungs, and the rhythmic, fluid contracting of muscle as we move our bodies over the earth. Through it, we become whole again.

I don't know what running will be for me in the future. I don't know how many more races I will run or marathons I will finish or if I will even compete again, but running will always be there for time alone or time with friends. I will always run simply because it feels good and it opens the passage to my strength.

I hope this book will help you become the runner you want to be, whether you choose to run for fitness, fun, challenge, sport, friendship, personal growth, or all of these. Most of all, may you find the joy in running that I have.

—*Claire*

PART I

Why Run?

1 Running for the Body

WHY TAKE UP RUNNING? BECAUSE IT IS THE simplest, fastest, most accessible way to fitness and good health known to woman. You don't need a partner; you don't need equipment, a court, or a gym; and you don't need much time. A mere 20 minutes three or four times a week is enough to make you fit, although most of us find that 20 minutes isn't enough to satisfy our desire to run.

3

Those who say they haven't time for running are simply making excuses. The morning, before the family wakes or work begins, is free time for most of us. If not, how about during your lunch hour or after you come home from the office? Just 20 minutes. It might seem difficult at first—even the slightest changes in routine can take some getting used to—but before you know it, you'll be figuring out ways to find 30 minutes, 40 minutes . . . an hour for running.

Then there are others who say running is just too hard, too painful. They wrinkle up their noses at the mere thought of it. Running *is* hard, but that's one of the reasons we love it. We feel special as runners because we can endure. Besides, running gets easier. The reason many people say it's painful is because they go out for their first run and virtually sprint for as long as they can—which isn't very long—with their chest heaving, their tongues lolling, their muscles straining until finally they can go no farther. They stop and pant, hands on their hips, wobbly kneed. "I—*gasp*—hate—*gasp*—running," they say.

So would I if I ran like that every day. Running is not an act of will over body—the brain whipping the legs to go as fast as they can as long they can (except when you really are sprinting). When you're running, your mind and body work in tandem toward an enjoyable continuum of movement over the ground. In the beginning, when your body is not yet capable of blazing speeds, your mind should say, *Okay, slow down. Let's go at a pace that's comfortable for you.*

Now that you don't have any excuses not to start, here are several reasons to begin running if you haven't already and to continue running if you have.

Running Is the Quickest and Most Efficient Means of Weight Loss

Let's compare running to another popular and convenient fitness activity—walking. In 20 minutes of running at a relaxed 10-minute-per-mile pace, a 130-pound woman burns 200 calories. In 20 minutes of walking at 15 minutes per mile (a brisk pace), a 130-pound woman burns only 72 calories. Of the 200 calories burned running, roughly 100 come from fat and 100 from carbohydrates. The 20-minute walk burns 54 fat calories and 18 carbohydrate calories. Furthermore, studies show that running increases your resting metabolic rate (meaning you burn more calories even when you're

THE BEST CALORIE BURNER

If one of your goals is weight management, you can't find an easier and more efficient way to burn calories than running. The table below shows the calories burned in 30 minutes at several different activities for a 130-pound woman.

Activity	Intensity	Calories Burned
Running	9 minutes per mile	324
Basketball	General game	236
Bicycling	Moderate, 12–14 mph	236
Calisthenics	Vigorous (push-ups, pull-ups, sit-ups)	236
Cross-country skiing	Moderate, 4–5 mph	236
Snowshoeing	Moderate	236
Swimming, laps	Moderate, freestyle	236
Tennis	Singles match	236
Volleyball	Beach game	236
Racquetball	Moderate	206
Rowing, stationary	Moderate	206
Skiing, downhill	Moderate	206
Soccer	General game	206
Aerobics	General	177
Stairclimbing	Moderate	177
Weight lifting	Vigorous (power lifting, bodybuilding)	177
Calisthenics	Moderate home exercise	133
Volleyball	Gym game	118
Walking	Brisk pace (3.5 mph)	118
Weight lifting	Light to moderate	88
Sitting		30

Calculations made from data in "Compendium of Physical Activities: Classification of Energy Costs of Human Physical Activities," *Medicine and Science in Sports and Exercise* (the journal of the American College of Sports Medicine), 1993; 25: 71–80.

not active) and improves your body composition by reducing body fat. The clear result of all of this is a leaner, trimmer figure.

Vanity aside, managing your weight is one of the most important things you can do for your health, well-being, and longevity. Obesity is a heavy contributor to heart disease, high blood pressure, stroke, breast cancer, and diabetes.

Running Reduces Your Risk of Cardiovascular Disease, the Number-One Killer of Women

In the Nurses Health Study of 73,029 women aged 40 to 65, conducted by JoAnn E. Manson, M.D., of the Brigham and Women's Hospital and Harvard Medical School in Boston, the rate of heart attack was found to be 44 percent lower among the most active women compared with those who were sedentary.

Running has several effects that lower your risk of cardiovascular disease:

- Running strengthens your heart.
- Running reduces the risks of blood clot formation.
- Running lowers blood triglycerides (fat).
- Running lowers total cholesterol levels.
- Running raises levels of high-density lipoprotein (HDL) cholesterol, also known as "good" cholesterol.
- Running prevents the stiffening of arteries that comes with age.

High mileage seems to have the best effect on raising HDL cholesterol levels, whereas running faster is better for lowering triglycerides, according to a study by Paul T. Williams, M.D., of the Lawrence Berkeley Laboratory in California. Williams's research looked at 1,837 female runners who were grouped according to weekly mileage: 0 to 9, 10 to 19, 20 to 29, 30 to 39, and 40 or more miles. HDL cholesterol levels rose with mileage—those in the 40-plus mileage group showing the highest levels. Also, as mileage increased, heart rate and body mass index (BMI; a calculation of weight based on height) decreased. Williams concluded that women who run 40 miles or more a week decrease their risk of dying from cardiovascular disease by 45 percent. He pointed out, however, that significant benefits are accrued at lower levels of weekly mileage as well.

Running Lowers Your Heart Rate and Blood Pressure

Williams also noted in his study that running lowered blood pressure and heart rate. Though the women who put in more weekly mileage showed the lowest figures for blood pressure and pulse, Williams found that fast running seemed to have an even greater effect—a good reason to do speed training and take up racing.

Running Reduces Your Risk of Stroke, the Second Leading Killer of Women

Given that running helps lower blood pressure and keeps the cardiovascular system healthy, it's not surprising that it can also help prevent stroke. A study conducted by researchers at the University of Alabama at Birmingham and reported in the *British Medical Journal* (July 24, 1993) compared 125 men and women who had just had their first stroke with 198 men and women who had never had a stroke. In looking at the activity levels of these groups, the researchers concluded that vigorous exercise—defined as running, swimming, cycling, and other strenuous activities—"confers substantial protection against stroke. These effects were seen in both sexes and all age groups." The Nurses Health Study also shows that exercise prevents stroke, finding that active women have a 42 percent lower rate of stroke than do sedentary women.

Running Lowers Your Risk of Breast Cancer

For several years, health experts have suspected that physical activity may lower the risk of breast cancer, and recently a significant study reported in the *New England Journal of Medicine* supports this theory. Over a 13-year period, researchers in Norway studied 25,624 women aged 20 to 54. They grouped these women according to level of activity: sedentary, moderate exercisers ("those who spent at least four hours a week walking, bicycling or engaging in other types of physical activity"), and regular exercisers ("those who spent at least four hours a week exercising to keep fit and participating in recreational athletics" plus "those who engaged in regular, vigorous training or participated in competitive sports several times a week"). They found that the regular exercisers—the most active group—had a 37 percent lower risk of breast cancer compared with the sedentary group. The moderate exercisers showed a 7 percent lower risk.

When looking only at premenopausal women, the risks of breast cancer were even lower with physical exercise. "Our results support the idea that physical activity protects against breast cancer, particularly among premenopausal and younger postmenopausal women," the researchers concluded. The theory behind the protective effects of activity is that vigorous exercise, such as running, may suppress the secretion of estrogen and progesterone, which have been linked to breast cancer. Also, the lower levels of triglycerides seen in physically active women reduce the amount of estrogen in the bloodstream.

Running Enhances Your Immune System

Most runners rarely get sick, and the reason is that running boosts the immune system. Researchers have determined this by measuring blood levels of lymphocytes (white blood cells that attack disease-causing antigens) and finding higher concentrations during and after exercise. It seems your body reacts to running as if a foreign invasion were occurring, and it recruits an army of lymphocytes to allay the onslaught. (During extremely long runs, however, especially those of high intensity—such as the marathon—so many lymphocytes are called into action that the reserves become depleted. Your immune system then becomes depressed, and you become more susceptible to illness. This is why runners often come down with a cold after a marathon. You can also wear down your immunity by running too many miles at too high an intensity in your regular training.)

Running also prevents that natural decline of immunity that occurs as we age. In 1993, David Nieman, Ph.D., and colleagues at Appalachian State University in Boone, North Carolina, compared the immune systems of active elderly women (who had been exercising aerobically for more than an hour a day for several years), sedentary elderly women, and sedentary young women aged 19 to 25. They found that the activity of T-cells and natural killer (NK) cells—two types of lymphocytes essential to immune function—was significantly higher among the active elderly women than in the sedentary elderly group and comparable to that seen in the young women. "The T-cells of the elderly active women were functioning like those in women half their age," says Nieman. Other good news: a 1997 study of women, activity levels, and causes of death showed that those who were most active had a considerably lower risk of death from respiratory diseases than did sedentary women.

Running May Prevent Diabetes and Help Those with This Disease to Manage It More Efficiently

Running burns glucose (blood sugar) for energy, which helps prevent glucose levels from rising too high. This doesn't mean that diabetics don't still need insulin, but they may be able to use lower amounts. Running also improves circulation, which commonly deteriorates with diabetes.

Running Helps Keep Your Intestinal Tract in Good Working Order

Regular running can keep you regular. This, in combination with a diet rich in fiber, lowers your risk of colon cancer.

Running Enhances Your Respiratory System

When you run, your muscles require a quick delivery of oxygen. The more you run, the more efficient your respiratory system becomes and the easier breathing is. Though running can stimulate an asthma attack in runners who suffer from exercise-induced asthma, the fitter you become through running the less frequently you should experience such episodes. Some women have reported that running has enabled them to cut back on their use of asthma medications.

Running May Reduce the Symptoms of Premenstrual Syndrome

Scientists have no proof that exercise relieves the pains of premenstrual syndrome (PMS), but many women report that even though they may not feel like running when their period hits and they're bloated and suffering cramps, once they go for a run, they feel much better. If physical symptoms don't subside, the moodiness—irritability or depression—that some women experience may dissipate after a good run.

Running Improves Your Health and Well-Being During Pregnancy

We now know that most women can continue running safely during pregnancy (see chapter 10). Those who do gain less unnecessary weight, sleep better, have better appetites, and generally enjoy better moods than do women who are sedentary. Running may also help prevent gestational diabetes and may contribute to shorter or easier deliveries, although not all runners can attest to this.

Running May Reduce the Symptoms of Menopause

When you've stepped beyond your childbearing years, you may find that running eases the discomforts of menopause by improving sleep patterns and stabilizing erratic moods that often accompany this period of changing hormones. It also helps control weight gain associated with this time of life.

Running Prevents Muscle and Bone Loss That Occur with Age

Running keeps the muscles of your legs in good shape as you age, but you'll need to do some regular weight training to maintain strength in your upper body. As for your bones, the forces that running exerts on your skeletal system stimulate bone formation and increase density. The effects are greatest in the legs, hips, and spine, the latter two areas being the most common sites of osteoporosis and fracture later in life. You can use resistance training (weight lifting) to build the bones of your upper body.

GOOD FOR THE BONES

In 1982, the Melpomene Institute for Women's Health Research in St. Paul, Minnesota, began a study of the effects of long-term physical activity on bone density. They looked at 111 women between the ages of 46 and 80; 54 were classified as physically active and 57 as inactive. Their study revealed that the average bone density of the active women was 25.6 percent higher than that of the inactive women. Melpomene's research is ongoing and further results are to come.

Running Is Good for Your Joints

Contrary to what most people believe, regular running *does not* ruin your joints; rather, it improves their flexibility and range of motion. "Running doesn't cause arthritis; injury does," says Warren Scott, M.D., chief of sports medicine at Kaiser Permanente Medical Center in Santa Clara, California. "Exercise is good for osteoarthritis. It speeds the rate at which cartilage is replaced by your body, making it stronger."

Running Helps Prevent a Decline in Reaction Time

Regular exercise has been shown to keep your mind sharp and reaction time quick. As you get older, quick reactions, good muscle tone, and overall flexibility help prevent accidents, such as falls.

Running Leads to a Long and Happy Life

That running can help you live longer and feel happier comes as no surprise, since running helps prevent heart disease, stroke, cancer, diabetes, and osteoporosis and strengthens your immune system. In a study reported in the *Journal of the American Medical Association* (April 23/30, 1997), Lawrence Kushi, Sc.D., and his colleagues at the University of Minnesota School of Public Health looked at a group of 40,417 postmenopausal women between the ages of 55 and 69. They found that the most active women showed a 30 percent lower risk of death from all causes compared with those who were least active. Add to that the physical strength and emotional well-being that running gives us, and we can look forward to a vibrant and happy, long life.

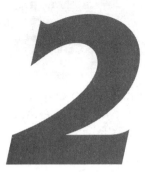

2 Running for the Mind

WE RUN FOR OUR HEARTS AND OUR bones, to melt away body fat and steel up strength, to prevent illness and to extend life. Besides the physical rewards, running also brings us mental benefits.

Running Helps You Feel Good About Yourself

In 1990, the Melpomene Institute for Women's Health Research in St. Paul, Minnesota, surveyed 600 women about why they exercise. Seventeen percent said that exercise helped them realize a positive self-image. A better body image is part of a positive self-image—not just because of the weight control that running provides but because of the fitness, endurance, and strength you gain. You feel proud of a body that can run for 3 miles, 5 miles, 10, 20— farther than most people can even walk.

How fast and how far you run depend solely on your individual ability and how well you've trained. Thus, every improvement in distance or speed is your own. Every improvement is an achievement, and with achievement comes self-respect and a feeling of self-worth. Running is hard. You have only to look at the great number of calories it burns for proof. It is continuous physical effort. There are no stops and starts or time-outs. You run and you keep running until you get to your finish line. You run in the heat, you run in the rain, you run in the snow. You run up mountains, down hills, over trails. To take on the challenge requires courage, and to continue demands a rare mental and physical fortitude. You gain the confidence to take on other of life's challenges.

Running Gives You Energy

Shortly after a friend of mine began running, she remarked with surprise about how much more energy she had since she started. Previously, she would come home from work and collapse on her couch until dinnertime. Running unleashed reserves of energy she never knew she had that kept her active until bedtime. My friend is not alone. Many women attest to a boost of energy and mental alertness after a run. You expend energy through running only to have it come back to you multiplied.

Running Relieves Stress

A *Runner's World* survey of female subscribers found that though most took up running to lose weight, their reasons for continuing had to do with stress reduction. Several studies have shown that exercise lowers stress, and not only does this benefit our psyches but it may also protect us from illness. More and more research is finding a link between mental stress and diseases, including cancer, and scientists suspect that stress may negatively affect a pregnant woman's fetus.

When you're anxious, frustrated, or angry, running provides a simple and effective release, one that won't get you into trouble the way a fight with your supervisor or spouse might. The accumulation of all the pent-up energy of negative emotions gets burned off with a good run—and can provide fuel for a pretty fast pace. Running, in fact, is a natural biological reaction to stress. You may have heard of the "fight or flight" response. When you are under stress, your body releases chemicals called catecholamines, which raise your heart rate and blood pressure. It's an instinctual reaction to situations that we perceive to be harmful—our bodies are preparing to fight or flee. This can be very helpful when you are faced with real danger, such as someone who intends you physical harm. When the stressful situation is an argument with your significant other or an overload of work at the office, though, neither fighting nor fleeing (at least in the usual meaning of the word) is recommended—but you can "flee" with a run. You'll use up those catecholamines, calm your beating heart, and temper your raging emotions.

Running Elevates Your Mood

Endorphins get a lot of credit for producing the "runner's high." Your body releases endorphins in response to stress—either emotional or physical—and one of the effects is to reduce pain. Levels of this natural painkiller rise measurably with running. The harder and faster you run (in other words, the more "stress"), the more endorphins your body produces.

Researchers have not yet confirmed that endorphins directly affect your sense of well-being, but they do agree that regular exercise can elevate your mood. Some psychiatrists and psychologists even prescribe exercise as treatment for patients with mild to moderate depression, and studies have confirmed a positive effect.

The harder you run, the better. Think about how good you feel after having completed a particularly fast run or long run, a speed session on the track, or a competitive race. It's not simply because the agony of exertion is over. It's the joy of accomplishment, the exhilaration of expressing your physical and mental toughness, and maybe, too, some extra endorphins.

You don't have to run hard or fast or long to experience a runner's high. There is joy simply in the rhythmic motion of the body. Babies are soothed by rocking, and children get great pleasure from play, which generally involves continuous movement. This applies to

ON RUNNING AND COURAGE

One day while I was running, I decided to take one of the braver steps of my life. I made up my mind to go skydiving. It was ironic that during running, which brings me so constantly and literally in touch with the ground at approximately 180 footstrikes per minute, I would decide I should take a leap into the air from a plane 11,000 feet above the earth, but I don't believe the decision would have come any other way.

I had spent the better part of a week interviewing the members of Sebastian 4NB, the best four-way women's formation skydiving team in the country, for an article in *Women's Sports and Fitness.* Each woman had spoken so passionately about skydiving and of course encouraged me to give it a try. "Yeah, sure," I said, while recalling uneasiness even at ascending the Eiffel Tower.

After one of my final interviews, I headed out for a run, one of the hilliest in my hometown. The air was cool, the sky was blue, my mind was going over the conversation I had just had. I think it must have been the exhilaration of climbing over those hard hills. I felt fit and strong, and I looked up at that blue sky and said to myself, "I'm going to do it. I'm going to try a jump." As soon as I got home, I called a drop zone and arranged to go that weekend.

The experience was one I will never forget, both exhilarating and surprisingly peaceful. Just as my skydiving friends had said, I will never look at the sky in the same way again. I am quite sure that without running, I wouldn't have made the decision to jump. Had I been a chair-bound journalist, I would not have been able to push through my fear. Charging up those hills and then skimming the down sides made me feel invincible that day and helped me find my courage.

—CLAIRE KOWALCHIK

adults, too. You know the joy that movement brings. In certain runs, it is exquisite. Your arms and legs move in synchronicity with the beating of your heart and lungs in a perfect unwavering rhythm. Running feels effortless. This is the way your body was meant to move, and you are certain it could continue like this forever.

Running Enhances Your Mental Power and Stimulates Creativity

Those same endorphins that possibly contribute to runner's high may positively affect your mental power. In fact, there's evidence that upswings in endorphin levels increase the ability to learn and remember. Certainly the energy we get from running and the fact that we sleep better because we run both contribute to mental alertness and make us more productive at home and work. Studies show that people who make a point of fitting an adequate amount of physical activity in their lives not only get more done in less time, but they're also better at handling stress and tend to be more imaginative when it comes to solving work-related problems.

Why? Perhaps it's because physical activity stimulates neurotransmitters or increases blood and oxygen flow to the brain. Science is uncertain of the mechanism. Though no one suggests that we can raise our IQs by becoming runners, many experts advocate exercise as a way to enhance mental and creative power. Many great artists and thinkers have been avid exercisers—Einstein, Thoreau, Wordsworth. Writer Brenda Ueland takes walks of 6 miles or more to free her creativity. Novelists Joyce Carol Oates and Mary McCarthy both run. Perhaps what running offers the thinker and the artist is an opportunity for time and solitude away from the distractions and disruptions of everyday life. Running makes us feel strong and gives us the courage to step into the sometimes-scary creative places in our minds. Maybe it is the return to innocence that opens us to free thinking. When we run, we become the blank slate and anything may be written upon us.

Running Brings Renewal

You know those days when you're just off? Your mind feels cluttered and disorganized, you can't seem to figure anything out, and it makes you cranky and fatigued? Then you go for a run. Just a 3-miler, because that's all you have time for, and you finish feeling like you'd spent a day at the spa—clear-minded, energetic, capable of tackling any task. There's something about a run that blows out the accumulation of mind dust, clears the windows of mental vision, and simply invigorates the workings of your mind. All of the mental benefits of running combine to keep us at our best for accomplishing the daily "to do" list, coping with difficult times, and creating and enjoying the happy, meaningful experiences of life.

3 Sex Differences

Once a woman decides she's going to do something, she'll probably stick to it. The only problem with women is if there's anything wrong with them, they won't tell you. They'll get out there and run on one leg. They don't moan and groan like a lot of men do.

—ARTHUR LYDIARD, New Zealand running coach

SHORTLY AFTER MY BOYFRIEND PORTER AND I started dating, we entered a 10-K together. Though he had been a marathoner and could boast a 2:40 for his best, he hadn't raced or run in several years. He had, however, kept active with calisthenics and stationary aerobic machines. Porter said he'd run by my side the entire race, but once the run started, his male competitive ego kicked in—he pulled away after the second mile and finished ahead of me.

In the years that followed, I remained dedicated to my running and he to his push-ups and rower. Then in the fall of 1996, friends invited us to the inaugural Old Chatham Hunt Club 5-K in Old Chatham, New York. Porter, curious to test his running prowess, decided at the last minute to enter. This time, there were no promises. May the best runner win.

That runner was me—with time to spare.

Sex doesn't always determine who will be the fastest. Winning depends on the amount and type of training you do, the specificity of training, and who has the best ability (speed, endurance, and mental toughness) on a particular day. Look at any race and you'll see that the best women beat most of the men. With the exception of ultra-runs of 50 miles or more, however, women don't win races outright. On an absolute level, sex does make a difference. Men have certain biological advantages and may have an edge psychologically and sociologically as well.

Body Composition

One of the factors that most influences the difference in men's and women's performances is body composition. Men have a higher proportion of muscle to fat than women do. Muscle does all the work of running; fat just goes along for the ride. It slows you down. Imagine the extra effort it would take if you ran wearing a weight vest.

The average college-age man carries 15 percent body fat; the average woman, 27 percent. Some fat is essential to the proper physiological functions of the body, and women require even more padding for pregnancy and childbirth. Though we can reduce our levels of body fat, this should not be the focus of training. Women who become too concerned with body fat are more susceptible to developing eating disorders. Furthermore, dieting can do more to ruin your performance than improve it. Consume too few calories and your body thinks there's a famine going on—it slows down its metabolism to conserve calories. Also, with dieting, you lose muscle, which is precisely the body tissue you need more of in order to perform better. Nutritionists recommend that to preserve muscle, weight loss should be slow—0.5 to 1 pound a week.

Rather than try to reduce fat, put your efforts toward building muscle by doing strength training regularly—two or three times a week. In the long term, increased muscle mass raises your metabolism and will burn some unnecessary fat. When you focus not on fat but rather on following healthy guidelines for training and nutrition, your body will find its best weight and composition for optimum running performances. Keep this in mind: in a test of the body fat of 30 elite women runners, Joan Benoit Samuelson's was found to be the highest. Joan holds the American record for the women's marathon (2:21:21 at Chicago in 1985), which is the third fastest women's marathon time ever.

Aerobic Capacity

When you run, your muscles use oxygen to burn glucose (blood sugar) for energy. The more efficiently this process occurs, the better your running performance can be. Maximum oxygen consumption, or $\dot{V}O_2$ max, is the maximum amount of oxygen that your muscles are able to use per minute. This is affected by how much oxygen is carried in your blood, how quickly it gets to working muscles, and also by the efficiency of the chemical reactions in the muscles that use oxygen to create energy.

Men have some advantages here, too. Their high levels of testosterone significantly increase the amount of hemoglobin in their blood. Hemoglobin is the protein that carries oxygen in red blood cells. On average, women have 10 percent less hemoglobin, which means we transport 10 percent less oxygen from our lungs to our muscles than men do. Furthermore, women have smaller hearts than do men, so we pump less blood with each heartbeat. The more you run, however, the more you'll increase the strength and function of your heart and the efficiency with which your muscles use oxygen, thus improving your overall aerobic capacity.

Anaerobic Capacity

Not all the energy you use during running comes from the metabolic process of burning blood sugar in the presence of oxygen. Your body has a faster way of creating energy. Your muscles contain stored carbohydrate called glycogen, which can be burned for energy by certain enzymes in your muscles. No oxygen is required. This is called anaerobic metabolism, and it's a process that becomes especially important when you are running fast and need energy ASAP. Here again, men appear to have an advantage because of larger muscle fibers and better muscle enzyme activity, but you can improve your anaerobic capacity through speed training. Because fast running requires your body to use anaerobic metabolism to create energy, weekly speed workouts will help your body become more efficient at producing energy this way. Practice makes perfect.

Running Economy

Running economy is defined by the amount of energy you use to run at a certain pace. The less energy required, the higher your economy. This is one of the most important factors affecting performance in distance runners and is one area where men and women are equal.

The more training you do, especially fast-paced training, the more efficient you will become in all ways. You will develop better form. The interactions of nerves and muscles will become more efficient, and your body will improve in its ability to use oxygen and create energy to keep your muscles moving.

Muscle Strength

On average, men are bigger and stronger than women, exceeding us in upper body strength by a margin of 40 percent to 50 percent. We come closer in lower-body strength, however, where the difference is only 20 percent to 35 percent. The reason for these differences has to do primarily with greater muscle mass in men and their higher ratio of muscle to body fat. If you were to isolate a woman's muscle tissue and a man's, they would be equivalent in strength.

More muscle doesn't translate into faster running times for distance runners, however. The petite bodies of many of the world's best marathoners—men and women—prove that to be true. Because men have a better ratio of "working" muscle to "do-nothing" body fat than do women, however, they are stronger and faster overall.

Skeletal Structure

Women's wider pelvises, built so for childbearing, result in a greater Q-angle, or quadriceps angle, formed by the position of the outside of the hip relative to the knee. This can result in overpronation (excessive inward rolling of the foot during footstrike), which can lead to injuries, including knee problems, shinsplints, and stress fractures.

Neither Q-angle nor overpronation detract from running performance, unless, of course, you become injured. Fortunately, most cases of overpronation can be corrected with proper shoes.

Joint Laxity

Women tend to have looser joints than men do, and our joints become even looser during pregnancy, when our bodies produce the hormone relaxin to "relax" the pelvis in preparation for childbirth. Researchers suspect this may make women more vulnerable to injuries, especially of the knees. There are no studies that confirm this, however.

Fuel for Energy

Chalk one up for women. During endurance activities like running, we burn more fat than carbohydrates or proteins for energy, compared with men. This means our glycogen stores (our premium carbohydrate fuel) will last longer. Then again, maybe this simply evens the playing field: it appears that men can store more glycogen in the

ENDURANCE EXPERTS

Ann Trason is one of the best ultra-distance runners in the world—female or male. Her greatest achievement came in 1997 when she won the Comrades Marathon in South Africa, a 54-mile race, for the second year in a row and then just a few weeks later finished first among women in the Western States 100-Mile Endurance Run for the ninth consecutive time. Ann places in the top 10 (men and women combined) in almost every competition she enters, has twice finished second overall at Western States, and has won first place outright in some 50-mile trail races. She is not the only woman to win overall in an endurance event; a few others have as well.

Does this mean women may, in fact, equal or perhaps even exceed men in endurance? Many have speculated just that. Perhaps our extra body fat may finally give us a performance edge in long distances, providing a constant supply of fuel, and there's the fact that we tend to burn fat for fuel more than men do, thus stretching our reserves of glycogen (which is the only fuel our brains can use). Plus, women are often regarded as having extraordinary inherent mental endurance, as evidenced every time a woman gives birth. Whether all of this adds up to make us better endurance athletes than men hasn't been proven. As with all questions we have about sports and performance, researchers will continue to look for an answer.

first place. Researchers have found that during carbo-loading (increasing consumption of carbohydrates in order to pack muscles with glycogen for use as fuel during a long-distance event), women store the same amount of glycogen whether they eat a diet containing 60 percent or 75 percent carbohydrates. Men, however, will store *more* glycogen on the higher-carbohydrate diet, giving them greater reserves of fuel for the long run.

Competitive Qualities

It is often assumed that men are more competitive than women, but as a society in which men's participation in sports has dominated for so many years and continues to be the focus, we tend to define competitiveness by the way men compete—aggressively. Just think of the language we use: a competitor is one who has the necessary "killer instinct" to "go for the jugular" and "crush his opponent" to "take" the victory. There are women who exhibit these qualities, too, but in general, competitiveness in women may simply have a different expression—less aggression toward the opponent and more assertiveness of personal athleticism. We don't *take* victory; we *earn* it.

Diane L. Gill, a professor in the Department of Exercise and Sport Science at the University of North Carolina at Greensboro who has done considerable research in the social psychology aspects of sport, has found that competitiveness differentiates athletes and nonathletes, not men and women. Both men and women are competitive, but styles and motivation may differ. Gill developed a sport orientation questionnaire to help her evaluate men's and women's orientation toward achievement in three areas: (1) competitiveness, "an achievement orientation to enter and strive for success in competitive sport"; (2) win orientation, "a desire to win and avoid losing in competitive sport"; and (3) goal orientation, "an emphasis on achieving personal goals in competitive sports." She found that men scored higher than women on competitiveness and win orientation and women scored higher than men on goal orientation. Other researchers have seen similar patterns.

Experts believe these differences grow from patterns of socialization developed in childhood. In a group of boys, order and hierarchy become established rather quickly. Among girls, the emphasis is on forming relationships and on cooperation. Boys risk offending others to prove themselves the stronger ones of the group. Girls prefer not to risk the bonds of friendship; relationships take priority over overt superiority.

This doesn't mean that deep down inside, we're not competitive. I belong to a women's running group, Making Strides, which once a week brings together women of all abilities in their early twenties to early sixties for speed workouts. It's been interesting to observe that when we are asked to line up in order of fastest to slowest for the purpose of dividing into different groups, there's much shuffling around at the front because no one wants to be first. It feels as though it would be somehow too prideful or too arrogant. Later, when we line up to start a fast interval, there's more hesitancy about approaching the start and who will lead. Once we begin running, however, that demureness burns off, our competitiveness kicks in, and we're all pushing and striving to run our very best and, yes, to beat others of our ability.

I also find a great deal of support and cooperation among these women. Each of us wants to be the best runner, but we all also support and encourage others to achieve their best. I believe we are all thinking, *I want to run better than you, but I also want you to run well and do your very best.* When someone else does run better, we offer congratulations, and the disappointment isn't that we didn't "win" but that we didn't perform better ourselves.

Although the demureness many women express in sport may be due in part to socialization and the importance we place on relationships, it may also be influenced by a lack of confidence ingrained in us through years of living in a culture that believes boys and men are better at sports than are girls and women. Not only can this social attitude dampen our confidence and inhibit our competitiveness, it may affect our performances, too, as Diane Gill states in *Women and Sport* (Champaign, Illinois: Human Kinetics, 1994): "More girls than boys expect to do poorly at sports and competition, and more women than men believe they cannot develop sport skills or maintain an exercise program. Indeed, this gender influence on expectations and confidence is one of the most important considerations for achievement, particularly in the realm of physical activity." Gill goes on to point out that in areas where there is no sexist bias, women display as much confidence as men. "If the task is not male-linked, females are just as likely as males to exhibit achievement-oriented cognitions," she states.

Clearly, the goal for the future of women's sports is to work toward erasing societal expectations about participation and performance, which will allow women equal opportunity in athletics. We can begin by encouraging our daughters as equally as our sons to play outside, climb trees, ride bikes, hit baseballs, kick footballs, risk cuts and bruises and broken bones. We can learn to love the tears and grass stains on our daughters' jeans, knowing that this is part of a world changing toward equal acceptance of men's and women's athleticism.

Participation and Achievement

History has certainly seen differences in men's and women's participation in sports and also in what we've been able to achieve. Sports psychologists believe that societal encouragement of boys' and men's sports participation may influence everything from the way women compete and approach sports to how well we perform to even our injury rates. Some say men who have been physically active since boyhood may be better conditioned and less prone to injury when they reach their adolescent and adult years, as compared with women, who might not have been encouraged toward sports during girlhood.

Certainly the centuries of men's sports participation has enabled the sex as a whole to advance their achievements. Women have come later to the game, but we're catching up rapidly. Improvements in women's race performances have led many to speculate that we might someday be as fast as men. Most likely, the gap has narrowed because we are now running in increasing numbers and with increasing intensity and focus on competition and athletic achievement. Because of our physiologies, we probably won't run as fast as men over most distances, but we can train just as hard and with the same passion for excellence.

Man or woman, each of us has only our own mental and physical limitations to contend with. As we move toward our athletic dreams, gender differences and sexism need to be stored in our histories—not to be forgotten, because their lessons can help us change the future for our daughters, but to be moved out of the way of our footsteps. To push our individual boundaries farther, we must be in the present. We must take these bodies and minds that we have, train them according to the knowledge available to us and the instinct within us, and drive them with our passion toward our individual goals. In that process, we find equality with all others who strive toward their dreams and we achieve the excellence of realizing our very best.

Saying Is Being

BY DAWSON WINCH

THE ROAD STRETCHES BEFORE ME, ENDLESS, ROLLING THROUGH farmland. Cornfields rush by on both sides. My breath comes steady and strong, cloudlike in the cool air. My legs and arms move together smoothly and rhythmically. The world, my mind, my body are in sync.

Unfortunately, this picture exists in my mind more than in reality. I experience such "flow" during some runs, but others are downright painful. When I run in winter, my asthma kicks in, and hills—in any season—zap my strength. I imagine long, enjoyable strengthening runs, but I am having difficulty reaching the point where a 10- or even an 8-mile run feels comfortable. Sometimes I feel as though I have one speed and one speed only, like my old red Schwinn bicycle.

But my stubbornness keeps me from quitting. I keep trying—striving to lengthen my runs, doing speed work to quicken my pace, lifting weights to build strength, visualizing myself running smoothly and strongly down the road.

Someone once asked me if I was a runner. It took me a minute. My answer, surprisingly, was no.

I run, but am I a runner? At what point does an activity become an integral part of your personality, your identity? I do see myself as a hiker, a biker, a backpacker—even an athlete—so why not a runner? Is it my expectations of the qualities runners possess? I think of runners as ultra-athletes, competitors who race regularly and run marathons.

Is it an issue of body type? When I look in the mirror, I don't see a runner—a tall, thin, muscular individual. I see a woman with hips (thanks to genetics), and despite a healthy diet and daily exercise, a woman who can well afford to lose a couple pounds, a woman who has difficulty finding running shorts that fit well and who experiences chafing in hot, sticky summer months. If I were in a lineup and someone were asked to pick out the runner, I sincerely doubt I'd be picked.

25

Still, I try.

I see the women I consider runners on the treadmills at the gym. They clock miles and miles at speeds that would leave me flying off the back end. I don't know if or when I'll ever reach that level, but I'm definitely making strides, because I'm still there. I no longer mind running next to someone who's taking one stride for my two and whom I know could do twice the distance in half the time. I'm there doing my best, and I'm proud of that.

I even joined a Tuesday-night running group for women last year to try to improve my speed. I was so nervous the first night, hoping I wouldn't fall too far behind. I didn't. There were others who were faster than I and those who were slower. I stuck to it throughout the summer. Although I didn't feel like I was getting any faster or that running was getting any easier, I ran a 5-K that fall (the same one I had run the year before and that was my first race ever) and improved my time by 2 minutes.

It made me realize that I am more of a runner than I've given myself credit for being. Perhaps I've been going about this backward. If I say I'm a runner, then I'll be one, rather than the other way around. You are what you believe you are. It's taken me a while to see this, but you can be sure that the next time someone asks if I'm a runner, I'll answer quickly with an affirming and resounding *yes!*

Dawson Winch is marketing manager for *Backpacker* magazine. She's also a backpacker, a cyclist, and a runner.

PART II

Becoming a
Runner

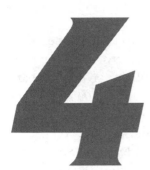 # The Mindset

A runner is real when she takes the first step.

—CLARISSA PINKOLA ESTÉS, PH.D.,
author of *Women Who Run with the Wolves*

KATHY DOUKAS HAS BEEN RUNNING FOR several years, primarily for fitness. Her current goal is simply to run 4½ miles 4 or 5 days a week consistently. "I've never been very fast," she says. "I can only run a 10-minute mile, but I don't care about that. I like to run first thing in the morning because it makes me feel really good and gives me more energy for the rest of the day. Some people say, 'Oh, you're doing only 10-minute miles; you're just a jogger,' but it feels like running to me," says Kathy. "If you say to yourself you're a runner, you feel more confident, more powerful."

29

And Kathy *is* a runner. As is the high-school girl who competes on her cross-country team or the 42-year-old executive who runs to relieve stress or the 25-year-old who runs for fitness or the 65-year-old grandmother who wins her age group in the marathon or the 37-year-old mother of three who runs to control her weight.

What does it mean to be a runner? Simply that you run.

"To move the legs quickly," says the *Oxford English Dictionary*, "(the one foot being lifted before the other is set down) so as to go at a faster pace than walking; to cover the ground, make one's way, rapidly in this manner." Now, consider what the dictionary says about jogging: "To move up and down or to and fro with a heavy unsteady motion; to move on at a heavy or labored pace, to trudge." Is that the kind of activity you see yourself doing? No. You don't jog—you run. It doesn't matter how fast, how far, or how often you run, if you're moving faster than you would if you were walking, you are a runner. Not all women believe this about themselves, however.

Amy Jones has been running for over a year. She trains 16 miles a week and has completed a 5-K in 31 minutes. Still, she doesn't consider herself a runner. "I do feel like a runner among people who don't run—like my family—but not around my friends who run. Part of it—and I'm embarrassed to admit this—is that I don't think I *look* like a runner. The ones you see in magazines or TV ads and my friends who run are all so thin. I don't have that body type, and I probably never will."

The Power of Positive Thinking

Why is it important to see yourself as a runner? As Kathy points out, you'll feel more confident and more powerful, and these feelings fuel your excitement for running. When you believe you are a runner, you naturally assume the responsibility of fulfilling that role. You'll be more motivated to run and thus more consistent in running. You'll be eager to take on the challenges necessary for improvement, such as increasing your mileage, picking up your pace every now and then, or running with friends who are a little faster than you. You might even decide to run a race.

Try this. Say to yourself, "I'm just a jogger." How does that make you feel? Maybe a little wimpish? Certainly it doesn't make you feel special in any way. Now say, "I am a runner." Say it again with conviction. Do you notice a boost in your attitude? Doesn't it make you feel proud to say you are a runner?

Within running is a self-fulfilling progression: when you feel confident, you train a little harder, you become a better runner, you become more confident. Even if your goal is to maintain a certain weekly mileage for fitness reasons, when you feel good about yourself and your running, you will be more excited by even the thought of it, and then running regularly will be easy. As Tim Gallwey states in his book *The Inner Game of Tennis* (New York: Random House, 1997), "I know of no single factor that more greatly affects our ability to perform than the image we have of ourselves."

Changing Your Image

Jerry Lynch, Ph.D., sports psychologist and author of *Thinking Body, Dancing Mind* (New York: Bantam, 1992), quotes the American philosopher William James as having said, "Human beings, by changing the inner beliefs of their minds, can change the outer aspects of their lives." Two techniques sports psychologists use very successfully to help individuals change their inner beliefs are affirmation and visualization. If your self-image could use a little boost—and whose doesn't every now and then—give them a try.

An affirmation is a positive statement that you repeat over and over. Print the words *I am a runner* (*I am an athlete* is another good one) in big letters on several index cards and tape them around the house in places where you'll see them often: the bathroom mirror, the refrigerator door, the television, the computer monitor. Say it out loud: "I am a runner. I am a runner. I am a runner." Eventually, you will come to believe it. (All right, it sounds corny, but it works!)

Visualization draws on your imagination to create positive images of you as a runner. "What you see in your mind's eye can strongly influence your beliefs and achievements," says Lynch. "Our central nervous system does not distinguish between real and imagined events: it sees and accepts all images as if they were real." To illustrate this, Lynch suggests a little experiment: close your eyes and imagine a lemon. See yourself cutting a wedge of it and biting into it. Taste the sour juice in your mouth. Are you salivating? Is your mouth puckering? Picture yourself as a strong runner, and your body and mind will respond as though you are one.

Here's how to practice visualization:

1. Find a quiet place where you won't be disturbed.
2. Close your eyes and take five deep abdominal breaths. You should be able to feel your abdomen rise with each breath.
3. Relax and clear your mind of distractions.
4. Now, imagine yourself running—down your street or on the path in your local park. Be specific. See yourself moving with good posture, arms close to your sides, swinging forward and back in relaxed good form. Your feet lightly touch the ground as your legs lengthen into a smooth stride. Your breathing is relaxed and comfortable. You are strong and swift and you feel as though you could run forever.

That is the runner you see in your mind; that is the runner you will become.

Practice visualization often—every day, if you can. You'll be pleased with the feelings of confidence and the improved performance that result.

Building on Your Image

Some of us, even though we have come to see ourselves as runners, may still, at times, disparage our level of ability. Do you ever find yourself saying, "Oh, I'm too slow to run with my friends"? Or if you do get up the courage to go out with a group that's a little faster than you, do you automatically put yourself at the back of the pack, saying, "I'm pretty slow. You can go on ahead whenever you feel like it. You don't have to wait for me"?

You've heard of the self-fulfilling prophecy? Speak something, and it'll probably come true. "The words you use to express yourself are the seeds of your future experiences," says Lynch. "The mind constantly searches for ways to confirm negative self-talk and sabotage the chances for successful athletic performance." If your friends invite you along on a run, don't disparage your running. Talk to them about your usual running pace and distance, and together you can plan a run at a pace that will be appropriate for everyone. The day before, visualize yourself running among your friends, running strong and staying with them to the end. Remember, they invited you. Draw confidence from the fact that they believe you are capable.

Nervous about your first race or going for a personal best in a 5-K? Use affirmations and visualization to give you confidence. In the week before the important event, say to yourself over and over again,

"I am prepared. I will run well." Picture yourself running the race. (If you can, drive over the course ahead of time.) Imagine all the details: starting relaxed and controlled, running strong up the hills, gliding the downhills, picking up your pace just a bit with every mile, and sprinting the last 200 yards for a strong finish. Then go do it.

Use challenges to build confidence. Rather than shy away from something you think you can't do, try something you think you can do . . . but that you're not certain you'll succeed at. It might be running 5 miles instead of your usual 3, or running 4 miles at a 9½-minute pace instead of 10 minutes per mile. Enter a race and make it your goal just to finish, running the whole way. The exhilaration of achieving something you weren't certain you could do is a runner's high unlike any other, and your feelings of confidence will soar.

The key is to pick a goal that's doable. Don't try to run a distance or a pace that's considerably farther and faster than what you're used to, because then you *might* fail, and failure will only make you feel bad about yourself. Choose little challenges. Succeed at them, and they will be like stepping-stones to a stronger self-image, more enjoyable running, and better performances.

Reaffirming Ourselves

A positive self-image is important throughout our lives as runners. Chances are, your running will take you in a variety of directions over the years and your running identity will change. You might have taken up running to lose weight but later find that running has become important to you for many other fitness reasons as well. You might try a 5-K and discover the excitement of racing. You may wander off onto some trails one day and find yourself seduced by the sport of ultrarunning. You may decide to enter an all-comers track meet and discover there's been a 400-meter runner hiding inside you. Then in your later years, you may return to running simply for fitness and pleasure.

Our lives change. We may switch jobs. We may find new homes. We may have children. And our bodies change. Eventually, we slow down and aren't able to achieve the running goals of our youth. Reexamine your running periodically. Redefine your identity as a runner and focus on that identity. Avoid comparing yourself with other runners or the runner you once were. Live and run in the moment and according to your needs and desires. And remember always: you are a runner.

5 The Elements of Running

RUNNING IS SIMPLE. THAT'S ONE reason we love it.

It doesn't require lots of technical equipment like cycling and backpacking do or the layers of expensive clothing that downhill skiing demands. In fact, in most seasons, very little clothing is required at all. You don't need a gym, a court, a pool, or snow, but you could run in any of them if you had to. You don't need a class, a team, or even a partner, but it's easy enough to find someone to run with if you want company. There's no scheduling a game or tee time, or signing up for a 3-nights-a-week 12-week class. You don't even need much time.

When the desire strikes, simply put on a pair of shorts and a T-shirt, lace up your running shoes (see chapter 14), and head down the road, up a trail or through an open field. I know runners who always have a bag packed with running clothes in their car so that if they drive by a scenic spot, they can hop out and go for a run.

And running doesn't require very much instruction. Still, there are some basic principles you should know—tips on form, pace, the best surfaces to run on—that will help keep running healthy and fun.

Running Form

For the most part, running form is a given. No two bodies are identical, and yours will move according to its inherent physics. Fortunately, you don't need ideal form to run well. No one would ever describe Joan Benoit Samuelson as a graceful runner, but she won the first women's Olympic marathon in 1984 and continues to hold the third-fastest time in the world for that distance. Still, some attention to form will help you run more comfortably, will help you run faster if that is a goal, and may prevent injury. All of us can make a few adjustments.

Running is about moving directly forward as efficiently as possible.

THE ELEMENTS OF FORM

Every now and then during a run, focus on your form from head to toe, especially toward the end of a long run when fatigue frazzles good form. Check for the following points and make adjustments accordingly:

- Good posture is the most important element of good running form. Imagine a big helium balloon attached to your head by a string and pulling your body straight up.
- Look ahead as you run, not down at the ground. This also helps you maintain good posture.
- Your arms should be bent at about a 90-degree angle. As you swing them, keep them relaxed but close to your body. On the backswing, your hands should pass your body at hip level. As your arms swing forward and up, they should cross your torso to about the midline of your chest (drawn vertically).
- Your hands should be relaxed, not clenched in a fist, palms facing your body and thumbs upward. Imagine you are holding an egg in each hand as you run.

You don't want to waste energy and motion bouncing up and down or twisting sideways. Too much side-to-side motion is more common among women than men—a result of our proportionately wider hips. To correct this, simply monitor your arm movements. Keep your arms relaxed but close to your body, and as they swing in front of you, don't let them cross over the vertical center line of your torso. Pay attention to this and a few other points (see The Elements of Form on page 35) and you'll be moving down the road in fine form.

The main thing to keep in mind about running form is not to struggle with it. If you try to force your body into the stride and posture of your most-admired Olympian, you may end up running in a way that doesn't work for your particular body type and cause an injury. Relax. Occasionally check to see that you are following good general form and then get back to enjoying your run.

Form Enhancers

A strong upper body is important to good posture and hence good form, and though running uses the legs primarily, some of your power comes from your arm swing. Consider doing some strength training for your arms, shoulders, and back. Two or three times a week will do, and throw in some abdominal (ab) work, too; strong stomach muscles also contribute to good posture while running. (See chapter 18 for a complete strength-training program.)

Another way to develop better form is with faster running. When you pick up your pace, your form automatically changes to help you move more quickly. With regular speed training, your body will gradually adopt an improved, more efficient style for all paces. This doesn't mean you have to take up a regimen of intense and measured speed sessions, as you would if you were training to race. Just run a little

GO GENTLY INTO THE MORNING

If you're like most women, you run first thing. A 1996 *Runner's World* survey showed that many of us are up and running even before the crack of dawn in order to fit running into our busy lives. If that includes you, remember that muscles are stiff in the morning and thus more susceptible to strains and pulls.

Take a little extra time to warm up. Walk and/or jog slowly at the start of your run and gradually ease into your usual pace. You can also add some light stretching to your warmup, but do so after a few minutes of slow running when your muscles have loosened up some; stretching muscles that are too tight can cause injury.

faster than usual once or twice a week or do a run in which you alternate a few minutes at a fast pace with a few minutes of slow running.

With a little strength training and some speed and regular running, your form will gradually improve on its own. I remember after I had been running for a few years, my friend Jane Serues, who is quite an accomplished runner, passed me on the road one afternoon. Later that day, she came up to me and said, "You looked good out there. You actually look like a runner now." Geez, what must I have looked like those first couple of years? Fortunately, we can't see ourselves running. What I found most interesting was that I hadn't specifically worked to change my form at all. It came naturally as I became a better runner.

Stride

The one element of running form that we all secretly wish for is a longer stride. Don't you sometimes find yourself, on a run, drifting into a mental reverie, imagining that you are bounding gracefully over the earth? (I know I do.) That's a nice image, but leave it to your imagination. Stride length is something you don't want to mess with. Many runners think they'll be not only more graceful but faster if they take long leaping strides. Leave it to Mother Nature. As with trying to dramatically alter any other element of form, changing your stride length can lead to injury if it's not appropriate to your biomechanics or your level of ability.

What you should focus on is your stride *rate*. Jack Daniels, Ph.D., sports scientist and head track and cross-country coach at the State University of New York at Cortland, studied the stride rate of runners at the 1984 Olympics. He found that almost every runner there took about 180 steps a minute. Daniels, who also works with

> ### *RAISING YOUR RATE*
>
> Do some downhill running to help increase your stride rate. Gravity promotes quicker leg turnover, and good form on downhills requires a slightly shorter stride and quick, light steps.

beginning runners, notes that they take only 150 to 160 steps a minute, which costs more energy. "A slow stride rate means you spend more time in the air and thus land harder," he points out. "With a quicker turnover, you will land lightly, which lessens your risk of injury."

Next time you go for a run, count your stride rate for 1 minute, which means count every footstrike: right, left, right, left—1, 2, 3, 4. If it's less than 180 steps per minute, practice taking quicker steps.

This does not mean running faster, it means picking your foot up more quickly after it hits the ground, which will require you to shorten your stride. Aim for between 180 and 190 steps per minute, no faster. As for bounding like a gazelle, your stride will naturally lengthen as you become a stronger and faster runner.

Running Pace

Women who say they hate to run or that it's just too hard probably run too fast. The effort of running should feel comfortable no matter what your fitness level. If you can't have a conversation while you're running, then you should slow down.

Don't let yourself get caught up in timing every run and calculating your daily minute-per-mile pace either. We've all seen those runners who set their sports watches at the beginning of a run and immediately check them at the end. Even the most serious runners don't need to do this except on the days they are focusing on speed work, and that should be only 1 or 2 days a week.

It is good to time yourself every now and then. Knowing your pace gives you a benchmark as to where you are in your personal range of running fitness. If you measure your speed every day, however, you can quickly become too focused on it. It's easy to get caught up in trying to run your regular route just a little faster each time and fret when the going's a little slow.

The best advice I ever received was to leave my watch at home. I enjoyed running more, and I didn't burn out worrying about keeping a certain pace every day. I believe that not measuring my every run was one of the keys to my becoming a better runner. By ignoring your watch, you'll run as your body feels—faster on days when you're feeling perky and slower on days when you're tired and *should* run slower. Becoming a slave to pace only sets you up to become overtrained and ultimately injured, and it turns running into a task. You'll enjoy running so much more when you run *with* your body, not against it.

Of course, if you plan to race or if you simply want to become a faster runner, you will need to do some running at speeds that will barely allow you to mutter a word, and you'll want to learn your paces so that you can improve on them. (You'll find details on training to race in part VII.) Even when you are training to be faster, though, 90 percent of your running should be at conversation pace.

Breathing

One way to judge your pace and effort is through rhythmic breathing. This involves coordinating your breathing with your stride cadence such that you inhale and exhale over an odd number of foot strikes. During a relaxed run, you want to inhale for three steps and exhale for two steps (a 3:2 ratio). Why inhale for more steps than you exhale? Because inhalation should be as relaxed and fluid as possible, whereas exhalation is naturally a bit shorter and more forceful. Breathing in this way helps prevent "stitches," those short, painful cramps in your diaphragm that sometimes occur during running. Here's how it works.

Footstrike	Breathing Pattern
Left	Inhale
Right	Inhale
Left	Inhale
Right	*Exhale*
Left	*Exhale*
Right	Inhale
Left	Inhale
Right	Inhale
Left	*Exhale*
Right	*Exhale*

At first, learning to breathe using the 3:2 pattern may be difficult (unless this is your natural rhythm). If you focus on maintaining this breathing pattern each time you run, however, it will become second nature within a week.

When you're running hard and fast, such as during a speed workout or a 5-K race, your breathing pattern will automatically shift to a 2:1 ratio of inhalation to exhalation. If you find yourself in this 2:1 pattern during a run that's meant to be relaxed and comfortable, you're running too fast—slow down.

Rhythmic Breathing and Injury Prevention

The greater value to learning these 3:2 and 2:1 breathing patterns has to do with injury prevention. During running, you hit the ground with the greatest force at the beginning of exhalation. If you inhale and exhale on an even number of footsteps—2:2, for example—you will end up always striking the ground with the same foot at the beginning of each exhalation. This means one side of your body will experience greater impact stress during running than the other. Experts believe this is one of the reasons runners often develop injuries on the same side of the body each time. With the 3:2 and 2:1 breathing patterns, which follow an odd number of steps, you'll begin exhaling first on one foot and then the other, which will distribute the impact stress evenly on both sides of your body.

When I'm running, should I breathe through my nose or my mouth?

You will naturally breathe through both your mouth and your nose. Some runners force themselves to breathe through their noses, but there's no advantage to this.

The Uphills . . . and the Downhills

Of course breathing isn't all that comfortable when you're running up hills, but that doesn't mean you should avoid them. Running uphill builds strength and power. On any incline, your stride will shorten, your pace will slow, you'll lean forward a little, and your arms will "pump" a little harder—all this happens naturally. One mistake some runners make is to slow their stride. By maintaining your normal rate, which should be between 180 and 190 steps per minute, getting up a hill will be easier. This shouldn't be difficult, as a shorter stride length on the uphills will allow you to maintain your stride rate without having to increase your pace.

Once you reach the top, it's time to celebrate. You've conquered a challenge, and now the fun begins—running downhill, where gravity's assistance lets you run faster with little effort. Downhill running offers real benefits to your legs, too. It works your muscles differently than running level or uphill does, and the result is that it strengthens your legs against the muscle soreness that you might feel the day after a hard run or race.

The downhills are a bit trickier than the uphills, though. You'll notice a strong impulse to lean back, lengthen your stride, and "brake" with your legs as your pace quickens. This increases the impact forces of running downhill. Instead, try to relax, stay forward, shorten your stride, and take quick, light steps. Keep your arms close to your sides—don't let them flail about—and simply "go with the flow." If a hill is very steep and you can't help but brake with your legs, run zigzag to the bottom. Downhill running can be lots of fun, but you increase your risk of injury if you don't follow good form.

Running Hot and Cold

What are a runner's favorite seasons? You guessed it—spring and fall. Sure, the long, hot days of summer are great if you're "lazy," but runners are far from lazy, and running in the heat can be deadly—literally. Subfreezing temperatures aren't very inviting, either, if that's what you face during the winter months. Still, it's much easier to get warm on a cold winter run than to stay cool in the heat and humidity. After all, running is a heat-generating activity.

Fortunately, manufacturers of sports apparel have designed clothing with exceptional properties for keeping you warm in winter and as cool and dry as possible under a sweltering sun (see chapter 15). Dressing right is the first and most important step in handling the elements, but there are several other steps you can take to keep you comfortable when the air around you is not.

Keeping Your Cool in the Heat

During your first couple of weeks running in a hot season or a hot climate, take time to acclimate, meaning gradually introduce and adapt your body to the change in temperature. Do not do speed work; limit your running to about 30 minutes (longer is okay during "cool" times of the day). In 10 to 14 days, you should be acclimated and can resume your regular routine. Here are several other bits of advice for hot-weather runs:

- Drink plenty of water or other noncaffeinated, nonalcoholic beverages throughout the day every day to keep your body well hydrated. Dehydration can lead to heat exhaustion or heat stroke. You know you're drinking enough when your urine is pale yellow. (For more information on hydration and sports beverages, see chapter 8).
- Run during the coolest times of day. Mornings are best; evenings, second best.
- If you'll be running for more than an hour, take along water or a sports beverage (see chapter 16 for water-carrying systems) or

plan a route that takes you past water fountains or a convenience store where you can buy something to drink.
- Run on trails or through parks where the shade—as well as the moisture released from trees and plants through transpiration—keeps you cool.
- If you're doing speed training on a particularly hot day, go at a slower pace than usual.
- Stop running if you feel dizzy or weak or experience headache, muscle cramps, or an upset stomach. These are symptoms of heat exhaustion and heat stroke (see chapter 27 for treatment of heat illness).
- Know that you are *not a wimp* if you take a day off when it simply feels too hot to run.

Keeping Your Heat in the Cold

Don't let the snow scare you. It's much easier to get comfortable in winter than summer. Remember, running *generates* heat. All you really need is the right clothing and you'll be cozy. Yes, that first blast of cold air out the door may be daunting, but give it a half-mile and you'll feel fine. In fact, you'll probably find that winter running is absolutely exhilarating. A few pointers:

- Drink plenty of fluids daily. Though hypothermia occurs rarely in runners, staying well hydrated is essential to its prevention.
- Wear a hat. Ninety percent of your body's heat is lost through your head, so forget about how silly your wool knit hat looks—put it on to stay warm.
- Mittens are warmer than gloves because they keep your fingers together. By separating your fingers, gloves allow cold air to circulate around them.
- When the windchill factor knocks the temperature below zero, think about taking a day off, using the treadmill, or pumping iron. If you must go out, put on a layer of petroleum jelly to help protect exposed skin or wear a ski mask to cover your face.
- If you do a lot of winter running on snow-packed roads and could use some extra traction, consider this tip: buy some ¼-inch or ⅜-inch screws and screw them through the bottoms of your running shoes. You may need to use a tack to start the hole, and then the screw should go through easily.

Where You Run

One of the great things about running is that you can do it anywhere. I've even heard of marines stationed for long periods of time on ships logging their daily miles on the deck. Not all running surfaces offer equal footing, however. Here's a review of the most common options.

Roads

Most of us put in a lot of miles on asphalt streets. Roads score big points for accessibility and abundance, and most offer even footing. Be careful of those with high crowns (the center of the road is higher than the sides); they force you to run on an incline, which can lead to injury if you overdo it. The biggest drawback to asphalt: it's hard. Softer surfaces definitely reduce the impact of running (although they have their own drawbacks), but for most runners, roads are fine. I do most of my running on the streets around my home, and in 13 years and eight marathons, I've only had one running injury. One thing is certain, asphalt beats the next option in this category—concrete.

Sidewalks

Avoid sidewalks at all costs. Concrete is one of the hardest surfaces you could ever run on. It's 10 percent harder than asphalt. "You can cut your risk of injury in half simply by staying off concrete," says John Pagliano, D.P.M. The high force of impact is not the only peril of running on sidewalks. Unless you run circles around a block, you frequently have to hop on and off sidewalks—potentially risky business. Older walks often have broken, uneven surfaces, making it easy to catch your toe and fall flat on your face. (I know; I've done this.) Use sidewalks only if running in the streets puts you in danger of being hit by a car.

Trails

They come in a variety of grades from level dirt paths to steep, rocky, tree root–strewn passageways that seem fit for mountain goats only. Trails can take you into the most beautiful landscapes you'll ever run—through woods and fields, up hills, around lakes, along mountainsides . . . As for footing, that obviously depends on the path you choose. Trails lessen the impact of running, which makes them easier on your legs, but the rugged ones will challenge your strength

FINDING TRAILS

If you want to locate trails in your area, check with your local running store. Someone there should be able to point you in the right direction.

and agility. You can get a terrific workout if that's your goal; you can also get terrific cuts and bruises if you trip on a tree root or rock. If you have weak ankles or knees, avoid the rough ones. Unfortunately, most of us don't have trails right outside our door, but off-road running is worth the drive.

Cinder Paths

One of the best surfaces for running, cinder trails are most common in city and town parks, where you can usually find a water fountain, too. The soft surface is easy on your legs, and you don't have to worry about tripping over rocks and tree roots. However, heavy rains can cut deep ruts and those trails that aren't well maintained may become very uneven. Cinder paths are popular among runners and walkers, so you won't be alone on your run.

The Track

Running's arena, the track is the best place to run if you want to know exactly how fast and how far you're going. Most outdoor tracks are 400 meters around, about a quarter-mile, measured on the inside lane. If you do speed work, you'll get the most benefit by doing it on the track. The surface is fast and even and you can time your pace precisely.

TRACKING YOUR KIDS

If you have children, take them to the track with you. They can play on the infield while you run.

Tracks are softer than the road and thus easier on your legs. Their only drawback is the constant turning they require, which places an uneven stress on your body, so change directions every 4 laps. Indoor tracks are even tighter than outdoor tracks, with 8 or 10 laps to a mile.

Cross-Country

Rolling hills, open fields, golf courses, and college cross-country courses are all great places to run. Grassy surfaces lessen the impact of running, and they're fun to run on. You blaze your own way, and you can go barefoot if you want, but watch for holes and ground that's uneven. The well-manicured greens of golf courses make them some of the best places to run; of course, there, you need to watch out for flying balls and angry golfers. Running on grass builds strength in your legs and feet because this surface isn't perfectly smooth and you have to work a little harder as your muscles make minor adjustments to accommodate the bumps and dips.

Beaches

Softer isn't always better. When you run on sand, your heels sink and your Achilles tendons stretch. This is no big deal unless you do too much of it—then you'll likely end up with Achilles tendinitis. The softness of the beach forces your muscles to work harder than if you were running on a firm surface. You'll run more slowly, but you'll burn more calories doing so. For the firmest footing on the beach, run near the water's edge.

The other drawback to the beach is that it slopes down to the water, which forces you to run on an uneven surface—one leg hits the sand higher than the other. Imbalanced running can cause strain but, again, you'll have a problem only if you overdo it. Simply keep your runs short—3 or 4 miles—and turn around midway to balance the effects of the incline.

All that being said, beach running is great fun. In your bathing suit and bare feet, running along the water's edge, in the sun, sand, sea breeze, salt air, cool water . . . it doesn't get much better.

A Week in the Life of a Runner

Where you run, when you run, and how often you run clearly depend on what your goals are and what fits your lifestyle. If you want to improve your race times, you'll probably run almost every day if not every day. If you run for general fitness and for the simple joy of it, you still might run every day, or you may run only a few days a week.

Do I need a stress test before I start a running program?

"If you're over 45 and beginning an exercise program for the first time, it's a good idea to get a stress test, especially if you have a family history of heart disease or if you have diabetes, high blood pressure, a high high-density lipoprotein (HDL) cholesterol level, or if you smoke or are considerably overweight."

—PAUL THOMPSON, M.D., CARDIOLOGIST

Whatever way you choose to pursue your running, keep in mind the importance of rest. Running is fun, but it's difficult. Rest days allow your muscles to recoup. Follow the "hard/easy approach" to running. Alternate harder days of running with days of light running, cross-training, or no running. For some, a hard day might be 3 miles and an easy day no running. A marathoner might run a 20-miler followed by 3 miles the next day. Maybe you want to mix running with other activities, such as swimming, cycling, or softball. Play around with different routines. Find what you enjoy. Imagine that your week is a blank canvas and that you hold a fitness palette. Paint your week with running, swimming, weight lifting, days off . . . in whatever pattern pleases you.

From Zero to 30 Minutes in 10 Easy Weeks

If you are new to running or if you are getting back to it after some time off, it helps to have a little direction at first. The schedule on page 47 was created by Budd Coates, a long-time runner, coach, and corporate fitness director. He uses this schedule every year with groups of new runners training to participate in the Chase Corporate Challenge, a national series of 3½-mile races. Everyone who has followed this plan has successfully completed the race. The program combines walking and running for a total of 30 minutes a session and progresses to 30 minutes of running, or roughly 3 miles. Before starting this schedule, you should be able to walk for 30 minutes 4 times a week.

Increasing Your Mileage

Let's say you've been running about 12 miles a week for a few months now, and you'd like to increase your mileage. You and your friends have decided it might be fun to try the Thanksgiving Day 10-K this fall, and you'd like to get in better shape. What's the best way to add miles to your weekly routine? Gradually.

If you increase your mileage too quickly, you'll get hurt. This is something even a lot of experienced runners forget in their quests for improved performance and faster times. You have to let your body gradually adapt to reasonable increments of additional miles. The rule of thumb is to make increases about every 3 weeks, and in increments of 10 percent to 15 percent of total weekly mileage. The idea is to add a few more miles and adapt to the increase over a cou-

Week	Sunday	Monday	Tuesday	Wednesday	Thursday	Friday	Saturday
1	Run 2 minutes, walk 4 minutes; repeat 4 times	Day off	Run 2 minutes, walk 4 minutes; repeat 4 times	Day off	Run 2 minutes, walk 4 minutes; repeat 4 times	Run 2 minutes, walk 4 minutes; repeat 4 times	Day off
2	Run 3 minutes, walk 3 minutes; repeat 4 times	Day off	Run 3 minutes, walk 3 minutes; repeat 4 times	Day off	Run 3 minutes, walk 3 minutes; repeat 4 times	Run 3 minutes, walk 3 minutes; repeat 4 times	Day off
3	Run 5 minutes, walk 2½ min.; repeat 3 times	Day off	Run 5 minutes, walk 2½ min.; repeat 3 times	Day off	Run 5 minutes, walk 2½ min.; repeat 3 times	Run 5 minutes, walk 2½ min.; repeat 3 times	Day off
4	Run 7 minutes, walk 3 minutes; repeat 2 times	Day off	Run 7 minutes, walk 3 minutes; repeat 2 times	Day off	Run 7 minutes, walk 3 minutes; repeat 2 times	Run 7 minutes, walk 3 minutes; repeat 2 times	Day off
5	Run 8 minutes, walk 2 minutes; repeat 2 times	Day off	Run 8 minutes, walk 2 minutes; repeat 2 times	Day off	Run 8 minutes, walk 2 minutes; repeat 2 times	Run 8 minutes, walk 2 minutes; repeat 2 times	Day off
6	Run 9 minutes, walk 2 minutes; repeat once; run 8 minutes.	Day off	Run 9 minutes, walk 2 minutes; repeat once; run 8 minutes	Day off	Run 9 minutes, walk 2 minutes; repeat once; run 8 minutes	Run 9 minutes, walk 2 minutes; repeat once; run 8 minutes	Day off
7	Run 9 minutes, walk 1 minute; repeat 2 times	Day off	Run 9 minutes, walk 1 minute; repeat 2 times	Day off	Run 9 minutes, walk 1 minute; repeat 2 times	Run 9 minutes, walk 1 minute; repeat 2 times	Day off
8	Run 13 minutes, walk 2 minutes; repeat	Day off	Run 13 minutes, walk 2 minutes; repeat	Day off	Run 13 minutes, walk 2 minutes; repeat	Run 13 minutes, walk 2 minutes; repeat	Day off
9	Run 14 minutes, walk 1 minute; repeat	Day off	Run 14 minutes, walk 1 minute; repeat	Day off	Run 14 minutes, walk 1 minute; repeat	Run 14 minutes, walk 1 minute; repeat	Day off
10	Run 30 minutes	Day off	Run 30 minutes	Day off	Run 30 minutes	Run 30 minutes	Day off

UPPING YOUR MILES

Here's a sample plan for a runner who wants to increase her mileage from 12 a week to 20. The basic principles to follow: increase mileage by no more than 10 percent to 15 percent at a time; take 2 or 3 weeks to adjust to your higher level of running before adding more miles; and if you feel fatigued at the end of a week, cut back on mileage for 1 or 2 weeks and then resume your buildup.

Week	Sun.	Mon.	Tues.	Wed.	Thurs.	Fri.	Sat.	Total
1	3	3	0	3	0	3	0	12
2	4	3	0	4	0	3	0	14
3	3–4	3	0	3–4	0	3	0	12–14
4	4	3	0	4	0–2	3	0	14–16
5	4	3	0	4	0–2	3	0	14–16
6	4	3	0	4	0–2	3	0	14–16
7	4–6	3	0	4	2	3	0	16–18
8	4–6	3	0	4	2	3	0	16–18
9	4–6	3	0	4	2	3	0	16–18
10	6	3	0	4	2–3	3–4	0	18–20

Note: This is only an example. You may choose to arrange your mileage differently. Just remember to follow a day of high mileage with a day off or a day of low mileage.

ple of weeks before doing more. See the box above (Upping Your Miles) for an example of how to approach a buildup in your running.

Setting Goals

Although there are several specific guidelines you can apply to your running, the essence of it is simplicity. Part of what makes running so simple is its versatility. You can run as little or as much as you choose, as slowly or as quickly as you desire. What you do with your running depends on what you want to get out of it and how it fits into your lifestyle.

You may choose to run for weight loss, cardiovascular health, or stress release. Perhaps the challenge of competing excites you, or maybe you like to run simply because it makes you feel good. If you run primarily for general health and fitness, Ken Cooper's guidelines still apply: 20 to 30 minutes of aerobic exercise three times a week is the minimum requirement. If you run for the sport of it—to race—running will require more of your time, physical energy, and mental energy.

Take a look at your lifestyle and find a way to run that's compatible. Running shouldn't be an added stress. Those of you who have jobs, a family, and community obligations may choose to run just a few times a week for fun, fitness, and the extra boost of energy that running provides. Others may have the time and energy to focus on training to compete.

Lately all my runs seem to be slow. I don't look forward to them anymore, and I'm feeling tired and irritable. What could the problem be?

You may be running too many miles or running them too hard. Try cutting back on mileage or intensity or both, even if you look at your schedule and think that it's conservative. Remember, running is one part of your life. What goes on in the rest of your life affects your running, too. If work or family has been requiring more energy, or if you have been under extra stress, you'll tire more easily on your runs. Try to find a balance that works. You might even take a break from running altogether and come back to it when you have more time and energy. If you cut back on your running but still feel tired and cranky, take a look at your diet and sleep patterns. You may need to make some adjustments in those areas.

Allow your running goals to change over time, too. It's easy to create a routine and never break out of it, but then we risk becoming stale as runners and individuals. If you've run primarily for fitness, challenge yourself to a race. You may be surprised at how fun competing can be. If training to race is all you're used to, give yourself a break. Put aside your training log and your sports watch and run with no purpose but the sheer joy of it.

A Few Words About Racing

If you've never raced before, why not give it a try? There are as many kinds of races as there are models of running shoes. "Sorry, I'm not the competitive type," you say. "Besides, I don't have the time or inclination to train hard." Well, you don't have to be competitive, and you don't have to train hard to participate. There are many races you can do just for fun—events such as the Bay to Breakers 12-K in San Francisco or the Lilac Bloomsday 12-K in Spokane. These races draw everyone from walkers to serious competitors, and they are *fun.* There's music along the course, runners dressed in costume, and no one cares how fast you cover the distance. Furthermore, the fun doesn't end at the finish line. Postrace activities involve lots of food, beverages, and socializing.

I think the best place to run your first race, however, is an all-women event. Though racing among men is fun, too, women's races have a special spirit of camaraderie and mutual support. The L'eggs Mini Marathon in New York City was the first women's race I ever ran, and I will never forget the special connection I felt to all the other women runners. You shouldn't have any trouble finding an all-women event near you. More and more women are running races every year. One of the newest and now largest all-women events, the Idaho Women's Fitness Celebration in Boise, grew from 2,300 to over 19,000 participants by its sixth year (1998), and the nationwide Race for the Cure series of 5-Ks, which took place in nearly 90 cities in 1998, is constantly expanding. In addition, the Road Runners Club of America (RRCA) organizes two race series: the RRCA Women's Distance Festival of approximately 80 events around the country and the RRCA Women's 5-K series, which is sponsored by Avon Products. For more information about these series, call the RRCA at (703) 836-0558.

Give some thought to taking on the *challenge* of racing, too. You don't have to be a talented runner to revel in the satisfaction of a race well run. The beauty of racing is that we can compete with ourselves, and the measure of our success is individual. We set our own standards to achieve, whether they be running a faster 5-K or completing a marathon. The final achievement of a goal that you've worked toward is a proud moment. It shows you that you are worthy, capable, and strong. It brings you joyous accomplishment.

Running Safely

You have to realize that bad stuff can happen to anybody, anyplace, anytime, but if you've got a plan of action, you won't have to fear.

—J. J. Bittenbinder, Chicago detective

YOU RUN FOR PLEASURE, FOR THE FREEDOM of it. It is your release. Then you read a story in the newspaper about a woman attacked in a park while running. In *broad daylight,* a man grabbed her, pulled her into the bushes, and raped her. The next time you go out for a run, you think of that woman and you feel a little afraid—but even more, you are angry because the freedom of running has been tainted. You are a woman, you are vulnerable, and you cannot run carefree through the streets anymore. The reality is you cannot run *carelessly,* but you *can* run without fear if you follow a few guidelines and know what to do to stay safe. Knowledge is our strongest armor, and best of all, it doesn't weigh an ounce.

Running Smart

One of the best things you can do is run with a friend or a group of friends. There *is* safety in numbers. If no one you know runs, join a local running club. Most have organized group runs once or twice a week for runners of all abilities, and you might meet someone you can get together with regularly.

Sometimes, though, you just want to go alone, have some time to think, or enjoy your own private space. That's fine, too. Just run smart, and you'll be safe. The following recommendations come from the Road Runners Club of America (RRCA) and experts who regularly instruct women on safety.

Leave Word of Your Whereabouts

Let a friend or family member know approximately how long you'll be gone and what route you'll be taking. If you don't return when expected, they'll know where to look for you.

Carry Identification

Write down your name, the phone number of someone to call in case of an emergency, and any necessary medical information (blood type, medications, drugs you are allergic to) on a piece of paper and stick it in your shorts pocket, jacket pocket, or in your shoe. This is especially important if you are running in an unfamiliar city. Also, take along a quarter for a phone call or some cash for a cab.

Avoid "Lonely" Roads

One of the joys of running is exploring rural roads and wooded trails, but it's best not to run alone through isolated areas or unfamiliar territory. Save these runs for times when you can get together with friends. When you're on your own, stick to your neighborhood, familiar and populated streets, or, for the back-to-nature experience, run in your local park during peak exercise hours when you'll be with cyclists, walkers, and other runners. Who knows? Maybe you'll meet a new running partner.

Rearrange Your Route

Don't be predictable. If you run the same roads at the same time on the same days every week, you become an easy target—and your running life becomes really boring.

Be Aware

Whether you're running alone or with a friend, run with awareness, especially if you're in new territory. Pay attention to what's around you so that know where to go if you do need help. Take note of the people around you, too. Don't avoid eye contact with strangers, and if you hear someone running up behind you, turn around to see who it is. Let him know you know he's there. A potential attacker is more likely to approach you if he thinks he can catch you unaware.

Do Not Wear a Headset

It's surprising how many women run with headphones when in just about every report of a runner attacked you learn that she was using a portable tape player. If you listen to music while you run, you invite attack. It's that simple. Wearing headphones blocks your awareness. You can't hear cars approaching and you won't notice someone coming up behind you. You are vulnerable, and an attacker knows it. Save the headset for the treadmill—that's when you'll need it most anyway.

Run in the Daylight Hours

Most assaults are committed between 6 P.M. and 6 A.M., according to statistics from the U.S. Department of Justice. Try not to run alone during these hours.

Don't Talk to Strangers

You're a nice person, so of course when someone stops his or her car and asks for directions, you want to help. Don't go up to the car; keep moving and call out directions or simply say you don't know.

Carry a Safety Device

Pepper sprays and an implement called the Persuader can help you escape attack if one should occur. You'll find more information about these later in this chapter under the heading "Tools of Self-Defense."

RULES OF THE ROAD

- Run against traffic so you can see approaching cars. The only exception might be when you reach a blind curve in the road; cross over well before the curve, and once the road has straightened, return to the left side of the street.
- Give cars the right of way at all intersections and road crossings. When you're running on a narrow street and traffic is coming from both directions, simply stop and wait until it has passed.
- Be alert when approaching just-parked cars. An unaware driver or passenger might open a door as you're running by.
- Never assume that a driver sees you. For example, if a car is backing out of a driveway, swing wide or stop and wait.
- Wear a reflective vest or clothing and light colors when running in the darkness of early morning or evening.

Woman's Best Friend

Dogs can make great running partners. Not only are they the most enthusiastic companions you can find, but they'll defend your life against any attacker. Full of love and loyalty for you, even the most docile pup can turn into a vicious protector if someone threatens you.

Best Breeds

The best running dog has a good temperament and is well trained. You want your dog to stay with you, not head off into the bushes after a groundhog, and you don't want him or her to go chasing after other runners or getting into fights with other dogs. Just because a particular dog seems "built for running" doesn't mean he or she will become a good running partner, but some breeds that may not seem runworthy can be perfect running companions. Dog lover and road runner Jon Sinclair has a friend who runs with a one-eyed toy poodle. Nonetheless, certain breeds are more likely to produce better runners than others. Dogs bred for sport or work are physically well suited to running, and they respond when you call them; however, hunting dogs—hounds in particular—are likely to go off on the trail of a rabbit or squirrel.

Robin Kovary of the American Dog Trainers Network in New York City recommends that you look for a dog with long legs and an athletic body, such as golden retrievers, Labradors, greyhounds, Dobermans, or salukis. German shepherds, collies, and shelties can become good runners also. Kovary cautions against breeds with pushed-in muzzles—bulldogs and pugs, for example—as they'll have a harder time breathing. "Also short, stocky, long-backed breeds, like bassett hounds or any big dog on short legs, will have a harder time running," says Kovary. "So will the very large breeds like mastiffs and Saint Bernards, which can overheat quickly." Most terriers are simply difficult to run with. "Many can be aggressive toward other dogs, and they tend to chase after squirrels and chipmunks," says Kovary.

Training

You might be lucky and own a pup who was born to please, but most of us need to take our dogs to obedience school. Keep in mind that no dog is too old to learn new tricks. If yours didn't go to obedience school as a puppy, it's never too late to enroll.

Don't begin running with your dog until he or she is fully grown. Running can damage the shoulders, hips, and knees when a dog's bones and muscles are still developing, which takes 6 months to a year or more, depending on the breed. The larger the dog, the longer the maturation period. Ask your veterinarian. It's also a good idea to have your dog checked for any orthopedic problems before beginning a running program.

Introduce your dog to running gradually. Just as you had to start slowly and with short distances, so does your dog, especially if you'll be running on the road. A dog's pads need time to toughen up—too much too soon, and they'll become sore and may crack and bleed. (Imagine yourself running barefoot down the street.) Begin with a block or a quarter-mile and gradually increase the distance. How many miles your pup will eventually be able to cover depends on the dog.

Running Safely with Your Dog

Use a leash, especially when running near traffic. You can purchase a special running leash that attaches around your waist, leaving your hands and arms free.

Keep an eye on your dog's level of fatigue. If you see signs of overheating (excessive lolling of the tongue and wooziness), stop and get water for the dog to drink and pour cool—not cold—water over his or her whole body if possible, or at least on the pads, says Kovary. In wintertime, you might need to cover your dog for warmth if he or she doesn't have a thick coat of fur. Also, avoid running over areas that have been treated with ice-melting chemicals and salts, which can burn a dog's paws. Be sensitive to your dog's needs and comfort as well as your own, and the two of you can share miles of healthy and happy running together.

When a Dog Is Not Your Best Friend

Dogs have a natural prey drive, meaning when they see something run, they'll chase it. That something could be you, and if the dog chasing you isn't a friendly one, you could be in big trouble. How do you know whether a dog might attack? "Raised ears, tail, and hair are signs that the dog is aggressive, and you need to be very careful," says Robin Kovary. "When a dog's tail is down, that indicates a fear-based aggression; the dog may or may not attack you." Kovary also points out that a wagging tail does not always mean a dog is friendly. Terriers, for example, wag their tails when they spot potential prey. You need to evaluate the whole situation.

Here's what to do if you think you might become potential prey to an unleashed dog:

- Do not try to outrun the dog. You won't be able to and you'll only encourage attack. Stop and walk, keeping the dog in your peripheral vision. Don't look directly at the dog; eye contact is considered confrontational.
- When you are safely past the dog, slowly begin running again.
- If the dog walks up to you, stay calm, stand with your side to the dog, and let it sniff you. It may just want to check you out and then leave you alone.
- If the dog does attack you, don't flail or scream, this will make the dog more aggressive. Protect the most vulnerable parts of your body: your neck, face, and stomach.
- If you do get bitten, locate the owner of the dog. You'll need to find out whether the dog's rabies shots are up-to-date. Then go to the emergency department. You may need a tetanus shot or other treatment.
- Report all unleashed dogs to the authorities.

Tools of Self-Defense

When you don't have a human or canine companion to run with, consider carrying a self-defense device as an extra precaution. Pepper sprays and a small implement called a Persuader are easily carried on a run and can help you protect yourself in a threatening situation. *Instruction in the use of these devices is essential,* however. If you don't know what you're doing, you may hurt yourself before you deter any attacker. Check for self-defense courses in your area and inquire if instruction in the use of safety devices is offered. If not, call your local police department. Many policemen and -women have training in the use of chemical sprays and Persuaders and may be able to recommend a class or instructor.

Sprays

Most people assume Mace when they think of self-defense sprays, but Mace is the brand name of one specific chemical spray—chloroacetophenone. It works by causing pain when sprayed on the skin or in the eyes or nasal passages. "The problems with Mace are that it doesn't act fast enough and it doesn't work on people who don't feel pain in the normal way—people who are drunk, enraged, or psychotic," says Lyn Bates, vice president of AWARE (Arming Women Against Rape and Endangerment), an organization that informs and instructs on self-defense.

"Pepper sprays are faster acting than Mace and they are more effective on people who have a high pain threshhold," says Bates. "They cause swelling of mucous membranes and can slam shut your attacker's eyelids or swell his throat enough to make breathing uncomfortable." Pepper spray (oleoresin capsicum) is not legal in all states, and where it is legal, you may be required to get a license or a firearm ID card to carry it. Check with your local authorities.

The Persuader

The Persuader is a lightweight 6-inch metal or plastic rod that attaches to your keychain and can easily be looped onto the waistband of your running shorts. You can use it to strike at an attacker or to pry yourself free if you are grabbed. But to use the Persuader effectively, you need training. "Training teaches you techniques, which you can use even with a pen or pencil," says Bates. "You learn different areas to strike and how to apply different levels of force." Persuaders cost $12 to $15 and can be purchased by mail order or in stores that sell other types of self-defense products.

What About Whistles?

Whistles seem like a good idea, but most safety experts agree that whistles are not effective at either deterring an attacker or calling for help. "Attackers are not afraid of a whistle," says Bates, "and furthermore, it's unlikely that someone will respond and come to your rescue. We have become so accustomed to hearing alarms—all sorts of alarms—that we disregard them." Experts also point out that you waste valuable time using one—grabbing it with your hand and blowing it with your mouth. You could be taking more effective self-defense actions, like running, kicking, hitting, biting. Besides, you have a natural sound alarm—your vocal cords. You can scream.

What to Do If You Are Attacked

Running is one of your greatest assets in a threatening situation. Even if your attacker points a gun at you, run. If you're grabbed, fight back. Kick, bite, scream. "Most criminals don't expect resistance because so many women give in," says Bates. "An attacker has a plan, and the only scenario in his mind is to carry out that plan," adds Bates. "If you do anything unexpected to upset that scenario, the attacker can't deal with it and takes off. Act, immediately and with 100 percent commitment, and you'll most likely scare him away."

Whatever you do, never let your attacker take you anywhere. Chances are, you won't come back. "If someone is trying to get you to go with him, you should do everything in your power not to go," says Bates. "Even if he has a gun or knife, he isn't necessarily prepared to use that gun on you right there." Remember, his *plan* is to take you somewhere—upset his plan.

Again, the key to safety is preparation. Be *prepared* to put up a fight. Take a self-defense class. Bates recommends finding a course in which you train one-on-one with another person so that you will be prepared for a real-life situation. It's not likely you'll ever have to fend off a punching

SAFETY SOURCES

For more information on safety, the Road Runner's Club of America (RRCA) publishes brochures and a safety video, *Women Running: Run Smart. Run Safe.* Contact them at 1150 S. Washington Street, Suite 250, Alexandria, VA 22314; phone: (703) 836-0558.

Also, you'll find lots of information through AWARE (Arming Women Against Rape and Endangerment). Their mailing address is P.O. Box 242, Bedford, MA 01730; phone: (617) 893-0500. Their web-site address is **www.aware.org./index.html**.

bag. AWARE recommends these classes: Model Mugging, Impact, and Bamm, which are taught in many cities across the country. Another good program is Campus Confidence (call 800/850-7237 for more information).

It's unfortunate that we have to consider our vulnerability when we run, especially when we run alone. By acknowledging that vulnerability, taking the right precautions, and knowing what to do in an unsafe situation, though, you can run without worry.

7 Finding Motivation

IT HAPPENS TO ALL OF US. YOU'VE planned a run, just a simple 5-miler, but you just plain don't feel like running. Doesn't matter that the sun is shining and it's a perfect 62° out. It's not that you have a zillion other pressing tasks to accomplish or obligations to meet. There are no excuses. You just don't want to go. Of course, more often, there *are* lots of reasons not to run: it's raining, it's too cold, you don't have the time, you're just too tired . . . but you really do love running. It makes you feel good. It's an important part of your life. You know that if you go for that run, you'll feel better. You just need a little help getting out the door.

Quick Fixes

Following are some tactics you can try right now if you happen to be having one of those days.

Think About How Good You'll Feel

Most of us have never gone on a run we've regretted. Think about how you feel at the end of a run. Close your eyes. Imagine. Feel the flush in your face, the trickle of sweat, the deep breaths and beating heart—your whole body stimulated by activity, your mind high with the accomplishment of another run. You feel renewed, energetic, ready to take on any challenge.

Choose a Fun Route

If you're not feeling particularly motivated, don't even consider doing the usual straight, flat out-and-back. You'll have an easier time getting out the door if you think about doing a run that's varied and interesting.

Think about how you might design a unique run. Go for a "flowering gardens run" in spring, exploring the neighborhood for the prettiest gardens and blossoming trees. Plan a "historic sites tour" in which your route passes by the old churches and buildings of your town. Do a mini "duathlon" or "triathlon": ride your bike to a nearby park or scenic spot, then run a loop that brings you back to your bike and cycle home or to another location for another run. Mix up running on the beach with dips in the ocean, or if you live near a lake,

NATURE RUN

"My favorite run is my nature run. It's a long one where I'm running slowly and can look around. I record in my brain all the birds I see and hear, all the reptiles, the flowers. . . . I pass a horse pasture. I check out where my frogs like to sit. A salamander that I've been looking for I saw crossing the road the other day. It's amazing what I see. I'm up and down mountains and running along streams. Even though I do that run the same way every week, it's never the same. I'm never bored."

—CATHERINE ELWELL, RUNNER

you can combine running and swimming or cycling, running, and swimming.

I have the most difficult time motivating myself to run after work, even though I usually feel really good on my evening runs. One winter evening at Christmastime, I decided to take a tour of the light displays in my neighborhood. With no plan in mind, I headed out the door and down the road, checking out the lights, turning down whatever street looked most interesting. I was having so much fun I ran for nearly an hour.

Running doesn't have to be monotonous if you put a little imagination into your step.

Do Speed Work

"What?! Why would I want to run hard when I don't feel like running at all?" you ask. Because it's another way to put some variety into your running and make it fun. *Fartlek* is a fun type of speed work. The word is Swedish for "speed play," and it *is* play. After you've run easily for 10 minutes or so, pick a point in the distance—a tree, a telephone pole, a mailbox—and run fast to that point, then slow down. Once you're running comfortably again, pick another point and pick up the pace again. Continue to change pace randomly according to what you feel like doing. Finish with about 10 minutes of easy running.

Run like a Kid

Why do we think of running as obligation or exercise? Ever notice how the children in your neighborhood love to run? It comes so naturally, without thought, a spontaneous burst of energy born of a pure love of movement. It's play. Kids would rather run to their friends' homes than walk.

You were like that, too, once. Remember? You can get it back—just release yourself from all the constrictions you put on your running. Set no time, distance, pace, or route. Leave your watch on the kitchen table and go run—freely, like a child. Run down whatever street or trail entices you. Run fast and run slow. Stop to take a drink at a water fountain or to enjoy a scenic view you've happened on. Walk for a little while, and then when you feel like it, begin running again. There are no rules. Continue in your spontaneous meandering until you feel like stopping. Note: when you leave home on one of these runs, be sure to take a quarter—you might just stray so far from home, you'll need a ride back.

Bargain with Yourself

When all else fails, strike a deal with yourself. Say, "Okay, I'll go for a run, but if it feels crappy, I'm turning around and coming home." This takes the pressure off you to do a set distance. You've given yourself permission to run as little—or as much—as you want. Sometimes it's the thought of running 8 miles versus 3 to 5 that's got you less than enthused. Of course, be fair about this deal and give your body a chance to warm up before you call it quits. It may take a mile or two before you start feeling good. Not surprisingly, most times, you end up enjoying the run and going farther than you anticipated. If in fact you *don't* feel good and you do stop, it means that you really are too tired—you *should* take a rest day.

Long-Term Strategies

Okay, so there are several little tricks you can try to get you going on any particular day, but sometimes the running blahs can last for days, weeks, months. Some runners find they have seasonal motivation deficit disorder: they shiver at the thought of running through the winter or cringe at summer's heat. Of course, you don't have to run year-round, but if you do want to, there are several strategies you can use to make it easier to get out the door when the going gets tough. Remember, the toughest part is getting out there. Once you're running—whether through rain, sleet, or snow—the good feeling of it all returns and you wonder why you ever hesitated to run in the first place.

Pair Up with a Partner

Running with someone—human or canine—is a great motivator in many ways. It's easy to bag your own run but not so easy to cancel plans with a friend. Besides, who'd want to? Running with a friend is fun. You can talk the whole way and the miles just fly by.

Keep a Training Log

Whether in a special running log, a calendar, or your computer, write down what you hope to do for, say, every day for the next month. Then each day, record what you actually do in miles or time spent running. This is the guilt method of motivation. It's hard to look at a week of zeroes.

Keeping a training log can be helpful in other ways, too. If you make notes about your run—temperature, course, time of day, how you felt, how fast you ran if that's important—you'll be able to learn a lot about your running. You can even chart your running against your menstrual cycle to see how you are affected (more about that in chapter 11). When you've been running for a few years, it can be a lot of fun to revisit the experiences you've recorded.

Set Goals

Want to keep running? Chase a goal. It could be increasing your weekly mileage from 15 to 25 miles or completing a 10-mile run. Racing provides the perfect goal-setting opportunity. In fact, many runners use a marathon to maintain their motivation. The training can take anywhere from 3 months to a year, depending on your experience and level of fitness, and you can't skimp on your running if you want to complete a marathon. Training for short races can be motivating as well. Completing a race regardless of distance or how fast you run leaves you with a special feeling of satisfaction and accomplishment (see chapter 21). You can increase that satisfaction exponentially by running a little faster the next time you participate in a race of the same distance. Wanting to improve at running is one of the greatest motivators of all.

Mix It Up

If running is becoming a drag, take a look at a typical week in your program. Are you running the same 5 miles at the same pace every day? No wonder you don't feel like it anymore. Try to make every day different. It's easy. The options are many. There are long runs, medium runs, short runs, slow runs, fast runs, fast and slow runs, uphill runs, downhill runs, runs on the grass, runs on the track, runs on the trail, runs on the treadmill, runs alone, runs with a friend, runs with groups, races, and all the creative runs discussed earlier. Plus, you don't have to run every day. Mix in some cross-training—mountain biking, inline skating, weight lifting, soccer, tennis . . . your choices are endless. Also, take at least 1 day of total rest each week. It gives your body a break and leaves you feeling fresher for your next active day.

Sometimes you need to step back and take an even longer view of your running. For example, if you're always racing distances of 5 kilometers or longer, consider training to race a mile or look for a local track meet that's open to the public.

Become a Coach

Do you know someone who wants to take up running but isn't quite sure how to get started? Perhaps you have a friend or sister or brother whom you think might enjoy the sport. Consider offering your assistance as a "coach" and running partner. This shifts your focus away from your own training, providing a psychological and physical break while still keeping you active. More important, helping someone else find joy in running might renew your own.

Take a Break

If you just can't seem to find the joy in running no matter what you do, it's a sign that you should take some time off, especially if you find that when you do go for a run it's slow and sluggish and leaves you feeling more fatigued than energized. You may be experiencing symptoms of overtraining—running too much and/or too fast for too long. A period of complete rest will revive your body and mind. In fact, after you've stopped running for a while, chances are that you'll miss it. You'll become hungry to run again. You'll get edgy and fidgety, and the only way to resolve the anxiety of inactivity will be to run.

Sticking to It When You've Just Started

Let's be honest—running is hard, especially in the beginning. It just doesn't feel good at first—at least it didn't for me. It seemed during that whole first year, running was just exercise. I stuck with it because it relieved stress and I knew it would keep me fit. Rarely did I experience a runner's high. Looking back, I wish I had entered running gradually, through a walk/run routine. I think I would have enjoyed it more that first year. Instead, I'd just head out and run until it became too uncomfortable.

I don't know when exactly it happened, but eventually I had a "breakthrough" where running actually felt *good* and discomfort became the rarity. Before long, I could run 8 miles with ease and feel hardly fatigued at the end of it. Runner's high? I began to experience it often—that wonderful feeling when your whole body is in synch and you feel like you can run forever. I knew then I was hooked for life.

What got me to that point? Running with friends, setting goals, keeping a training log. Finally, it all comes down to patience and perseverance, being willing to put up with whatever discomfort and drudgery you might experience until your body learns to run again as it did when you were a child and running came naturally. That point does come, and to run for miles with ease is an extraordinary pleasure.

Making Time to Run

Not surprisingly, the number-one reason most women give for not running is lack of time. Going to college, developing a career, and raising children are each demanding in their own right, and many women balance at least two of them. Add to that trying to nurture a meaningful relationship with a partner, keeping up with household responsibilities, maintaining friendships, plus making time for interests other than running, and our lives fill up fast. Occasionally, we all could use some suggestions on how to fit in a run.

The Early Bird Gets the Run

Runner's World magazine once asked its women readers how they fit running into their busy lives. More than half of the respondents said they run early in the morning before work or before the family wakes up—some even before the birds start chirping.

Does the thought of getting out of bed early sound as feasible to you as pushing a boulder up a hill? Well, if you just can't seem to find time during the rest of the day, at least give it a try. Many women admit that the first week or two can be tough, but, like anything else, the more you do it, the easier it gets. You may surprise yourself and find you love to run in the morning.

Run—Don't Drive—to Work

Provided there's a shower in your office building and you can stash some clothes in your office the night before, consider running to work. Take the bus or train home or get a ride from a co-worker who lives near you. If you have a bicycle, you can cycle to work and run home; then reverse the routine the next day.

Run During Your Lunch Hour

Using your lunch hour to run may be the most efficient way to fit a run into your day, and it gives you an energy boost for the afternoon. Give yourself 10 minutes to get into your running clothes; 30 minutes to run; and 20 minutes for a quick shower, change of clothes, and touch-ups to your hair and makeup. You can eat lunch afterward at your desk.

Run Errands

Need to stop at the drugstore, mail some letters, deposit a check in the bank? Leave the car in the garage and do your errands on foot. You accomplish your tasks and get your run in at the same time. Simply get yourself a fanny pack or a lightweight knapsack for carrying around the items you need to take with you.

Involve Your Children

When you have children, it's much more difficult to find the time to run. Hopefully, you and your partner can make arrangements for one of you to be home while the other runs, but that's not always possible. If you know another running mom, perhaps the two of you can arrange to trade baby-sitting.

When no one's available to be with your children, consider taking them with you. You can push your littlest one along in a running stroller or take your toddlers to a nearby track, where you keep an eye on them while they play inside the oval. Some women have devised creative strategies, such as setting a baby monitor outside while they run laps around their house or up and down the driveway. Older children can bike, skate, or run alongside you. Involving your children will make your run more fun. It's a great way to spend time with them, and it shows them the importance of staying active and fit.

TIME TO RUN

"I believe the key 'strategy' for finding the time to run is priority. There is *always* something else to do. If you make running a priority, then it isn't difficult at all to 'find the time.' "

—ALICE BERNTSON, RUNNER

"Finding time to run continues to be a challenge as my children get older. We have soccer practice, ice skating, piano lessons, and numerous school activities, but as my life gets busier and more complicated, I find I need and enjoy running more than ever. It is *my* time. It's something I do just for me, and I cherish it. The house isn't always clean—there is always more to do than any one person could get done in a day—but it all seems easier to face when I've made time to run."

—KIM HARTMANN, RUNNER

Get a Treadmill

Running on a treadmill isn't the most fun way to run, but it's awfully convenient, especially if you have a family and need to be at home. And it doesn't have to be boring (see chapter 20).

Be Spontaneous

Always have a sports bag, packed with running clothes, shoes, and a towel, in your car so that you can take advantage of any opportunity to run.

Getting Back to Running After a Layoff

Many of us take a break from regular running at some point. It could be that an injury has you off your feet for a while, or you moved and started a new job that temporarily interrupted your routine. Perhaps you decided to stop running during your pregnancy or maybe for 3 or 4 years while your children were young. Whatever the reason for the break, your life has settled into a new order now, and your thoughts have turned to running again.

To go out for a refreshing 5-miler would feel so good. The reality is, however, that you've lost your fitness, and even 5 minutes of running seems daunting. You just know you will labor through your first run in months, huffing and puffing and slogging through whatever distance you cover.

Although it's true you can't go out and clip off a quick 5 miles, you don't have to suffer either. Just start slowly and gradually ease your way back into running. If you've been inactive for a few months or more, begin with walking—20 to 30 minutes every other day for a couple of weeks. Then start mixing in some running—walk for a few minutes, run for a few, walk, run. Each week, run a little more, walk a little less. Use the schedule in chapter 5 (page 47) as a guide. Having a program to follow helps you stay focused and makes it easier to stick to your comeback. You may find that you can progress faster than the recommendations given; that's fine. Just be sure you are running comfortably. You should be able to carry on a conversation; if you can't, slow down. By making a gradual return to running, you'll enjoy it more, you'll stick with it, and you'll prevent injury, which you are more susceptible to during a comeback. Hey—before you know it, you'll be running a brisk and easy 5 miles again and loving every minute of it.

Out the Door—Twice

BY PATRICIA LOCKHART

SUNDAY IS MY DAY FOR MY LONG RUN—USUALLY—BUT THIS WAS the Sunday of the New York City Marathon, which kept me glued to my TV until well into the afternoon. It was almost 2:00 before I even began thinking about suiting up for my weekly 12-miler, in fact, and my thoughts were straying toward the slothful. "Should I or shouldn't I?" I debated. It sure would be easy just to drift mindlessly into a juicy grade-B movie or cozy up with the novel I was reading, but no, I needed something to rouse me from my lethargy, I decided, so I donned my tights and my Nikes and headed out the door.

Only to head straight back. It was windy, foggy, drizzling, and cold—certainly not a day capable of making for a run I'd care to remember, I thought as I sat unlacing my shoes in the kitchen.

But then my "other" voice began chirping away, the one that had gotten me out the door in the first place. "How are you going to feel if you don't run?" it asked. "Are you really going to enjoy that brain-numbing movie or be able to concentrate on your novel, feeling like a wimp?"

Before the second shoe dropped, the answer became obvious. "I'll just do a quickie," I thought, as I rummaged through my closet for a windbreaker. "Just enough to silence my guilt."

My front door swung open for a second time, and I was off.

At first, I felt sluggish and stiff, and the weather certainly wasn't making things any easier. Gradually, though, I began to loosen up, and the weather slowly started to clear, and by the time I reached the turnaround for what would have been my "quickie," I was in gear. Maybe I'd make my 3-miler a 6-, I thought as the fog began to lift, revealing brilliant crimson and amber November foliage. I turned onto a cinder path that ran alongside a creek and eventually into the rich aroma of a quiet woods, my feet sounding like hand claps on the fallen leaves, applauding my every step.

I kept running, eventually coming into a clearing just as the late-afternoon sun finally broke free of its clouds, almost blinding me with its brilliance. *And I came close to* missing *this,* I thought.

From the woods, I broke into an open field recently harvested of its corn. I felt childlike as I hurdled over rows of fallen stalks. I felt such energy, such happiness, such peace. *Will I be able to stop at all?* I thought. *And why should I want to?* I was in awe of the sheer ecstasy of my movement.

Of course I did stop, though not because of fatigue. It was one of those magical experiences when I felt I could have run forever—and almost did, in fact, as my "quickie" turned out to be an 18-miler. I couldn't believe I almost missed out on one of the most truly memorable experiences of my running life.

Patricia Lockhart is a writer and musician living in Woodbury, Connecticut.

PART III

Calories, Carbos, and Weight Concerns

8 The Nutrients You Need

WHEN WE THINK ABOUT WHAT IT MEANS to run, and what comes to mind are mileage, pace, form, strength, and when we seek to improve, these are the aspects of training on which we focus. Also essential to running, however, are carbohydrates, protein, iron, and other nutrients. To enjoy the fullest benefit of running, we need to pay attention not only to the outer mechanical aspects of running but to our internal nutritional requirements as well. What we give our body directly affects what it will give back to us in both health and performance. This is especially true of women. We have broader nutritional needs and more specific requirements than men do.

The foundation of good nutrition is a well-balanced diet high in carbohydrates and low in fat. Specifically, a runner's diet should include 60 percent to 65 percent carbohydrates, 10 percent to 20 percent protein, and 20 percent to 30 percent fat, all from a wide variety of foods that will supply the vitamins and minerals you need. Along with those foods, you need lots of water.

Water

Water is one of the most important elements of nutrition and yet perhaps the least recognized. We tend to focus so much attention on getting enough carbohydrates and vitamins to keep us healthy and energized for running that many of us neglect our need for water. It has no calories, carbohydrates, proteins, fats, or vitamins; however, its significance to our health and our running is great.

We can live for weeks without food but only days without water. Comprising 50 percent of a woman's body, water is present in every cell and is necessary to just about every bodily function: digestion, absorption of nutrients, energy metabolism, and excretion of waste products. It lubricates the joints, intestines, the heart. It cushions the brain and spinal cord, and it is essential to temperature regulation, especially when you're running in hot weather. Running generates a lot of heat, and sweating is the best and quickest way to cool off. When sweat evaporates from your skin, cooling occurs and water is lost.

Most of us are pretty good about drinking up after a long, sweaty run. It's the prerun fluid intake that needs more attention. By making sure you are always well hydrated, you can avoid dehydration during exercise and ensure that all your body's systems—including sweating—function properly and efficiently.

Dehydration

If you don't take in enough fluids regularly or replace water lost during exercise, you will become dehydrated. At low levels, your health may not be affected, but your running performance will deteriorate. Even small deficits—a water loss of only 1 percent of body weight—can have adverse effects on your performance, raising your heart rate, reducing your sweat rate, and increasing core body temperature. As you continue to lose fluid, your ability to run declines even further and you begin to experience such physical symptoms as chills, nausea, and a more rapid pulse rate. Severe dehydration leads to heat exhaustion, symptoms of which include headache, dizziness, disorientation, and possibly vomiting. As soon as you begin to notice *any* signs of dehydration, stop running, get yourself to a cool place in the shade, and drink water or, better yet, a sports beverage, which will be absorbed more quickly. If you don't feel better within 30 minutes, go to the hospital.

Dehydration is not only a summertime phenomenon. You sweat during winter running, too, and if you are not well hydrated, loss of too much water can lead to hypothermia. Whether it's winter, spring, summer, or fall, keep a water bottle close at hand. Active women who are not careful to drink regularly can develop a level of chronic dehydration, which won't kill you but will lessen your endurance, lower your running performance, and leave you fatigued throughout the day.

Hydration

How much water you need depends on your height and weight, how active you are, your level of fitness, how much you sweat, and other factors. Therefore, there is no one recommendation that's right for everyone except to drink fluids throughout the day. You'll know you're getting enough if you urinate frequently (at least five times a day) and your urine is pale yellow to clear. The only time this color test won't work is shortly after you've taken vitamin supplements, which turns urine bright yellow.

One of the easiest ways to get plenty of fluid is to carry a water bottle around with you all day and sip from it regularly. Water isn't your only option, though. Juices, sports drinks, decaffeinated sodas, and milk all count toward your daily hydration efforts. Fruits and vegetables contain lots of water, too, so it's not like you have to go through a gallon of H_2O every day to be well hydrated.

H_2O TIP

Put a little zip into your glass of tap water by adding a bit of cranberry juice, lemon, or lime. Even a hint of flavor will make that water taste better, and you'll drink more.

Is bottled water better than tap water?

Bottled water may taste better, depending on how water is treated in your municipality, but public water supplies are carefully regulated—even more strictly than the content of bottled waters. You can rest assured that what comes out of your faucet is as safe as or safer than what comes out of the bottle you pay for at the supermarket. Nonetheless, if you enjoy bottled water more for its taste or convenience, buy it. Whatever makes it easier for you to meet your fluid needs is best.

Rehydration

It's especially important to drink fluids after a run or race to replace what you've lost through sweat. Your body will probably feel like a wrung-out sponge after a summer run, and it will act like one, too, soaking up fluids about as fast as you can swallow them. You can actually figure out exactly how much water you need by weighing yourself immediately before and after a workout. For every pound lost during running, drink at least 2 cups of fluid. You can also use this guideline to determine fairly precisely how much you need to drink *during* a long run or a race to maintain maximum performance. Let's say that after a 1-hour run, you've lost 2 pounds. That means you need to replace approximately 4 cups of fluid. On this basis, you can assume that you will need to drink 1 cup of water every 15 minutes to maintain hydration. You'll have to recalculate for each season as you sweat away a lot more water during the summer months. If you don't want to go to the trouble to figure out how much water you need, the general guideline for drinking on the run is to take about 8 ounces of fluid every 15 minutes.

Sports Beverages

You can't miss sports beverages. They line the supermarket shelves in just about every hue of the color spectrum, from chartreuse to

BEVERAGES TO BEWARE

Just because it's liquid doesn't mean it will help you hydrate. Alcoholic and caffeinated beverages rob water from your body. They are diuretics, which means they encourage loss of water through urination—definitely not good choices when you are trying to saturate your body with water before a run or race or replace lost fluid afterward. Drink these beverages moderately and try to drink a glass of water for every glass of wine or beer.

turquoise, and every flavor imaginable, from plain old orange to Alpine Snow. (How could you not try a drink called Alpine Snow?) Gatorade is the original and best-recognized sports beverage, but in recent years, the industry has simply burst with brands—All Sport, Cytomax, Endura, Exceed, Hydra Fuel, PowerAde and many more— all promising to replace lost nutrients and improve running performance.

Do we need them? Won't water do just as well? Yes and no. Water is its own best replacement during runs or races of an hour or less— it's free, it doesn't cause gastrointestinal distress, and it's quickly absorbed by your body. To say that you need sports drinks to replace sodium lost in sweat simply isn't true. Though you do lose sodium and potassium and other nutrients through sweat, the amount is minimal and is easily replaced by the foods in your daily diet. Loss of salt becomes an issue primarily for ultramarathoners.

When it comes to runs or races that will last 90 minutes or more, however, sports drinks are preferable to water for most runners because they contain carbohydrates: at about 90 minutes of running, your stores of carbohydrates (read: energy) start to run low. The sports drink will replace some of those spent carbos, plus the sodium speeds fluid absorption. You don't have to drink sports beverages to get through a marathon, but it certainly helps. Though formulated for quick and easy digestion, sports drinks don't sit well in every runner's stomach. Therefore, it's important to test these beverages in training, not during a race.

You have many options when it comes to sports beverages. There are only two guidelines to follow when choosing one. First, it should contain between 50 and 80 calories per 8-ounce serving; a higher concentration of carbohydrates slows down absorption of the fluid (high-carbo drinks do have a purpose, though, which we'll look at later in this chapter). Second, avoid sports drinks made with fructose only, which can cause gastrointestinal problems for some people. Then it's up to you. Try different brands and see which one works best.

Carbohydrates

Sports beverages have only a minimal role in providing energy to help fuel running. The bulk of the energy you use during a run comes from the carbohydrates you eat. Your body also burns fat and protein, but when you're running, your muscles need energy fast, and carbohydrates are easily and quickly converted. The harder you run, the more your body relies on carbos for fuel. Here are some quick carbohydrate facts.

- There are two major groups of carbohydrates: simple and complex.
- Simple carbos include the sugars glucose, fructose, sucrose, galactose, and lactose.
- Complex carbohydrates—the kind found in grains and pastas as well as in beans, vegetables, and fruits—are many simple carbohydrates linked together.
- Carbohydrates are stored in muscles as glycogen.
- All carbohydrates are converted to glucose before they can be used as energy.

Your body can store only a limited amount of carbohydrate (unfortunately, we can stockpile lots of fat), and this amount is smaller for women than for men. Since you are constantly burning carbohydrates to fuel your running as well as all daily activities, you must regularly replace them, hence the recommended high-carbohydrate diet for athletes.

Which Carbos Are Best?

Ask a group of runners to list sources of carbohydrates and they'll say pasta, bagels, rice, potatoes . . . We have come to define carbohydrates as starchy foods; although these are indeed excellent low-fat sources, so are fruits, vegetables, and dairy products (a glass of skim milk contains 54 percent carbohydrates). Athletes who fill up on breads and pastas and leave little room for fruits and vegetables, which are packed with vitamins and minerals, may fall short on certain key nutrients. The best way to get your carbohydrates is by eating a wide variety of grains and grain products, fruits, vegetables, and low-fat dairy products.

Carbos Before and After You Run

When it comes to eating before and after running or racing, there are certain high-carbohydrate foods that are better choices than others. Some foods are very easily and quickly broken down into glucose in your body; these foods are said to have a high glycemic index. Other foods break down more slowly and are released more gradually into your bloodstream; these foods have a low glycemic index.

Before you run or race (especially longer than an hour), you are better off eating foods with a low glycemic index. These will provide a prolonged and steady supply of glucose (energy) for your working muscles. Because high-glycemic foods break down quickly, they don't provide energy for a sustained period of time. *During* a run, however, a high-glycemic food is a good source of quick energy, which your muscles can use right away. High-glycemic foods are also the best choice for quick refueling after you've run or raced, especially if you plan to exercise again within 8 hours. For a list of foods' glycemic indexes, see The Glycemic Index on page 82.

Make Room for Fruits and Veggies

Fruits and vegetables arc thc gems of a well-balanced diet. Brilliant in color, taste, and texture and rich in carbohydrates, vitamins, minerals, and fiber, they can play a significant role in preventing cardiovascular disease, cancer, and diabetes.

Recent research has discovered that plant foods—fruits, vegetables, legumes, grains, nuts, and seeds—contain phytochemicals, which may offer significant health benefits. Phytochemicals are substances in plants not classified as vitamins, minerals, fats, or proteins. Broccoli contains indoles, isothiocyanates, and sulforaphane, which research shows may help prevent cancer. Garlic and onions contain allylic sulfides, which appear to enhance the immune system, and the isoflavonoids in soy have been shown to reduce cholesterol levels.

Scientists have only begun to discover and name these substances. Many more phytochemicals have yet to be isolated and identified and their benefits confirmed, but the American Dietetic Association (ADA) sees significant potential in the power of these substances to prevent disease. In their 1994 position paper on phytochemicals, the ADA states: "Phytochemicals . . . have been associated with the prevention and/or treatment of at least four of the leading causes of death in this country—cancer, diabetes, cardiovascular disease, and hypertension—and with the prevention and/or treatment of other medical ailments, including neural tube defects, osteoporosis, abnormal bowel function, and arthritis."

If that isn't reason enough to make sure you're getting your fruits

THE GLYCEMIC INDEX

Foods are assigned a glycemic index on the basis of how quickly they pass through the digestive system and are broken down into usable forms of energy. The higher the index, the faster the food becomes available. Before a run or race, eat foods with a low (under 40) to moderate (40–60) glycemic index; they will provide energy to your muscles on a steady, prolonged basis. During or after a run or race, choose foods with a high index (60 or higher), which quickly convert to glucose and replace spent carbohydrates.

Food	Glycemic Index
Glucose	100
Gatorade	91
Potato, baked	85
Cornflakes	84
Rice cakes	82
Cheerios	74
Cream of Wheat, instant	74
Graham crackers	74
Bagel, plain	72
Bread, white	70
Bread, wheat	69
Raisins	64
Oatmeal	61
Ice cream	61
Moderate glycemic index	
Muffin, bran	60
Bran Chex	58
Orange juice	57
Rice, white long-grain	56
Rice, brown	55
Sweet potato	54
Banana, ripe	52
Lentil soup	44
Orange	43
Spaghetti (no sauce)	41
Apple	36
Pear	36
Low glycemic index	
PowerBar	30–35
Yogurt, low-fat fruit	33
Milk, skim	32
Apricots, dried	31
Banana, underripe	30
Lentils	29
Kidney beans	27
Barley	25
Grapefruit	25
Fructose	23

Reprinted by permission from Clark, N., 1997, *Sports Nutrition Guidebook*, 2nd ed. (Champaign, IL: Human Kinetics), 110–111.

and vegetables, I don't know what is. The leading cause of death among women is cardiovascular disease, followed by stroke (related to hypertension), followed by cancer. Neural tube defects can occur in the fetuses of pregnant women who don't get all the nutrients they need, and of course, osteoporosis afflicts women primarily. If you're taking a One-A-Day, don't use it as an excuse to skip the broccoli and carrots and opt for dessert. Supplements don't include all those magical phytochemicals you get when you eat vegetables and fruits.

> ## FABULOUS FRUITS AND VIRTUOUS VEGETABLES
>
> Some of the most nutritious fruits you can eat include kiwi, papayas, mangoes, oranges, grapefruits, bananas, raspberries, strawberries, and blueberries. As for veggies, broccoli, brussels sprouts, carrots, greens, red and green bell peppers, potatoes, spinach, winter squashes, sweet potatoes, and tomatoes are all packed with nutrients.

Okay, you're convinced, right? How many fruits and vegetables should you eat? You need three to five servings of vegetables and two to four servings of fruit daily, according to the new Food Guide Pyramid issued by the United States Department of Agriculture (USDA) in 1992. Sounds like a lot, doesn't it? As if you'll be eating nothing but fruits and vegetables. It's not—serving sizes as determined by the USDA are small.

FRUIT:
- 1 medium piece of fruit—an apple, banana, orange
- 1 cup of fruits, like strawberries, grapes, cherries, blueberries
- ½ cup of cooked fruit
- ¼ cup of dried fruit
- 6 ounces of fruit juice

VEGETABLES:
- 1 cup of raw leafy vegetables (spinach, lettuce, greens)
- ½ cup chopped or cooked vegetables
- 6 ounces of vegetable juice

Protein

Filling up on too much pasta can also push protein-rich foods off your nutrition plate. Though most of us get all the protein we need in our diets without even thinking about it, sports nutritionists report that many women athletes whose calorie intake is below what they require or who restrict meat in an effort to reduce the fat in their diets may not be getting enough protein.

Your body uses protein to build tissue and repair tears to muscle fibers that occur with running, but proteins have many other functions. The proteins of your immune system fight illness. The proteins in red blood cells carry oxygen. Enzymes and hormones are made of protein. And, though protein is not a primary source of fuel for endurance, some protein is burned for energy during such endurance exercise as distance running. Your body will also resort to burning protein when your caloric intake is low.

Proteins are composed of amino acids, many of which your body can make. There are several, however—called essential amino acids—that can be obtained only through foods: isoleucine, leucine, lysine, methionine, threonine, phenylalanine, tryptophan, valine, and histidine. Signs that you may not be getting enough protein include loss of hair and splitting or breaking of fingernails. A deficiency of protein can result in illness or injuries that take a while to heal, and for some women, it can contribute to loss of menstruation.

How Much Protein Do You Need?

The recommended daily allowance (RDA) for protein is 0.36 grams per pound of body weight. As a runner, you need more for muscle repair and to replace protein used up during exercise—between 0.50 and 0.75 grams per pound of body weight. The higher your mileage or the harder your training, the more protein you should consume. Marathoners and competitive athletes who train at high mileage and intensity should aim for the high end of the protein range.

Here's an example: A 130-pound woman who doesn't exercise needs 0.36 grams of protein per pound of body weight (0.36 × 130) daily. That's 47 grams. A 130-pound woman who runs needs approximately 0.60 grams of protein per pound (0.60 × 130), or 78 grams. Meat is an obvious source; a small 3-ounce portion of chicken breast contains 27 grams of protein, but protein pops up in most foods, even in vegetables (one medium baked potato contains 5 grams). Strive to include a variety of protein-rich foods in your diet, such as lean red meats, poultry, fish, skim milk, low-fat dairy products, egg whites, legumes, and soybeans or soybean products.

Misconceptions About Meat

For years, meat was considered the best source of protein, and athletes of all kinds made meat the mainstay of their diets, believing it would make them stronger. We now know that training is what builds muscle. With that knowledge and our concerns over the health risks of a diet high in cholesterol and saturated fat, many runners have cut back on the amount of meat they eat, particularly red meat. That's a good move, certainly, but those who have eliminated meat from their diet may not be getting enough protein. Women are more likely than men are to fall short of their protein requirements, in part because we need fewer calories than men, generally speaking, and we eat less food. In addition, women—especially runners—tend to be more weight and health conscious than men are and can be more dedicated to following a low-fat, low-cholesterol diet.

Good for us, but if we shun meat for these reasons, we eliminate not only a good supply of protein but also an excellent source of iron, zinc, and B vitamins, particularly B_{12}. These nutrients are available in plant foods but in smaller amounts, and they are less easily absorbed. Furthermore, meats contain the MFP factor, which increases the absorption of iron and zinc from vegetables and beans, another benefit of eating a little meat with your veggies. According to sports nutritionist Nancy Clark, M.S., R.D., active men and women who eat red meat have better iron stores than those who don't eat meat. She recommends that active women, who are at a higher risk of anemia than men or sedentary women, consider consuming lean red meat two to four times a week. Though fish and poultry contain iron, zinc, and B vitamins, the amounts are lower.

You *can* get all the protein and nutrients you need through a vegetarian diet, as we'll discuss a little later in this chapter, but you must be conscientious about searching out foods that contain all the amino acids, vitamins, and minerals that meat so generously supplies. You may simply find it easier to eat a little beef and pork regularly. Besides, not all red meats are high in fat (see Lean Red Meats, page 86), and because they pack significant amounts of protein, iron, zinc, and vitamin B_{12}, you don't have to eat large servings. A mere 3 ounces of beef—the size of a deck of cards—deals you a good portion of those valuable nutrients.

Fat

Fat, too, isn't quite the enemy it's made out to be. For one thing, though fat is not as important as carbohydrates, it is a source of energy during running, especially on long runs of 10 miles or more or during a marathon and other endurance events. Fat also performs many neces-

LEAN RED MEATS

Red meat is an excellent source of protein, iron, zinc, and B vitamins, yet many women shun it for fear of its fat content. Well, check out these cuts. (All servings are 3 oz. cooked.)

Food	Protein (grams)	Fat (%)	Calories
Venison	26	18	135
Veal leg	24	20	130
Top round	27	25	150
Eye round	25	26	140
Pork tenderloin	25	26	140
Lamb, foreshank	26	29	160

Data from United States Department of Agriculture Nutrient Database for Standard Reference.

sary functions in the body. It pads the vital organs, protecting them from injury, and provides a layer of insulation under the skin to keep you warm. It's needed to transport vitamins A, D, E, and K through your body. And fat can actually be an ally in your weight-management efforts. A little fat in a meal slows digestion and keeps you feeling satiated so that you don't go diving into the cookie jar 30 minutes after dinner.

A lot of fat on a regular basis, however, leads to obesity, high blood pressure, stroke, diabetes, heart disease, and cancer. Nutritionists recommend that you limit your fat intake to 20 percent to 30 percent of total calories. In addition to the *amount,* it matters what *type* of fat you consume. Fats fall into one of three groups: saturated, polyunsaturated, and monounsaturated. Fats from each of these groups are not purely saturated or unsaturated but are a combination. For example, butter is 65 percent saturated fat, 30 percent monounsaturated fat, and 5 percent polyunsaturated fat.

Saturated Fats

Saturated fats are the most solid of the three types of fats and the least healthful, raising cholesterol levels and increasing your risk of heart disease. Primarily from animal sources, saturated fats are found in butter, lard, cheese and dairy products, and meat. They are also present, however, in coconut, palm, and palm kernel oils. In fact, coconut oil has the highest percentage of saturated fat (90 percent) of all the foods listed here.

Polyunsaturated Fats

Found primarily in vegetables, nuts, and grains, polyunsaturated fats are liquid at room temperature and include corn, safflower, sunflower, and soybean oils. Less harmful than saturated fats, some of these oils can help reduce cholesterol in the blood. Furthermore, the two polyunsaturated fats linoleic acid and linolenic acid are needed by your body but cannot be manufactured by your body, so you must get them through your diet.

Monounsaturated Fats

Olive, canola, and peanut oils fall into the category of monounsaturated fats. These are the "heart healthy" fats that have been found to lower blood cholesterol levels. In fact, a study reported in the *Journal of the American Dietetic Association* found that of two diets—one 10 percent fat and the other 26 percent fat but primarily from olive oil—the higher-fat diet produced a better effect on levels of blood cholesterol. Both diets lowered total cholesterol effectively, but the one with monounsaturated fat preserved more high-density lipoprotein cholesterol (HDL)—the "good" cholesterol—which helps prevent heart disease. Just because monounsaturated fats lower cholesterol, however, doesn't mean you can pour on the olive oil. One tablespoon contains 120 calories, as many as in 1 tablespoon of corn oil.

Omega-3 Fatty Acids

Omega-3 fatty acids are found primarily in fish. Studies have shown that omega-3 fatty acids can lower the amount of fat circulating in your bloodstream, thus preventing the formation of blood clots and lowering the risk of heart disease. One or two servings of fish a week provides a good supply of this heart-healthy oil. Salmon, tuna, and lake trout are three fishes high in omega-3s.

The Final Word on Fat

Keep the calories from fat in your diet at a level of between 20 percent and 30 percent. Though monounsaturated fats have a better health record than do polyunsaturated or saturated fats, a smattering of fat from each group is appropriate: monounsaturates for health, the polyunsaturates for the fatty acids your body needs and can't make, and the saturated fats for the healthful and flavorful foods they come with—dairy products and meats.

I've heard that a high-carbohydrate diet can be more fattening than a diet lower in carbohydrates and higher in protein—like the Zone Diet. Is this true?

"No. Carbohydrates are not fattening—*excess calories* are fattening," says sports nutritionist Nancy Clark, M.S., R.D. "The mistake many people on high-carbohydrate diets make is to eat too many low-fat or fat-free refined food products, which contain a lot of calories leading to excess. The Zone Diet [popularized in *The Zone* by Barry Sears, Ph.D. (San Francisco: HarperCollins, 1995)], which calls for more protein and fat [40 percent carbohydrate, 30 percent fat and 30 percent protein], produces satiety—leaves you feeling full longer—but the better guidelines to follow are those given in the Food Pyramid, which calls for a diet of 60 percent carbohydrates, 15 percent protein, and 25 percent fat."

Keep in mind, too, that you are an athlete, and by consuming 60 percent of calories from carbohydrates versus the 40 percent recommended by the Zone Diet, you'll be able to store more glycogen for energy and good performance.

I read that too little fat can alter metabolism such that fewer fat calories are burned during exercise and that a diet of 30 percent fat is better for fat burning and ultimately weight loss. Is this true?

"No, lowering your fat intake will not alter your metabolism," says Clark. "Furthermore, fat burning is not the same as losing fat. You're burning fat when you are sitting in front of the TV, but that doesn't mean you're losing body fat."

Vitamins and Minerals

Pasta, potatoes, rice, barley, seven-grain breads . . . lentils, pinto beans, limas, carrots, squash, broccoli, and asparagus. Oranges, papayas, apples, strawberries, currants, blackberries . . . chicken, turkey, red snapper, salmon, roast beef, and pork tenderloin. Yogurt, milk, low-fat cheeses, an ice cream cone. A little butter on your toast, a little olive oil on your salad. There are so many healthful, flavorful foods available, it's amazing we eat any one food twice in the same week—or month, for that matter.

By choosing a variety of foods from all families in the edible kingdom, you can plan meals that titillate your taste buds and deliver a healthy dose of nutrients. Forget the supplement pills. You can get all the vitamins and minerals you need through your diet, but put a star next to these in your daily nutrition planner: calcium, iron, zinc, folate, and the vitamins riboflavin and B$_6$. These nutrients are especially significant to a woman's health and running performance, and it's easy to fall short of your necessary dietary requirements. Let's take a closer look at each and its role in our active lifestyles.

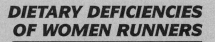

DIETARY DEFICIENCIES OF WOMEN RUNNERS

Nutritionist Jaime S. Ruud, M.S., R.D., has looked at various studies of the diets of female athletes, and in her book *Nutrition and the Female Athlete* (Boca Raton, Florida: CRC Press, 1996), reports the following most common nutritional problems among runners:

- Too few calories overall
- Low intake of calcium
- Low intake of iron
- Low intake of zinc
- Low intake of vitamin B$_6$

Calcium

Essential to strong bones and the prevention of osteoporosis, calcium also may help protect you from high blood pressure and certain cancers. According to nutritionists, however, many women do not meet even the minimum requirement of 800 milligrams a day, because they believe dairy products to be high in fat. Calcium needs are higher for teenagers, amenorrheic women, pregnant women, lactating women, and women going through menopause, which is just about all of us, so simply make a point of getting between 1,200 and 1,500 milligrams of calcium a day. The best sources are low-fat dairy products, such as skim milk and nonfat and low-fat yogurt. (See The Calcium Cache on page 91 for other calcium-rich foods.) A calcium-rich diet is important throughout life but especially during adolescence when bones absorb this mineral most readily and achieve greatest gains in density. On through adulthood and into old age, calcium helps protect against bone mineral loss and fractures.

Getting enough calcium isn't as simple as consuming plenty of dairy products and dark green leafy vegetables. You also want to make sure you're getting enough of the nutrients that help you absorb calcium and avoid foods that block absorption. Vitamin D promotes calcium absorption. Fortunately, milk and milk products are fortified with vitamin D, and when you're out under the sun,

READING MATERIAL

By becoming familiar with different foods and their content of carbohydrates, fats, proteins, vitamins, and minerals, you'll have an easier time planning meals and snacks that provide your daily nutritional requirements. Head to the bookstore and buy yourself a guide that lists foods from every food group and provides a nutritional breakdown of each. My favorite is *Prevention Magazine's Nutrition Advisor: The Ultimate Guide to the Health-Boosting and Health-Harming Factors in Your Diet* by Mark Bricklin (Emmaus, Pennsylvania: Rodale Press, 1994).

absorption of sunlight through your skin helps your body manufacture vitamin D. Diets high in sodium and/or protein reduce absorption of calcium, and too much caffeine may also get in the way. Follow dietary guidelines for sodium and protein, and if you're a coffee drinker, become a milk drinker, too. In other words, consume more than the daily requirement for calcium.

Oxalate, a substance found in vegetables, can inhibit calcium absorption if present in high amounts. Spinach and rhubarb are both high in oxalate, so though they contain a fair amount of calcium, you won't be able to count much of it toward your daily requirement. These veggies will also limit your absorption of calcium from other foods, so avoid eating them with dairy products or other high-calcium items.

I'm lactose intolerant and can't have dairy products. What's the best way to get calcium in my diet?

Though such vegetables as broccoli and kale are good plant sources of calcium, they don't contain nearly the amounts you can get in low-fat dairy products. Include in your diet calcium-enriched products, such as calcium-fortified orange juice or calcium-enriched soy milk, or drink Lactaid milk.

Iron

Iron helps carry oxygen through the blood to your muscles, where it is needed for the chemical process that transforms carbohydrates into available energy. Fall short on iron and you'll fall short on energy. When you're running, you'll feel like you're moving through glue, and when you're not running, you'll just feel tired.

Women runners are more likely to develop iron deficiencies than

THE CALCIUM CACHE

To build strong bones and prevent osteoporosis, try to get between 1,200 and 1,500 mg of calcium a day. Here are several excellent dietary sources.

Food*	Serving	Calcium (mg)	Calories
Yogurt, plain nonfat	1 cup	450	125
Yogurt, plain low-fat	1 cup	415	145
Milk, skim	8 oz.	350	100
Ricotta cheese, part skim	1 oz.	340	170
Yogurt, low-fat fruit	1 cup	315	225
Milk, 1%	8 oz.	300	100
Orange juice, fortified	8 oz.	300	110
Milk, 2%	8 oz.	295	120
Buttermilk	8 oz.	285	100
Cheese, Gruyère	1 oz.	285	115
Cheese, Swiss	1 oz.	270	105
Salmon, chum, canned	3 oz.	210	120
Cheese, cheddar	1 oz.	200	115
Tofu, firm	3 oz.	165	120
Edensoy fortified soy milk	8 oz.	160	130
Greens, turnip	½ cup cooked	100	15
Chicory	½ cup raw	90	21
Soybeans	½ cup cooked	90	150
Kale	½ cup cooked	85	20
Chinese cabbage	½ cup cooked	80	10

*Note: You do not absorb as much calcium from vegetable products as you do from dairy products. For example, though ½ cup of turnip greens contains 100 mg of calcium, your body will take in only about half of it, whereas you will absorb nearly all the calcium in milk.

Data from the United States Department of Agriculture Nutrient Database for Standard Reference.

men are partly because of blood loss during menstruation but also because we consume fewer calories and eat less red meat, which is the best source of absorbable iron. "Studies show that more than 50 percent of all women runners are deficient in iron," says nutrition expert Liz Applegate, Ph.D.

There are various stages of iron deficiency. The mildest shows up in laboratory tests as low levels of serum ferritin, a protein that stores iron. Anemia is indicated by significantly low levels of hemoglobin (the protein that carries iron to the tissues of the body) in your blood. Early stages of iron deficiency neither produce fatigue nor negatively affect your running performance. Still, if you should learn through a blood test that you are low in iron, eat more iron-rich foods to correct the deficiency and prevent it from progressing to anemia.

When should I consider getting tested for iron and exactly what tests do I need?

"If you are very white under the fingernails, are white in the lips, have a blue-gray tint to the whites of your eyes, and if you have a hankering for chewing ice, you should talk to your physician about the possibility of anemia and whether you should be tested," says sports nutritionist Nancy Clark, M.S., R.D. "If the decision is to go ahead with tests of your iron status, request that a test for serum ferritin be included."

Signs that you may be anemic include the following:

- Fatigue when you're not exercising
- Sluggishness, lack of endurance during running
- Becoming easily chilled in cool or cold temperatures

There may also be a link between lack of iron and injuries. Some researchers have observed higher rates of injuries among runners whose iron levels are low.

The RDA for iron is 15 milligrams a day for women. In the United States, women consume an average of 10.6 milligrams a day, according to experts. The best sources of iron are meats—red meat, poultry, and fish. They contain heme iron, which is more easily absorbed by your body than the iron found in vegetables, grains, and fruits, and meat generally has a higher iron content per serving than most plant foods do. Vegetarians need to make an extra effort to get enough iron. The best non-meat sources of iron are fortified cereals, soybeans, and lentils. Despite the fact that spinach contains a fair amount of iron (21 percent of the RDA for women), it's actually not a good source. Of that 21 percent, less than 2 percent can be absorbed by your body. For foods that will help you meet your iron requirements, see Iron Supplies on page 93.

Speaking of absorption, as we saw with calcium, certain substances hinder absorption of iron and others help. Caffeine, cal-

IRON SUPPLIES

The Recommended Daily Allowance (RDA) for iron is 15 mg a day. The following foods offer you a good supply. Foods shown in italics are sources of heme iron, which is absorbed more easily by your body.

Food	Serving	Iron (mg)	Calories
Clams, steamed	3 oz. (20)	25	130
Clams, canned	3 oz.	25	125
Tofu, firm	3 oz.	8	120
Cream of Wheat	¾ cup, cooked	8	100
Liver, chicken	3 oz.	7	130
Liver, beef	3 oz.	6	140
Mussels	3 oz.	6	145
Oysters, Eastern, raw	3 oz. (6)	6	55
Soybeans	½ cup, cooked	4	150
Pumpkin seeds	1 oz.	4	155
Quinoa	¼ cup, raw	4	160
Venison	3 oz.	4	135
Lentils	½ cup, cooked	3	115
Pot roast	3 oz.	3	185
Tuna, light, canned	3 oz.	3	110
Potato	7 oz., baked	3	220
Pinto beans	½ cup, cooked	2	115

Data from the United States Department of Agriculture Nutrient Database for Standard Reference.

cium, and bran can interfere with iron uptake, while vitamin C improves it. You'll also absorb more iron from vegetables and grains if you eat them along with a serving of fish, poultry, or red meat or with fruits high in vitamin C. So drink a glass of orange juice with your soy burger instead of a cola, and add some beef to your bean chili.

Zinc

If you're not a meat eater, you may also fall short of your requirement for zinc, which, like iron, is more prevalent and more easily absorbed from beef, poultry, and fish than from plant foods. Zinc has various roles in the body. It's an important component of many enzymes, it fights viral and bacterial infections, and it helps heal wounds.

ZINC UP

For a healthy body and a hearty immune system, be sure to get 12–15 mg of zinc a day. Here are some top food sources. Keep in mind that too much fiber and coffee can interfere with absorption of zinc.

Food	Serving	Zinc (mg)	Calories
Oysters	6 medium	76	60
Beef shank	3 oz.	9	170
Beef blade roast	3 oz.	9	215
Pot roast	3 oz.	7	180
Wheat germ	¼ cup	5	110
Turkey, dark meat	3 oz.	4	160
Crab, blue	3 oz.	4	90
Yogurt, nonfat	1 cup	2	125
Pumpkin seeds	1 oz.	2	155
Yogurt, low-fat	1 cup	2	145
Lentils	½ cup cooked	1	115
Milk, skim	8 oz.	1	100

Data from the United States Department of Agriculture Nutrient Database for Standard Reference.

Running and other intense exercise increase zinc loss through sweat and urine, and women athletes are more likely than men are to have low levels of zinc primarily because of their lower caloric intake. A deficiency in this mineral can stunt growth in adolescents, affect fertility, slow wound healing, and make you more susceptible to illness. The recommended intake of zinc for active women is 12 to 15 milligrams a day (see Zinc Up above for food sources). Too much zinc (six times the RDA), however, can interfere with absorption of iron and copper and may lower levels of high-density lipoprotein (HDL), or "good," cholesterol and raise levels of low-density lipoprotein (LDL), or "bad," cholesterol.

Folate

Also known as folic acid or folacin, folate is one of the B vitamins. Your body uses this vitamin to make genetic material, RNA (ribonucleic acid), DNA (deoxyribonucleic acid), and protein.

Dietary intake of folate in this country is low. Deficiencies of folate in pregnant women have been linked to neural tube defects in their babies. Research also indicates that women and men who don't get

FULL OF FOLATE

You may know the B vitamin folate as folic acid or folacin. Aim for 400 mcg a day.

Food	Serving	Folate (mcg)	Calories
Liver, chicken	3 oz. cooked	655	135
Liver, beef	3 oz. cooked	185	140
Lentils	½ cup cooked	180	115
Mung beans	½ cup cooked	160	105
Pinto beans	½ cup cooked	145	115
Pink beans	½ cup cooked	140	125
Lima beans, baby	½ cup cooked	135	115
Spinach	½ cup cooked	130	20
Black beans	½ cup cooked	130	115
Kidney beans	½ cup cooked	115	110
Wheat germ	¼ cup	100	110
Chicory	½ cup raw	100	20
Asparagus	½ cup cooked	90	25
Lettuce, Romaine	1 cup raw	75	10
Orange juice	8 oz.	75	110
Papaya	½ (5½ oz.)	60	60
Blackberries	1 cup	50	75
Parsnips	½ cup cooked	45	65
Brussels sprouts	½ cup cooked	45	30
Beets	½ cup cooked	45	25
Orange	1 (4½ oz.)	40	60
Broccoli	½ cup cooked	40	20

Data from the United States Department of Agriculture Nutrient Database for Standard Reference.

enough of this vitamin may be at an increased risk of heart disease. Though the RDA for folate is 180 micrograms, the United States Food and Drug Administration (USFDA) recommends that women get 400 micrograms daily, especially prior to and during pregnancy. This shouldn't be too difficult, as folate is found in many foods—meats, fruits, and vegetables. (See Full of Folate above for some of the best sources).

Riboflavin

Also known as vitamin B_2, riboflavin is important for good vision and healthy skin. It's also needed to convert carbohydrates and fats into energy during exercise. This means that as you run, riboflavin is being used to provide energy to your muscles. The longer you run,

RICH IN RIBOFLAVIN

The recommended daily allowance (RDA) for riboflavin is 1.3 mg, but it won't hurt to err on the high side, as this vitamin is crucial to energy metabolism. Riboflavin is found in lots of foods, but here are some of the richest sources.

Food	Serving	Riboflavin (mg)	Calories
Liver, beef	3 oz.	3.0	140
Liver, chicken	3 oz.	1.5	135
Milk, skim	8 oz.	0.5	100
Yogurt, low-fat plain	1 cup	0.5	145
Yogurt, low-fat fruit	1 cup	0.4	225
Clams, steamed	20 small	0.4	135
Clams, canned	3 oz.	0.4	125
Mussels, blue	3 oz.	0.4	145
Mackerel, Atlantic	3 oz.	0.4	220
Squid	3 oz., fried	0.4	150
Tuna, fresh	3 oz.	0.3	155
Soybeans	½ cup cooked	0.3	150
Lamb, leg	3 oz.	0.3	160
Pork, tenderloin	3 oz.	0.3	140
Veal, leg	3 oz.	0.3	130
Bagel, small	2 oz.	0.2	16
Wheat germ	¼ cup	0.2	110

Data from the United States Department of Agriculture Nutrient Database for Standard Reference.

the more you use, so it's important to regularly replace your supply by eating riboflavin-rich foods. Nutritionists suggest that active women may need more than the RDA for riboflavin (1.3 milligrams), but specific recommendations haven't been determined. Get *at least* the recommended amount. (See Rich in Riboflavin above for specific foods high in this important B vitamin.)

Vitamin B₆

According to nutritionist Jaime Ruud, studies indicate that female athletes may not be getting enough vitamin B_6. One study in 1992 of female cross-country runners found their intake was 65 percent of the RDA.

Vitamin B_6 breaks down and builds up amino acids; it helps synthesize hemoglobin, which carries oxygen in red blood cells; and it aids in metabolism and energy production for working muscles.

BEST SOURCES OF B₆

Getting enough vitamin B₆ shouldn't be difficult, but studies have shown that women runners often fall short on this nutrient. Include a few of the following foods in your diet and you'll meet your needs (1.6 mg per day) easily.

Food	Serving	Vitamin B₆ (mg)	Calories
Banana	1 (4 oz.)	0.7	105
Potato, baked	1 (7 oz.)	0.7	220
Chickpeas	½ cup	0.6	140
Prune juice	8 oz.	0.6	180
Chicken, breast	3 oz.	0.5	140
Turkey, breast	3 oz.	0.5	130
Tuna, fresh	3 oz.	0.5	155
Tuna, canned white	3 oz.	0.4	115
Wheat germ	¼ cup	0.3	110
Avocado	½ (3 oz.)	0.3	160

Data from the United States Department of Agriculture Nutrient Database for Standard Reference.

Some studies have reported that vitamin B₆ supplements relieve symptoms of premenstrual syndrome (PMS); however, large doses of this vitamin have been linked to neurological disorders, so it's best not to take megadoses without the advice of your physician.

Deficiencies of B₆ can cause depression, irritability, and skin rashes, among other symptoms. Fortunately, it's easy to get enough of this vitamin. The RDA is 1.6 milligrams, and one 3-ounce serving of chicken or turkey breast supplies 0.5 milligrams, nearly a third of your requirement. For other sources of vitamin B₆, see Best Sources of B₆ above.

Some Special Nutrients

Scientists are continually studying the properties of vitamins and minerals and certain foods as they search for health-enhancing or disease-fighting substances. Antioxidants, for example, have been and continue to be studied for their potential benefits in preventing cancer, cardiovascular disease, and such degenerative conditions as arthritis. Phytochemicals, as we've already discussed, are also the focus of much research. Conclusive evidence has yet to be reached regarding the effects of many of the foods and nutrients now being studied, but the findings thus far are intriguing. The following two items should be especially interesting to you as a woman and a runner.

Antioxidants

The hottest of the antioxidants are vitamins E and C and beta-carotene. What is an antioxidant and how does it work? Under exposure to pollution, cigarette smoke, radiation, and stress and during such strenuous exercise as running, your body produces chemicals called free radicals. Free radicals can cause irreversible damage to cells through a chemical process called oxidation. Vitamins E and C and beta-carotene may protect your cells from this damage, or oxidation—hence, they are called *anti*oxidants.

Researchers are looking into whether antioxidants might prevent or lessen muscle damage during running and other strenuous forms of exercise. In addition, some studies have shown that individuals whose diets are rich in *foods* containing these nutrients show a lower risk for heart disease and several types of cancer. Interestingly, research has yet to find significant benefits from taking supplements of vitamins C and E or beta-carotene.

Soy Foods

Soybeans contain phytoestrogens, which behave very much the way estrogen does in the body and may help alleviate some of the discomforts of menopause caused by the loss of estrogen. More important, phytoestrogens raise blood levels of HDL ("good") cholesterol and lower blood levels of LDL ("bad") cholesterol and may protect against heart disease, the leading cause of death among women. Studies have also shown that women whose diets are high in soy foods, such as soybeans and tofu, have a lower risk of breast cancer. Soybeans and tofu are high in fat (47 percent and 57 percent of total calories, respectively), however.

Another way to get these phytoestrogens is by using powdered soy protein (check the label to make sure Supro is listed as the main ingredient) available in health-food stores. It comes in a variety of flavors and is perhaps most palatably consumed in fruit juices or fruit smoothies.

Vegetarian Diets

Soy's protective effects against heart disease and breast cancer comes as good news to the many vegetarians who eat tofu or other soy foods for their protein. This may be one of several aspects of a vegetarian diet that helps prevent disease. Studies show that, in general, vegetarians are healthier than meat eaters and have a lower risk of heart disease and certain cancers. Though this may be partly due to a healthy lifestyle, diet has its influence, too.

Vegetarian diets tend to be low in fat and cholesterol; therefore, vegetarians tend to be lean and are less likely to develop high blood pressure, heart disease, or diabetes. The high fiber of a diet based on fruits, vegetables, and grains may also help prevent diabetes and protect against colon cancer.

Although a vegetarian diet can be a very healthy diet, it's also a challenging one. You must be conscientious about getting all the nutrients you need, some of which are difficult to come by in plant foods. Consuming enough protein is not a problem, especially if your particular diet allows dairy products, but even if you are a strict vegan, the protein in soy foods is nutritionally equal to the protein in meats. Plus, you can get all the amino acids you need by eating a variety of whole grains and beans, and you do not have to combine complementary sources of amino acids to create perfect protein at any given meal, as was once thought.

It's those nutrients found primarily in dairy products and meats—calcium, iron, zinc, and vitamin B_{12}—that vegetarians have to make extra effort to include in their diets. Calcium, iron, and zinc are found in many vegetarian sources, but they are not as easily absorbed from plant foods as from meats. You need to be vigilant about eating foods high in these minerals (see the boxes on pages 91, 93, and 94 in this chapter for good sources). Try to consume them with other foods that are high in vitamin C, which improves absorption. Vitamin B_{12} occurs only in meats, so you need to eat foods to which this vitamin has been added, such as cereal or fortified soy drinks.

Running demands that we maintain a high nutritional status. That becomes more challenging on a vegetarian diet, but it can be done.

Eating on the Run . . . and Before the Run . . . and After the Run

One of the questions runners most frequently ask at running clinics is "What should I eat before I run?" The concern often isn't over which foods will improve performance so much as it is over which ones will inhibit performance—cause stomach cramps, indigestion, or, worse yet, diarrhea. The answer has more to do with when you eat rather than what you eat.

If possible, morning runners should eat an easily digestible snack worth 200 to 300 calories about an hour before running. Blood sugar drops overnight, so eating a couple slices of toast, a bagel, a sports bar, or some fruit will give you the energy you need for your run. If you run so early that you essentially jump out of bed, into your running shoes, and out the door, then have a snack before you go to bed the night before.

If you run in the afternoon or evening, you'll need to time your meals and runs so they don't interfere with each other. Nutritionist Nancy Clark recommends that you allow 3 to 4 hours between eating a full meal and running. You may need to give yourself more time, or you may run well on less. After a light meal—say, a breakfast of cereal and fruit or a bagel and yogurt—you may be able to run within 2 to 3 hours.

I've heard that drinking milk or eating dairy products before running can cause stomach cramps. Is that true?

Yes, it's true for those who are lactose intolerant, but most runners will do just fine with dairy products. If you experience stomach distress after you've consumed milk or yogurt, you may want to check with your doctor to see if you are lactose intolerant.

At prerun or prerace meals, eat foods that are high in carbohydrates and low in fats and proteins. Fats and proteins take longer to digest and may still be hanging around inside your stomach when you go out for a run. Such light, lean protein foods as low-fat yogurt or cottage cheese or a turkey sandwich probably won't cause you any problems, but forgo the cheeseburger.

As mentioned earlier, good foods to eat before running are those with a low to moderate glycemic index (see the box on page 82 in this chapter), such as rice dishes, pasta, cereal, bananas, and yogurt. These foods digest easily but steadily, supplying a controlled amount of carbohydrates to your muscles.

Everyone responds to foods differently. I once knew a woman who could run 20 minutes to the doughnut shop, eat a doughnut, and run

POSSIBLE FOOD CULPRITS

If you experience gastrointestinal distress during or after a run, the following foods might be the cause. Experiment with limiting them before running.

- High-fat foods: cheese, burgers, bacon, fried foods, and pastas with cream sauces digest slowly and can feel heavy in your stomach during running.
- High-fiber foods: bran cereals, fruits, and beans that are especially high in fiber can cause gastrointestinal problems and possibly diarrhea.
- Caffeine: too much caffeine can also cause stomach problems and diarrhea. (I've found that if I drink a mug of strong coffee too close to a run, I'll begin to feel a little woozy after a few miles.)

back. Some women find they can't eat anything in the hours before running. You need to figure out the foods and timing that work best for you. Experiment with different foods and different meal or snack times. If eating before running consistently causes problems, try a blended meal, such as a smoothie made from fruit, yogurt, and juice. You may find that a sports bar, such as PowerBar, or one of the high-carbohydrate sports beverages, such as GatorLode, is easy on your stomach. Pay attention to the time of month, too. Hormonal changes during menstruation can affect your gastrointestinal tract and may cause looser bowel movements.

Sports Foods

The proliferation of scientifically formulated sports foods, which are now available in all kinds of textures, colors, and flavors, can make you feel like you're on the set of a Star Trek show, but such items aren't meant to replace the foods in your daily diet. These products have been designed to help you achieve optimal performance during races, particularly longer events such as the marathon. They are formulated to digest easily and provide a good supply of carbohydrates to muscles during running.

ENERGY BARS

Energy bars may contain anywhere from 110 to 250 calories and a supply of 25 to 50 grams of carbohydrates, along with some vitamins, minerals, protein, and fiber. They are designed to be eaten an hour before competition along with extra water to help digestion and absorption. Some runners carry them on long runs and marathons for refueling along the way. PowerBars are probably most familiar. Some other brands are Clif Bar, Exceed, Gatorbar, PRBar, and VO2 Max.

ENERGY GELS

Energy gels have the consistency of frosting or pudding. They come in small packets that you can carry in a pocket and rip open for quick carbos in the middle of a long run or race. Gels contain 70 to 100 calories and 17 to 25 grams of carbohydrates, along with small amounts of caffeine or amino acids. As with energy bars, you should take these with extra water. GU, Squeezy, and Power Gel are a few of the brands available.

CARBO-LOADING DRINKS

Carbo-loading drinks are not to be used during a run. They have a much higher carbohydrate concentration than the fluid replacement beverages mentioned in the beginning of this chapter. These beverages are meant to be consumed 2 to 4 hours before a long run or race or afterward and may be particularly useful to runners who have difficulty digesting solid foods close to a run. Examples are GatorLode and Ultra Fuel.

Any of these products can be a good source of carbohydrates before running and racing, and both bars and gels have been found to improve performance during a run or race. What you choose simply depends on personal preference. Find one that tastes good and digests easily. If you can't stomach any of them, don't think you'll be at a disadvantage compared with runners who do use these products. You can get all the carbohydrates, fluids, and nutrients you need for good performance from real foods, too. We'll talk more specifically about eating and drinking before races in part VII in the book.

Eating After the Run

Running and racing burn up the glycogen (stored carbohydrates) in your muscles. The longer or harder you run, the more spent your muscles will be afterward. The fastest way to fill them up with glycogen and get them ready to run again is by drinking fluids and eating high-carbohydrate foods as soon as possible after you stop running, especially if you will be exercising again within 8 hours.

Several studies have shown that athletes recover fastest from exercise if they begin to eat and drink within 15 minutes after a workout or competition. This is when the enzymes that turn carbohydrates from food into glycogen to replace depleted muscle stores are most active. Consume a high-carbohydrate snack containing between 200 and 300 calories. This is a good time to choose from the high-glycemic foods listed in the box on page 82, since they can quickly be broken down and stored as glycogen. You may prefer a sports bar or a high-carbohydrate drink instead.

Recent studies have shown that getting some protein along with carbohydrates speeds recovery even more. A bowl of cereal with milk, a banana or bagel with yogurt, a peanut butter–and–jelly sandwich, or a fruit-and-yogurt smoothie are good postrun snacks. Eating for recovery is most important after a race, after a run of 90 minutes or more, or if you run every day. Women who do maybe 30 minutes of running three or four times a week have less need to refuel immediately after their runs.

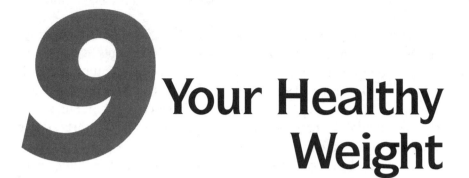

9 Your Healthy Weight

IT SEEMS FEW OF US ARE CONTENT with our weight. We want to either lose it, redistribute it, or avoid gaining it. Then there are those with such speedy metabolisms that they struggle to *put* flesh on their figures.

We have become a nation of weight watchers, most of us trying to prevent the health hazards associated with obesity but also trying to pare our bodies down to the unrealistically slim figures that are held as the standard of beauty. We try diet after diet, hoping that the next one's promise will finally hold true. We skip meals—breakfast or lunch, usually, the two most important of the day—and we stock our pantries with "foods" made from synthetic sweeteners and fake fats that promise flavor with no calories. Yum. As sports nutritionist Nancy Clark, M.S., R.D., points out, "so many women see food as the enemy." And we've waged war against it.

Exercise? It, too, becomes a means to an end—a way to burn off the brownie "snuck" before dinner, to tame our rounded tummies, to "whip our bodies into shape." With that attitude, it's no wonder that so many of us abandon our fitness routines.

Ironically, for all the effort we put into eating and exercising, we are a nation fatter than ever. Perhaps even more ironic, if we wouldn't work so hard at it, we'd have an easier time maintaining a desirable weight. Weight management isn't a project you take on; it occurs as a result of a healthful lifestyle. It begins with acceptance of what is an appropriate weight for your body type and genetics and is carried out through healthful eating and regular physical activity. Run for the pleasure of it, and you won't have difficulty with motivation. Enjoy eating, for deprivation leads to excess. And be glad for your body despite its imperfections, because it has many more exceptional qualities, one of which is that it can run for miles.

Body Weight

The weight that's best for you depends on your height, bone structure, and body type and is also partly determined by other genetic factors. Thus, guidelines for weight are given in ranges to allow for differences among individuals.

The issue of what's a healthy range often comes into debate, and many charts have been put forth over the years. You may be familiar with the Metropolitan Life Insurance Company Desirable Weight Tables, which have gone through several revisions and have been the standard most people have followed. A more recent weight chart was published in 1991 by the United States Departments of Agriculture (USDA) and Health and Human Services (USDHHS).

However, the American Dietetic Association (ADA) and new medical guidelines from the federal government say that body mass index (BMI) is a more accurate indicator of healthy weight. You can determine your BMI by dividing your weight in kilograms by your height in square meters. An easier way to figure your BMI is to locate it in Find Your Body Mass Index on page 107. A BMI between 19 and 25 is "acceptable," according to the ADA, which goes on to specify that a "desirable" BMI range for women is 21.3 to 22.1. Anything higher than 27 may mean you are at increased risk of heart disease, high blood pressure, and diabetes. One point to note: body mass index doesn't tell you anything about body composition—how much fat and muscle you're made of. A very muscular woman might have a higher BMI than would a woman who carries more fat.

Body Composition

The best indicator of health with regard to weight is body composition. It matters less what you weigh than how much fat versus how much muscle you carry. This is true for both optimal health and optimal performance.

As a runner, you are probably well aware of the very low body fat percentages of elite runners, which may be as low as 11 percent among female marathoners. Therefore, you might say to yourself, *Well, I am not an elite runner. Eleven percent is probably unrealistic, but since I run regularly, my body fat must be under 20 percent.* Many women runners I know would cringe at having a body fat percentage that's much higher than 20. The truth is very few women can attain a body fat level below 22 percent.

What's healthy? Again, it's a range. According to sports nutritionist Nancy Clark, a normal, healthy body fat level for women can fall anywhere between 18 percent and 25 percent, with more active women falling between 18 and 22 percent. Higher than 27 percent is creeping toward an unhealthy level. Above 31 percent, you are at an increased risk for cardiovascular disease and other health problems associated with obesity.

You can change your body composition somewhat with regular weight lifting to build muscle, but keep in mind that genetics also plays a role in how much fat your body stores. In the end, your body will let you know what your best weight is. It gets pretty stubborn about giving up pounds below a certain point. You can work hard at trimming down, even going below your body's set point, but you'll find that in no time, your body bounces back up to the weight it prefers. That's the key signal that you've reached your body's lowest acceptable weight. If you have to expend lots of effort dieting and

FIND YOUR BODY MASS INDEX

Use this chart to determine your body mass index (BMI). If it's between 19 and 25, your weight is within an acceptable range. If it's lower or higher, take a look at your lifestyle and make sure you are following healthful eating and exercise habits.

BMI	19	20	21	22	23	24	25	26	27	28	29	30
Height		**Weight (lb.)**										
4'10"	91	96	100	105	110	115	119	124	129	134	138	143
4'11"	94	99	104	109	114	119	124	128	133	138	143	148
5'	97	102	107	112	118	123	128	133	138	143	148	153
5'1"	100	106	111	116	122	127	132	137	143	148	153	158
5'2"	104	109	115	120	126	131	136	142	147	153	158	164
5'3"	107	113	118	124	130	135	141	146	152	158	163	169
5'4"	110	116	122	128	134	140	145	151	157	163	169	174
5'5"	114	120	126	132	138	144	150	156	162	168	174	180
5'6"	118	124	130	136	142	148	155	161	167	173	179	186
5'7"	121	127	134	140	146	153	159	166	172	178	185	191
5'8"	125	131	138	144	151	158	164	171	177	184	190	197
5'9"	128	135	142	149	155	162	169	176	182	189	196	203
5'10"	132	139	146	153	160	167	174	181	188	195	202	207
5'11"	136	143	150	157	165	172	179	186	193	200	208	215
6'	140	147	154	162	169	177	184	191	199	206	213	221

Reprinted by permission from Lutter, J., and L. Jaffe, 1996, *The Bodywise Woman,* 2nd ed. (Champaign, IL: Human Kinetics), 60.

exercising to maintain a particular weight, give it up—that's not the right weight for you. Have some respect for your body; allow it to be the weight it wants.

What's the best way to measure body fat?

There are four common methods of measuring body fat: underwater weighing, skin fold measurement (which uses calipers to take measurements at several sites of the body), bioelectrical impedance (in which a computerized system uses an electrical current to measure body fat), and near infrared reactance, or the Futurex 5000 method (which determines body fat by measuring tissue absorption and reflection of light). None of these methods is 100% accurate. Factors that affect readings include the quality of equipment, the expertise of the practitioner, the formula used to calculate body fat, and, in some cases, the density of your bones or your level of hydration.

Skin fold measurement and bioelectrical impedance are the most available, easiest, and least expensive methods. What's more important than the method is finding someone who's very experienced in administering the test. Experts recommend that if you do get your body fat measured, find an experienced technician, a registered dietitian, or an exercise physiologist, and have it measured—by the same practitioner using the same equipment—every 2 months over 1 year to look at a how your body fat changes. If you get your body fat measured at a health fair, you can't be sure of the precision of the equipment or the technician, so don't take the number too seriously.

The Weight Equation

Weight management is really very simple. It all comes down to calories consumed versus calories burned. To maintain weight, you must burn the same number of calories that you take in through food and drink. If you eat 2,000 calories a day and burn 2,000 calories a day, your weight stays the same. Eat more than you burn and you'll gain weight; burn more than you eat and you'll lose weight.

Your body burns a lot of calories just to maintain its daily internal functions; this is your resting metabolic rate. It varies from person to person, depending on height, weight, and genetics. Some people are born burning a lot of calories even when they sit reading a book. You have friends like this—they fidget a lot and eat monstrous meals and lots of snacks and never gain a pound. Others are very sedentary and have only to taste food, it seems, to soon find several extra ounces on their frame. Resting metabolism can be raised somewhat by developing more muscle, which burns calories even during inactivity, but then it's back to the calories in–calories out equation.

If You Are Overweight . . .

To lose weight, you must either burn more calories than you consume or consume fewer calories than you burn. If each day, you consume 2,000 calories and increase your activity so that you burn 2,500 calories, that's 500 calories' worth of weight loss. If you burn 2,000 calories a day but reduce the number of calories consumed to 1,500, that's also 500 calories' worth of weight loss.

Now, here's the deal: 1 pound of fat equals 3,500 calories. Dietitians recommend that you lose weight gradually at a rate of 0.5 to 1 pound a week—more than that and you begin to lose muscle along with the fat. You don't want to lose muscle tissue because it burns calories even when it's not doing anything, but let's get back to losing fat. To lose a pound a week, you need to "lose" 3,500 calories a week, or roughly 500 calories a day. The easiest way to do this is through a combination of exercise and diet.

Let's say you maintain your weight on 2,200 calories a day. If you were to add another 10 minutes of running each day, you'd burn an additional 100 calories. Then you'd need to cut 400 calories from your diet every day. Does 400 calories sound like a lot?

It's not. Leave the cheese (100 calories per slice) off your sandwich, have 1 cup of grapes (60 calories) instead of oatmeal cookies (160 calories for two Nabisco) for your afternoon snack; use low-calorie Italian dressing (30 calories) instead of oil and vinegar (140) on your dinner salad; and for dessert, indulge in Ben & Jerry's Chocolate Fudge Brownie frozen yogurt (180 calories per serving) rather than New York Super Fudge Chunk (290 calories). The total cut: 420 calories; the amount of food stayed the same (minus a slice of cheese). You don't have to eat *less* food—simply the *right* foods. Pretty painless, huh? And you don't have to precisely hit a 500-calorie deficit each day. Aim for a weekly total decrease of 3,500.

If You Are Underweight . . .

A sure sign that you are underweight is amenorrhea. If you are amenorrheic, cut back on your activity, consume more calories, or follow a plan that incorporates some of each to return to a healthy weight and normal menstrual status. For most women who have dropped too many pounds from perhaps overzealousness in their weight-loss efforts or because their intake of food didn't increase with their mileage, regaining normal weight should not be difficult. Some women do have difficulty gaining weight, however. Take a look at your parents and siblings. If they're all rail thin, you, too, are probably genetically predisposed to thinness, and running may have made you smaller still.

To gain weight without giving up your running, consume an additional 500 calories or more each day following the same percentages of carbohydrates, fats, and proteins in your regular diet, advises nutrition expert Nancy Clark, who also recommends choosing foods that are calorie dense so that you don't have to eat volumes and volumes of food to get the calories you need. Some suggestions are fruit juices, dried fruit, meats, beans, potatoes, breads, desserts, and starchy vegetables such as peas and corn.

The Healthy Way to Lose Weight

If you want to lose weight, don't diet. Most diets usually involve dramatic changes in the kinds and amounts of foods you eat. They may work in the short term, but as soon as you go off your diet and begin eating the foods you enjoy, the pounds pile on again.

Also, dieting for many people involves a substantial reduction in caloric intake. Not only is this torturous but it usually backfires, ultimately resulting in weight gain. When you go on a low-calorie diet, your body doesn't realize that you're just trying to lose a few pounds; it thinks that maybe there's a famine. To prevent you from starving to death, it slows your metabolism down a notch or two so as to hold on to calories.

You can boost your metabolism some by returning to an appropriate caloric intake; however, if on your low-calorie diet you've dropped more than 1 pound a week, you've lost muscle tissue along with some fat, and without that muscle, your metabolism won't speed up to normal. You go off your diet, your metabolism is slower than when you started dieting, and you gain fat easily. Don't diet. Simply adjust your caloric intake and output as described above to lose weight gradually or maintain the weight you are at.

I'm 5′7″ and I weigh 200 pounds. I eat a low-fat, high-carbohydrate diet of 1,800 to 2,000 calories a day. I run or bike for an hour each day and lift weights three times a week. All my family members are big, so I know I'll never be thin, but I'd like to lose a few pounds. The only time I lost weight was when I was eating 500 to 700 calories a day, but then when I returned to a normal diet, I gained all the weight back. Have I totally screwed up my metabolism somehow? What can I do?

"You have not screwed up your metabolism. Metabolic rate can be slowed down through dramatic weight loss and the consequent decrease in muscle mass, but it can't be permanently affected. It's possible that you have reached your set point and are thin for your genetics. Look at your family members. Are you the thinnest? If you are still concerned, meet with a registered dietitian who specializes in nutrition and weight management for active women. You can find one by calling the American Dietetic Association's referral hot line at (800) 366-1655."

—NANCY CLARK, M.S., R.D., AUTHOR OF *NANCY CLARK'S SPORTS NUTRITION GUIDEBOOK*, 2ND ED. (CHAMPAIGN, ILLINOIS: HUMAN KINETICS, 1997)

The best way to lose weight is by exercising regularly and making healthy food choices. Following are several suggestions that will help make weight management a piece of cake.

Know What You're Eating

Food is fascinating and the more you know about the content of various foods, the easier it will be to follow a healthy diet and manage your weight wisely. I happen to like *Prevention Magazine's Nutrition Advisor* (Emmaus, Pennsylvania: Rodale Press, 1994). The data was compiled from the United States Department of Agriculture Nutrient Database for Standard Reference. It has calorie counts and nutritional breakdowns for everything from carambola fruit to lobster thermidor. Plus, it's full of fun facts. For example, did you know that carrots were originally purple? Another good reference is *Bowes & Church's Food Values of Portions Commonly Used,* 17th edition, by Jean A. T. Pennington, Ph.D. (Philadelphia: Lippincott-Raven, 1997).

Eat Snacks

That's right: by eating healthy snacks between meals, you'll prevent overeating during meals. Plus, this keeps your blood sugar level at an even flow throughout the day, which helps maintain steady energy.

Don't Cut Out Your Favorite Foods—Cut Down on Them

If you deprive yourself of foods you love because they're too high in fat or calories, you'll be miserable and you'll be more likely to develop a craving for that food or for a similar calorie-laden treat and then binge on it. Are you a cookie monster? Eat two instead of four and you've saved yourself anywhere from 100 to 200 calories, depending on the cookie. With dinner, have one glass of wine rather than two—a savings of 70 to 100 calories, depending on how you pour. If frozen yogurt just doesn't do it for you, go ahead and have ice cream and limit yourself to ½ cup.

If you find, however, that you can't seem to stop until you've finished the whole pint of Ben & Jerry's or if you just can't keep your hands out of the cookie jar or the bag of potato chips, consider limiting their quantities in your cupboard and fridge. Then take a look at why you overindulge—are you eating out of depression or anxiety?—and make efforts to address that issue. Food isn't the problem; overindulgence is.

Make Trade-Offs

Having a healthy low-fat diet doesn't mean clearing out all fat from the pantry. It's okay to eat some high-fat foods; just balance them with low-fat or no-fat items. For example, if you use half-and-half in your coffee, use skim rather than whole milk on your cereal. Ever notice how people make fun of you when you have a diet soda with your hamburger? Well, a 12-ounce can of regular soda contains 150 empty calories versus zero empty calories in the diet version. It's your choice, based on your day's total intake of calories.

Reconfigure Your Portions

Double the vegetables and halve the meats and fishes. A serving of broccoli (½ cup, plain) contains a mere 20 calories. Eat two servings and you're up to only 40. Now for the broiled salmon. Your fishmonger will tell you to plan for ½ pound (8 ounces) per person. That's 300 calories—not bad, but you'll find 4 ounces is enough, and that comes to only 150 calories.

Follow a Low-Fat Diet . . .

Though weight management is a calorie-balancing act, not all calories are *exactly* equal. Excess fat calories are very readily stored as fat, whereas carbohydrates and proteins must be converted to fat. Read labels, educate yourself about the fat content of foods, and aim for a diet in which only 25 percent of calories come from fat. Translate this to grams per day. If your daily intake comes to 2,000 calories, 25 percent is 500 calories of fat. Since each gram of fat contains 9 calories, you should aim for roughly 55 grams of fat.

. . . But Don't Be Fooled by Low-Fat Foods

Low-fat products may be the biggest scam the food industry has come up with. Why? Many of us fall prey to thinking that because a

HOW TO TRIM CALORIES PAINLESSLY

Cutting calories doesn't mean eating less or depriving yourself of foods you love or tastes you treasure. The secret to creating a lower-calorie meal plan that you can live with, and better yet *enjoy*, is to search out substitutes for high-fat foods that satisfy your taste buds with fewer calories. When it comes to rich foods that you just can't resist, don't cut them out—just cut them down. Here are several suggestions for trimming the fat from your daily menu, beginning with breakfast and finishing with dessert.

Eat . . .	Instead of . . .	Calories Saved
Breakfast		
1% cottage cheese (1 oz.)	Cream cheese on bagels (1 oz.)	80
1 slice French toast plus		
1 cup strawberries	2 slices French toast	130
2 pancakes	3 pancakes	175
2-egg omelet	3-egg omelet	100
Lunch		
Ham, 5% fat (4 oz.)	Ham, 11% fat (4 oz.) in sandwich	60
Pastrami, turkey (4 oz.)	Pastrami, beef (4 oz.) in sandwich	240
Turkey breast (4 oz.)	Turkey roll (4 oz.) in sandwich	45
2 oz. turkey, lettuce,	Turkey (4 oz.) in sandwich,	
tomato, mustard (1 tbsp.)	mayonnaise (1 tbsp.)	85
Chicken McNuggets	McChicken sandwich	220
Hot dog, turkey	Hot dog, beef	40
Snacks		
1 oz. pretzels	1 oz. potato chips	50
2 Oreo cookies	4 Oreo cookies	100
1 cup grapes	2 Nabisco oatmeal cookies	100
Dinner		
Low-calorie Italian dressing		
(2 tbsp.)	Oil and vinegar (2 tbsp.) on salad	100
Plain yogurt (2 tbsp.)	Sour cream on potatoes (2 tbsp.)	45
Salt and pepper or		
lemon juice	Butter (2 tsp.) on veggies	70
Pork tenderloin (3 oz.)	Spareribs (3 oz.)	195
3 oz. filet mignon	6 oz. filet mignon	180
Dessert		
Chocolate ice cream, low-fat,	Chocolate ice cream, Häagen-Dazs	
Häagen-Dazs (1/2 cup)	(1/2 cup)	110
1/2 cup strawberries,		
1/4 cup vanilla yogurt	Low-fat strawberry ice cream	70
Dole fruit-juice bar, orange	Fruit ice, Häagen-Dazs (1/2 cup)	70
Pumpkin pie, 1/8 pie	Pecan pie, 1/8 pie	190
Strawberry pie, 1/8 pie	Cherry pie, 1/8 pie	124
Other		
1 tbsp. olive oil	2 tbsp. olive oil in cooking	120
Whipped butter (2 tsp.)	Stick butter (2 tsp.)	25
1% milk (1 cup)	Whole milk (1 cup)	55
Skim milk (1 cup)	2% milk (1 cup)	20

food is low in fat, we can eat more of it. We devour a bag of low-fat cookies in half the time it took us to eat a bag of regular cookies and then we buy another. The food companies get rich and we get fat.

Pay Attention to Serving Sizes

Pasta, bread, rice, and potatoes are all nutritious high-carbohydrate, low-fat foods, but they will put fat on your body if you overindulge. It's easy to eat too much of *any* low-fat food. Read labels, find out what a serving is and how many calories it contains, and you'll be less inclined to overdo it.

Allow for Some Fat and Protein

You need protein and some fat in your diet, but besides need, there's want: they help keep you satiated. It takes more time to digest fats and proteins, so they "stick" with you better than if you eat just carbohydrates. By eating balanced meals that include some protein and a little fat along with the carbos, you'll prevent hunger attacks that can lead to oversnacking between meals.

Flavor Foods the Low-Fat Way

By using less butter and oil when you cook and fewer cream- or cheese-based sauces over foods, you can cut back on lots of calories. This doesn't mean your meals have to be bland. Here are a few ways to add flavor without adding fat:

- Sauté foods in low-sodium broth or half the butter or oil recommended.
- Cook fish or chicken fillets on the stove in fruit juices. Orange and grapefruit work well; experiment with others.
- To liven up veggies, sprinkle them with lemon or lime juice, herbs, or balsamic vinegar. Even a touch of salt won't hurt.
- Most vinaigrette salad dressings are two-thirds oil. Given that 2 tablespoons of olive oil contains 240 calories and 1 tablespoon of vinegar has only 2 calories, consider using half the oil and a little more vinegar.
- Balsamic vinegar isn't just for salads. It can be used in sautés and reduced in sauces to add low-fat zing to dishes.
- Opt for tomato-based sauces rather than those made with cream or butter. Remember, though, don't deprive yourself. When you're really craving some fettucine alfredo, go ahead and have some.

Eat Slowly

It takes 20 minutes for your brain to receive the signals from your stomach that it's full. If you eat quickly, you might eat more than you need or ultimately want. This is why people tend to overeat when they've let themselves become too hungry. Intense hunger simply drives you to eat fast to satisfy the pang. Literally before you know it, you've eaten too much, and when your brain finally does catch up with your fork, you're left feeling uncomfortably full.

Trick Your Tummy with Optical Illusion

If you fill up a small plate with food, you'll think you're eating lots even though the portions are not that large, and you'll feel more satisfied than if you put those same portions on a large plate.

Balance, Balance, Balance

The age-old nutritional advice to eat a well-balanced diet is still the best advice for health and weight management. It's much easier to maintain weight or lose weight by eating a variety of foods—fruits, vegetables, grains, breads, pasta, meats, fish, poultry, and yes, a treat every now and then.

Many runners, with their minds set toward carbohydrates, develop a one-track diet of breads, bagels, pretzels, and pastas. All of these foods are excellent sources of fuel for running and are low in fat (provided you don't slather them with high-fat spreads and sauces). A high-carbohydrate diet can lead to a high-*calorie* diet if you overdo it, however.

Exercise and Weight Loss

Running is one of the best means of managing weight. It burns more calories per minute than does almost any other activity, making it extremely efficient. It's the busy woman's best choice for not only weight control but overall fitness. Moreover, with just a few tweaks to your running routine, you can turn up the heat in its fat-burning furnace.

Run Faster to Burn More Calories

A 130-pound woman running a 10-minute-per-mile pace will burn 295 calories in 30 minutes. Up that to a 9-minute-per-mile pace for 30 minutes and she'll use 325 calories. This doesn't mean you should try to do *all* your running faster. That's too difficult and will

THE WELL-BALANCED MEAL

Here are two sample meals. Notice that the one composed of a variety of foods is lower in calories and supplies whopping amounts of certain important nutrients.

Carbo Meal	Calories	Balanced Meal	Calories
Salad with 2 tbsp. Italian dressing	155	Salad with 2 tbsp. Italian dressing	155
Spaghetti with red sauce (2 cups)	530	Spaghetti with red sauce (1 cup)	265
2 slices Italian bread, plain	165	1 slice Italian bread, plain	80
4 oatmeal cookies	235	1 cup broccoli	40
		½ cup cooked carrots	30
		1 cup strawberries with ½ cup low-fat vanilla yogurt	160
Total calories	1,085		730

Nutritional Analysis (% of Nutrient Type)
Carbohydrates	65	62	
Protein	10	12	
Fat	25	26	

Nutrients (% Recommended Daily Allowance)
Vitamin C	40	280	
Vitamin A	20	225	
Iron	90	56	
Folate	55	85	
Calcium	0	20	

lead to overtraining. You'll eventually become tired and possibly injured and you'll hate running and quit. Instead, pick 1 day a week to do a "tempo" run at a pace that requires more effort than your usual pace yet still feels relatively comfortable. The effort should fall somewhere between easy and difficult. Start with 5 to 10 minutes of easy running to warm up and then pick up your pace for 20 to 30 minutes. Finish with a few minutes of slow running.

Lift Weight to Drop Weight

One of the reasons men can eat more than women without gaining weight is that they have a higher percentage of muscle than we

LEAN TREATS

Here are some low-fat choices among high-fat indulgences. Remember, low-fat doesn't mean low-calorie. Read labels to find out exactly what you'll be biting into.

- Cakes and pies: angel food cake, Boston cream pie, gingerbread, sponge cake, strawberry pie
- Candy: hard candies, jelly beans, mints, chocolate-covered mints
- Cookies: animal crackers, Fig Newtons, gingersnaps, graham crackers, molasses cookies
- Frozen desserts: fruit-juice bars, fruit ice, frozen yogurt, Jell-O pudding pops, low-fat ice cream, sorbet
- Other desserts: rice pudding, tapioca pudding
- Snack foods: popcorn, pretzels, rice cakes, saltine crackers

do, and muscle burns calories all day long—even when you're sitting in front of the TV. You can increase your muscle mass by weight training. Two or three sessions a week is all you need (see chapter 18 for a complete program).

The caveat: At first, you might actually gain a couple pounds because muscle weighs more than fat, but give it a little time and you'll begin to see the fat pounds drop away. *The bonus:* Not only does strength training increase your resting metabolism and fat-burning abilities, it tones your muscles and strengthens your bones.

Exercise After You Eat

Studies show that taking a walk within 30 minutes after eating can boost metabolism and increase your postmeal calorie burn by 10 percent.

An Activity Plan for Weight Management

For a healthy exercise plan that can help you maintain a healthy weight, design a schedule around the following:

- Run regularly.
- Do a tempo or *fartlek* run once a week.
- Lift weights two or three times a week (see chapter 18 for a complete program).
- The rest of the week, relax and enjoy yourself.

CALORIES BURNED RUNNING

Use the table below to determine approximately how many calories you burn running. Find your weight in the left-hand column, then find your average pace and you'll have the number of calories burned in *10 minutes of running* at that pace. Example: If you weigh 130 lb. and you run a 9-minute-per-mile pace, you'll burn 108 calories in 10 minutes, which comes to 324 calories for 30 minutes of running or 432 calories for 40 minutes.

Your Weight (lb.)	12-Min.-per-Mile Pace	11:30-Min.-per-Mile Pace	10-Min.-per-Mile Pace	9-Min.-per-Mile Pace	8-Min.-per-Mile Pace	7-Min.-per-Mile Pace	6-Min.-per-Mile Pace
100	60	68	76	83	95	106	121
110	67	75	83	92	104	117	133
120	72	82	91	100	114	127	145
130	79	88	98	108	123	138	157
140	85	95	106	117	133	148	170
150	91	102	113	125	142	159	181
160	97	109	121	133	151	170	194
170	103	116	129	141	161	180	206

Calculations are based on data from the "Compendium of Physical Activities: Classification of Energy Costs of Human Physical Activities," *Medicine and Science in Sports and Exercise* (the journal of the American College of Sports Medicine) 1993; 25:71–80.

Being relaxed about your weight will help you manage it more successfully. It's often when we fret and struggle the most that we achieve the poorest results. When we stop worrying about weight and simply eat healthy foods and run regularly, our bodies find their own best weight and shape.

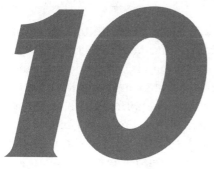# **10** Body Image

Seek not outside yourself, heaven is within.

—MARY LOU COOK, educator and environmentalist

MANY WOMEN TAKE UP RUNNING TO LOSE weight—with good reason, since running is one of the most efficient and best calorie-burning activities around. What often happens, though, is that once a woman begins running, she discovers many rewards she didn't expect. Running relieves her stress. It gives her more energy, makes her feel good physically. Weight loss becomes secondary. She continues to run and to improve, and she loses a few pounds, even though that's no longer the focus. She feels good about her body and about herself.

Now she runs simply for the pleasure of it and to feel good, and her weight and fitness naturally achieve their healthy best.

For a few women, though, running and weight loss become entangled in an unhealthy pattern of behavior, especially among those who place a premium on their running performance. The association between low body fat and faster race times can provide the impetus for a woman runner to eat less and less as she strives to improve her speed. This, plus societal pressures to be thin, can lead to overconsciousness about body weight and possibly even eating disorders. As the running community and society in general confront these issues and educate girls and women that skinny does not equal athletic excellence or beauty or success, we can hope that fewer women will feel so pressed to become so thin.

Beauty and a Beast: Weight

We have become obsessed with our bodies, and the focus of that obsession is our weight. It's not just women; men, too, fret endlessly

THE 1997 BODY IMAGE SURVEY

In March 1996, *Psychology Today* issued its third survey asking readers how they perceive their bodies. Of the roughly 4,500 responses received, the first 4,000 (from 3,452 women and 548 men) were tabulated and analyzed. The results appeared in the January/February 1997 issue. Here are some of the findings of that study:

- Among women, 56% were dissatisfied with their bodies.
- Among adolescent girls between the ages of 13 and 19, 62% were unhappy with their weight; 67% of women over the age of 30 thought they weighed too much.
- *Psychology Today* asked its readers how many years of their lives they would willingly give up to be the weight they desire. A shocking 24% of women and 17% of men said they would give up more than 3 years of their lives to be the weight they wanted. Fifteen percent of women and 11% of men said they'd sacrifice more than 5 years.
- Of the survey respondents, 159 women were extremely *underweight,* yet 40% of them still wanted to lose weight.
- Pregnancy is increasingly being seen not as a normal body function but as an encumbrance to body image. Some women said they are choosing not to have children for this reason.
- Almost half—43%—of women said that "very thin or muscular models" made them feel insecure about their weight.

about their figures. (See The 1997 Body Image Survey on page 120.) We loathe fat.

And there *are* good reasons. Obesity causes heart disease, the number-one killer of women and men, and it can also lead to diabetes, cancer, and numerous other ills. We *should* be concerned about fat as it affects our health, but many have taken this concern far beyond the issue of fitness. We've let our obsession with weight run into our definition of beauty.

These days beauty equals thin—very thin. And we have raised up before us goddesses of thinness: supermodels who pose in the pages of magazines and clothing catalogs and saunter across TV ads, reminding us again and again that we're "fat."

Compared to them we are fat. It is the rare woman who can attain such proportion of length and leanness, and still keep her breasts. Yet that is what we want. That is what we believe will make us pretty, desirable, successful, happy. But we can make ourselves miserable trying to achieve it—and in the end, never succeed. We work so hard to lose weight that sometimes it is our selves we lose.

Running

As a Solution

Women who don't feel good about their bodies can come to love their bodies through running. In the *Psychology Today* 1997 Body Image Survey, respondents said that exercise was the best source for positive feelings about their bodies. Running in particular can lead to a positive self-image. As we progress, we gain endurance, develop strong legs, acquire better muscle tone. We notice that our hearts and lungs are stronger, and many of us *do* lose weight.

Running also improves our inner images. There is such a feeling of accomplishment in completing however many miles we run. Running is a difficult sport, and we feel good about what we are able to do.

"Running has helped me with my body image because I know I am doing all I can to have the best body possible," says Lesley Leonessa. "The combination of running and very healthy eating allows me to forgive myself for not having a perfect, skinny body and to not beat myself up that there's more I could be doing."

As a Pressure

Though running helps most women feel good about themselves and their bodies, for a few, running steers them into a path of obsession with weight and thinness. A female runner faces greater pressures to lose weight than most women do. Not only is she bombarded by the typical societal attitudes toward thinness, but within her running world, she sees constantly—in magazines, advertisements, in television coverage of races, at races—an image of the female runner as superthin.

Add to this the association between low body fat and improved performance and it's not surprising that many women runners—and not just the superfast elite—become obsessed with their weight. Even those who do not develop distorted body images or, in the most severe cases, eating disorders, can become inordinately concerned with maintaining a particular weight.

What also can fuel an obsession with weight is the refined body awareness that you gain as a runner. Running is such a pure physical activity. It forces you to pay attention to your body. You develop a sensitivity to your breathing, to the workings of your muscles. You learn your paces and can tell when you're doing a 10-minute-per-mile pace versus a 9-minute-per-mile pace. You become so attuned that you quickly notice a difference of just a few extra pounds.

All these factors don't necessarily lead to dissatisfaction with body image or an obsession with weight. Many women are perfectly content with the way they are. They see images of thin women and skinny runners but have no desire to attain their shape. They take their running seriously, but they do not choose to try to hone their speed by paring their bodies. Why? Because they feel good about themselves, and they know that training, not dieting, improves running performance.

It is a need for acceptance that underlies a woman's obsession with body and weight—acceptance from herself and others. It's when you don't feel good enough about the person you are that you become caught up in trying to achieve superficial, arbitrary standards of beauty and performance that will make you feel good about yourself. If you feel unworthy, then you must assume that others see you as unworthy, too. Rather than trying to look to themselves to discover their own talents and beauty, many women grasp at society's definition of what's good and beautiful and try to remake themselves in that image. For many runners, an important part of the image is thin and fast.

What's Your Image?

Do you feel good about the way you look? Are you satisfied with the size and shape of your body? Are you comfortable with your weight? If you answer yes to these questions, then you probably have a healthy body image. The real test, however, is how much you *dwell* on your shape, size, weight, and all matters of lifestyle that can affect your physical geometry.

Some women may be thin and think their weight is okay, yet they live in steady fear of gaining a pound or two. They may feel a need to maintain a certain weight in order to keep their thighs thin or their stomachs flat or their hips narrow. Such a need sets them on guard against any action that might put on a few pounds, like cutting back on their running mileage or indulging occasionally in dessert. These women expend a lot of energy checking their figures and policing their lifestyles for any behavior that might lead to weight gain. Then there are those who go a step further—who are thin and even underweight but see themselves as fat. These women have a distorted image of their bodies, which can, and often does, lead to eating disorders in an effort to become even thinner.

RACE DIFFERENCES

Several studies have shown that African American women have a healthier body image and worry less about their weight than do white women. In a 1994 survey of girls attending YWCA summer programs, conducted by the Melpomene Institute for Women's Health Research in St. Paul, Minnesota, 40% of black girls considered themselves attractive or very attractive, compared with 9% of white girls.

The woman who doesn't feel daily compelled to examine her figure in the mirror or weigh herself on the scale, who doesn't waste time worrying about whether her waist will expand if she misses a week of running or enjoys a Thanksgiving meal with all the trimmings, is someone who is truly comfortable with herself. This woman loves herself from the inside out and knows she is a fine person regardless of how thin she is.

Refocusing a Distorted Image

Perhaps as you've read through this chapter, you've come to realize that, yeah, you are dissatisfied with your body even though your weight and shape are appropriate for your height and genetic history.

Such self-disparagement weighs heavily on your mind. Think about how much mental energy you expend worrying about what you eat, fretting about missed workouts, criticizing your figure in the mirror every day, agonizing over which outfit will best hide your rounded tummy or your "thunder thighs."

Imagine what it would be like to feel good about your body even though your proportions don't match the stick-figure ideal. Imagine loving that little bit of roundness in the tummy, the curves of your hips, the softness of your thighs, because these are what makes you a woman. Imagine being able to trust that with your regular running and good eating habits your figure will remain at its finest. What a relief to let go of a poor body image and all the negative behaviors associated with it.

How do you change the way you see yourself? Experts tell us simply to accept our bodies the way they are, to focus on the parts of us we do like, to stop comparing ourselves to others. It isn't quite that simple, though. You need to *work* at refocusing, at changing the way you see yourself. It takes time, and at the heart of the matter isn't how you feel about the way you look, it's about how you feel about who you are. If you feel good about yourself, you'll have an easier time accepting your body with all its imperfections.

Here are some points to contemplate that may help you gain a better perspective on your body, weight, and self-image.

It's Your Body—Be Proud of It

You inherited your basic body shape, structure, metabolism, and weight tendencies from your parents. Yes, you have some control over weight and muscle tone, but ultimately, you are what you are. Look at your mom, your dad, your aunts, your siblings. You'll see that certain features run in the family—could be big thighs, full hips, a large overall bone structure. You've probably inherited the same. You also may have inherited beautiful breasts or a regal nose or slender hands.

"I feel quite comfortable with my body," says Kay Nagel. "Yes, there are things I don't like (my poochy stomach), but then I look at my mom and throw up my hands, saying, 'It's genetics.' "

Women Are Supposed to Have Extra Fat

We see fat unequivocally as the enemy, but it is essential to the proper functioning of the body, our nervous system in particular.

Some fat pads inner organs and insulates us against the cold. Women also store adipose tissue in their thighs, hips, and breasts, which helps nourish a baby if we become pregnant. To rail against body fat is in essence to deny your womanhood.

"One of the things that helped me become more accepting of my body was the realization that it was okay to be female," says a 67-year-old woman from Ohio. "It sounds hokey, but watching old movies starring Sophia Loren and Ava Gardner helped. These women had shoulders, and breasts, and hips, and are some of the sexiest women I have ever seen" (quoted in *Psychology Today*, 1997, 30:80).

You Do Have Many Beautiful Body Parts

Stop focusing on the areas of your body you dislike. Try this: whenever you notice yourself becoming critical of, say, your hips, shift your attention to your great legs, your pretty face, your infectious smile.

You Have Many Exceptional Inner Qualities

What really matters? That you can fit into a size 8 dress or that you have the courage to be who you are? Would you trade your intelligence, creativity, and kindness for thinness or a new figure? If you had to choose between being an empty-headed, cold-hearted beauty or an average-looking intelligent, loving woman, which would you choose?

It's your character that ultimately defines whether you are beautiful or ugly. It is the person you are inside that lasts a lifetime. Beauty fades. Concentrate your efforts on being the best that you can be. Running will help you in this.

Beauty Is in the Eyes of the Beholder

Who are you trying to please with your body anyway? When we attempt to achieve some societal standard of beauty, it's as if we are making ourselves attractive to some invisible deity of glamour. Look at the people around you—your friends, family, your partner. To them, you are beautiful. They love you as you are. Let their acceptance help you accept yourself, because it is most important that *you* love you as you are.

"Part of the reason I run is to *try* to be slim," says one woman runner, "but I am no longer obsessed with being slim. I eat what I want, cut out junk when my weight increases. I think part of the reason for being more secure about my somewhat fluctuating weight is because I have a husband who accepts me no matter what I weigh. I have tested him on this—being one hundred four pounds when we married and two hundred three pounds when I gave birth to our second child."

Skinny Is Not Sexy

The next time you look in the mirror and think you're too fat and you make it your goal to become skinny, try to dig up photos of very thin women—not supermodels dressed in fashion's latest finery and wearing perfectly painted faces. Find an average woman in average clothing, maybe 5′6″ and 110 pounds who could appropriately weigh 130 pounds. You'll see that her face is rather gaunt and her arms and legs are bony and her chest is flat. Is this attractive?

A Fit Body Is a Beautiful Body

Would you agree that volleyball star Gabrielle Reese is attractive? Her beauty doesn't lie in a layer of perfect makeup, hair, and clothing. It comes from her physical power and fitness and her self-confidence.

Gabrielle Reese is a big woman—6′3″ and 170 pounds. She unabashedly talks about ordering two dinner entrées when she eats

TRADING SKINNY FOR STRONG

"When I started running, I weighed about one hundred twenty pounds, not an unhealthy weight for a five-foot four-inch woman. Through training and eating a healthier diet, my weight dropped to one hundred three. This wasn't by design, but once I got there, I didn't want to go back up. I suffered a lot of injuries back then and had no strength to speak of other than in my calf muscles. I was just skinny.

"Since then, I became involved in climbing and strength training, and my weight went up while my body fat decreased. I'm actually a size smaller than I was as an unfit teenager who weighed 5 pounds less.

"I don't focus too much on weight, though I'd be lying if I didn't admit that there is a certain threshold that causes me a bit of concern—I start training a bit more and watching the junk food—but I realize that to be one hundred three pounds would mean that I would have to get rid of some shoulder, back, and arm muscles, and I don't want to do that. Besides, I feel better and healthier than I did as a superlightweight."

—Kristi Carlson, runner

out. Granted, Reese represents another extreme—the superfit woman, which many of us cannot realistically achieve, either—but she does show us that there's beauty in size and strength.

Thinness Is Not Defined by the Circumference of Your Body Parts

Being thin means having a healthy body composition, a good ratio of muscle to fat. Some women are stocky because they are muscular, not because they are fat.

Runners Come in All Shapes and Sizes

Next time you're at a race, look around you. You'll see thin women, heavy women, tall and muscular women, women with narrow hips, women with big hips. And don't be surprised when a woman 20 pounds heavier than you passes you. Think about how many times you've been at an awards ceremony and witnessed a "sort of pudgy" woman win her age group. You thought to yourself, *How'd she do that? She doesn't look like a runner!* The swiftest are not always the skinniest. Running performance depends on many factors: training, genetics, fueling, strength, and mental toughness.

Beauty Radiates from Confidence and Happiness

You look at a pregnant woman and she simply radiates beauty. She's prettier than she ever was before pregnancy, and she certainly isn't any stick figure.

If it's important to you to be loved, accepted, and beautiful to those around you, you need first to find inner happiness and confidence. When we feel good about ourselves, we smile more, our muscles relax, our skin has better color, we rest better so we don't have dark circles under our eyes, our mood becomes cheerful and giving, and people like being around us. The right shape, perfect makeup, fashionable clothes don't hide sadness or a bitter soul. Put your energy toward finding happiness in your life in what you do and who you love rather than how you look—then beauty will come.

Disordered Eating

When the desire to be thin becomes a psychological need, what was once a troubled body image and an overconcern with weight turns into an eating disorder—anorexia or bulimia or a combination of

ARE YOU THE TYPE?

Athletes who suffer from disordered eating tend to have similar personality traits that affect their attitudes toward food, exercise, and weight. The traits may be the result of growing up in a family in which a parent was suffering from alcoholism or in an otherwise dysfunctional family where a parent may have been unavailable for the child.

Characteristic	Example
Drive for perfection	Not missing a day of running in years
Desire for control	Never eating any food with more than 1 g of fat
Compulsive behavior	Exercising for 1–2 hours every day regardless of holidays, injuries, or other events
Feelings of inadequacy	Believing you could have raced faster if you weighed less
Difficulty having fun	Choosing to work rather than go out with friends
Trouble with intimate relationships	Neglecting family because of time spent exercising

Reprinted by permission from Clark, N., 1997, *Sports Nutrition Guidebook,* 2nd ed. (Champaign, IL: Human Kinetics), 276.

both. Eating disorders are deadly. They can quite literally consume you, mentally and physically.

Anorexia Nervosa

Women with anorexia lose themselves in a long fall into starvation. They severely restrict their eating in order to lose weight. They fear fat intensely and even though they are underweight, they see themselves as overweight, which drives their disorder even further. They eat less and less, becoming skinnier and skinnier. If the disorder is not treated, these women can starve themselves to death. Because runners can become very thin, it may not be apparent to the friends and relatives of an anorexic runner that she has an eating disorder. It may not even be obvious to the anorexic woman herself.

The American Psychiatric Association defines anorexia nervosa by the following criteria: a weight below 85 percent of minimum for an individual's age and height and the refusal to maintain weight at or above the minimum. Because of their insufficient caloric intake, anorexic women develop amenorrhea (the absence of at least three consecutive periods).

Here are several other signs of anorexia:

- Recurring stress fractures
- Dry hair and skin
- Loss of hair from the head
- Cold hands and feet
- Sensitivity to cold temperatures
- Growth of fine hair on the body
- Lightheadedness
- Difficulty concentrating
- An abnormally slow heartbeat
- Unusual food rituals, such as taking a few bites of a food and then saving the rest or cutting up a meal into small pieces on the plate, pushing it around with a fork, and eating only a little
- Wearing baggy clothing to hide the body
- Emotional sensitivity—crying easily, feeling restless or uptight
- Compulsiveness in running (distress about missing 1 or 2 days)
- Compulsiveness in other areas, such as work or school
- Bulimic behavior—bingeing on food and then purging

Ironically, many women with anorexia love to cook and often prepare elaborate and exceptional meals for friends and family even though they choose not to partake themselves.

Bulimia Nervosa

The bulimic woman rides a roller coaster of bingeing and purging. Compelled by stress, she turns to food, eating an excessive amount uncontrollably in a short period of time. To compensate for this behavior and control her weight, she purges by vomiting or using laxatives, diuretics, enemas, or a combination of these items. Some bulimics purge through fasting or excessive exercise.

It is more difficult to recognize bulimia than anorexia. Bulimic women usually do not become extremely thin, and they hide their behavior. They regularly sit down to meals and secretively throw up somewhere where you won't hear them. After a time, however, you may notice that the bulimic can eat a lot of food and never gain weight, that she always excuses herself after dinner to use the bathroom, and that she runs the water in the sink for an inordinately long time.

Here are other signs and symptoms of bulimia:

- Bloodshot eyes and "chipmunk cheeks" from vomiting
- Erosion of tooth enamel because of stomach acid
- Knuckle scars from self-induced vomiting
- Puffy face and ankles from water retention
- Fluctuations in weight
- Sore throat
- Fatigue
- Weakness
- Headaches
- Dizziness
- Chest pain
- Abdominal pain
- Diarrhea or constipation
- Irregular menstrual cycle
- Depression

The Female Athlete Triad

Eating disorders lead to *amenorrhea,* which leads to bone loss and *osteoporosis.* In 1992 at a meeting of the American College of Sports Medicine, scientists defined the interconnection of these three disorders as "the female athlete triad."

The Risks

When a woman becomes amenorrheic, her body produces less estrogen. Estrogen protects bones from mineral loss, so when estrogen levels are low, bone loss increases and the risk for stress fractures and osteoporosis rises substantially. Osteoporosis is a condition in which the bones have lost mineral content and become more porous. They are weak, thin, and very vulnerable to fractures and breaks. Areas most susceptible to damage include the spine, hips, and forearms.

The Resolution

Amenorrhea is the red flag signaling the triad. If you are not menstruating, it is imperative that you take action to resume normal periods. Since amenorrhea appears to be caused primarily by an energy imbalance—too much energy being expended through running versus too little energy being taken in through food—the solution is to run a little less and eat a little more.

Unfortunately, the athlete with an eating disorder will have difficulty with this because the disorder has hold over her willpower even when she knows she must change her behavior to save her life. Women with eating disorders should seek the assistance of a physician, psychologist, and nutritionist. The help of all three specialists ensures a successful recovery.

When Someone You Know Has an Eating Disorder

Individuals with anorexia or bulimia may not see their behavior as harmful, or they may catch glimpses of the reality of their situation only to have the wall of denial close up again over their vision. This makes it difficult to confront someone who has an eating disorder. She may quickly become defensive and simply deny that she has a problem.

The best approach is a gentle one. Don't talk about her weight or eating habits; this is too sensitive an issue. Focus your concern on other aspects: fatigue, injuries, poor race times. Offer to listen should she want to talk about anything that might be bothering her. If she does, listen sympathetically. Don't be surprised, however, if she turns away from any discussion regarding her health.

Finally, you can give her a list of resources that she can use when she does realize she has an eating disorder and wants to do something about it. You, too, can use these resources to become better informed about eating disorders and how to help women who have them (see Where to Go for Help below).

Don't neglect your own well-being. Your friend's suffering causes you pain, too. Check with local counseling groups or psychologists to locate a support group for friends and families of women with eating disorders.

Remember, you cannot solve your friend's problem. The best thing you can do for her is to offer your support, understanding, and love.

WHERE TO GO FOR HELP

If you or someone you know struggles with an eating disorder, the following associations can provide you with information and advice on what to do.

American Anorexia/Bulimia Association, Inc.
165 West 46th Street, #1108
New York, NY 10036
phone: (212) 575-6200
web site: **members.aol.com/amanbu/index.html**
Provides information for professionals, sufferers, friends, and family and general information about eating disorders.

Anorexia Nervosa and Related Eating Disorders, Inc.
P.O. Box 5102
Eugene, OR 97045
phone: (503) 344-1144
web site: **www.anred.com**
Provides general information on eating disorders, suggestions on how to help, first-person stories, a self-test, and much more.

Eating Disorders Awareness and Prevention, Inc.
603 Stewart Street, suite 803
Seattle, WA 98101
phone: (206) 382-3587
web site: **members.aol.com/edapinc/home.html**
Provides educational resources for individuals, schools, and health professionals.

National Eating Disorders Organization
6655 South Yale Avenue
Tulsa, OK 74136
phone: (918) 481-4044
web site: **www.laureate.com/nedointro.html**
Provides information about anorexia and bulimia, suggestions on how to help a friend or family member, and much more.

National Association of Anorexia Nervosa and Associated Disorders
Box 7
Highland Park, IL 60035
phone: (847) 831-3438
web site: **members.aol.com/anadzo**
Provides hot line counseling, support groups, referrals, and information packets.

Bigger and Better

BY SUSAN LINDFORS

WE WERE JUMPING ON THE TWIN BEDS IN RACHAEL'S ROOM—
Rachael, Laurie, and I—three 7-year-olds giggling with delight at our
forbidden activity. Then Rachael said, "Laurie and I will jump on this
bed; you jump on that one. That way, the weight will be even." So began
my concern with my body.

Even in the early years, society sets a high standard. I was not by
nature a frilly, "feminine" girl. In fact, I didn't even want to be a girl. I
spent afternoons climbing trees, building forts, racing the boys around
the neighborhood blocks. I even broke a window playing baseball once,
and I sobbed the day I had to strap on my first bra, with my mother
standing by helplessly.

Also, I was not by nature small boned. No matter how hard I wished
or how hard I played, I would never have a wispy-thin, lithe figure. It was
neither in the cards nor in my Scandinavian genes.

Then I discovered athletics.

In junior high, I joined a swim team. It suited my shyness, as we were
mostly underwater. Yet ironically, despite the hampered communication,
I suddenly had more friends than ever. They became my closest friends,
the bonds forged through pleasure, pain, sweat, and our love of water.
From bleachers to poolside, we cheered each other on during countless
swimming competitions, through the challenges, hardships, injuries, and
victories. We were individuals, and we were a team. We understood each
other without needing to explain.

The most comforting revelation: looks and body type didn't matter.
We thought nothing of standing around the pool in tiny Lycra swimsuits.
My self-consciousness about my medium-size build vanished with the
jubilant realization that the muscles I once considered bulky and
"unfeminine" were actually necessary and encouraged. It turned out that

my muscles weren't even big enough. I had found a world that made sense.

When I left the swim team, I turned to running. Twenty years later, I'm still at it. Through running, I have found exhilaration, challenges, strength, confidence, inspiration, and peace—and lots of friends. I have run in all directions—away from, toward, in circles. I have run through joy, sorrow, anger, pain, and confusion. I have challenged myself again and again and have emerged from each test a stronger, more confident woman.

Let them call me "thunder thighs." I wouldn't have it any other way.

Susan Lindfors is a folk singer, editor, and writer. She lives in Emmaus, Pennsylvania.

PART IV

Your Special Concerns as a Woman

11 Menstruation

WE'RE WOMEN. WE RUN THROUGH A changing tide of hormones. Estrogens, progesterone, luteinizing hormone (LH), and follicle-stimulating hormone (FSH) swell and recede in a regular rhythm each month. The ebbs and surges of these hormones can affect our energy levels, our appetites, our moods, and our running. In turn, our running can affect the rhythms of our hormones and in some cases even alter the pattern of our menstrual cycles.

Fortunately for most of us, the rhythms of our running and the rhythms of our bodies flow smoothly and simultaneously. So that you can maintain a steady course of health and peak running performance, it's helpful to understand the workings of your hormones and the relationship between running and your menstrual cycle.

Primer: The Menstrual Cycle

We all know that the average menstrual cycle lasts about 28 days, that day 1 is when bleeding starts (which usually lasts 3 to 7 days) and day 14 is when ovulation occurs. When it comes to the changing levels of hormones and what roles they play, though . . . well, I know I have difficulty remembering what happens when. So that you can understand the relationships among running and menstruation and health, it's important to know in detail what's going on during your cycle; let's review.

The menstrual cycle follows a hormonal cycle involving the hypothalamus (a part of the brain), the pituitary gland, and the ovaries. On average, a complete cycle lasts 28 days, but anything from 25 to 35 days is considered normal.

The Menstrual Phase

Day 1: menstruation begins. At this point, levels of estrogen are low, which signals the hypothalamus that another egg needs to be released. The hypothalamus increases gonadotropin-releasing hormone (GnRH), which stimulates the pituitary gland to release FSH, which then triggers the growth of several follicles in the ovary, only one of which fully matures to release an egg. As the follicles develop in the ovary, they secrete estrogens.

DETERMINING OVULATION

You can determine when ovulation occurs by charting your temperature for several months. Do this first thing in the morning before getting out of bed (any activity will raise your temperature). During the first half of your cycle, your temperature should be under 98° Fahrenheit. Right before ovulation, your temperature drops, then rises over the next 1 or 2 days; in the second half of your cycle, it will remain just above 98°. If you do not notice any change in your body temperature, it may be a sign that you are not ovulating. You can also use an ovulation kit.

The Follicular Phase

Also called the proliferatory or the postmenstrual phase, the follicular phase is the period between menstruation and ovulation (usually days 6 to 13 of the cycle). Estrogen levels continue to rise, stimulating the development of the lining of the uterus. At the same time, one follicle continues to mature as others are resorbed by the ovary. When that follicle, containing a maturing egg, reaches almost full development, it releases a burst of estrogen and progesterone. These hormones signal the hypothalamus to increase levels of GnRH, which stimulates the pituitary to release large amounts of FSH and LH, which then triggers the follicle in the ovary to release its egg. *Day 14: ovulation occurs.*

The Luteal Phase

Also called the secretory or the postovulatory phase, the luteal phase of the cycle begins after ovulation and continues for 14 days. The empty follicle, now called a corpus luteum, secretes increasing amounts of progesterone but less and less estrogen. Levels of FSH and LH drop as well. The high level of progesterone stimulates the uterine lining to secrete fluids that will nourish the egg if it is fertilized. If indeed fertilization occurs, the placenta releases a hormone that will signal the corpus luteum to continue to produce progesterone and estrogen to maintain the pregnancy. In the absence of fertilization, the corpus luteum does not receive the message to continue releasing estrogen and progesterone, and levels of these hormones decline. When the levels reach a certain low point, the hypothalamus begins releasing GnRH, and the cycle begins again. See Figure 11-1 for a visual representation of hormone fluctuations during menstruation.

The Effect of the Menstrual Cycle on Running

As our hormones surge and recede throughout the month, it seems our bodies, moods, and even appetites undergo certain fluctuations as well. Most of the changes we experience occur during the week prior to our periods and are grouped together and called premenstrual syndrome (PMS). Approximately 40 percent of all women who menstruate experience some degree of PMS. Symptoms may include abdominal cramps, water retention and bloating, breast tenderness, nausea, fatigue, headaches, depression, irritability, and increased

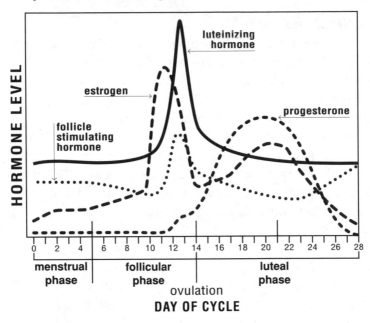

Figure 11-1. Hormonal changes during the menstrual cycle.

appetite. Given all these possible physical changes, it's reasonable to assume our running may be affected, too.

Many women runners do report that they feel sluggish and run slower in the week prior to menstruation and that they sometimes notice a surprising burst of energy in the first few days of their period. This has been my experience. The week before menstruation, I often have a harder time keeping up with my friends during a run. My breathing becomes more labored, and if I'm doing speed work, my times will be disappointingly slow. In the first few days of my period, however—even if I'm feeling like I really don't want to run—the running seems effortless once I get going. In fact, I ran my fastest and easiest marathon on the first day of my period one year.

"A couple of studies suggest that during the luteal phase of the menstrual cycle [days 14 to 28], running economy decreases, meaning it takes more effort to run at a particular pace," says Constance Lebrun, M.D., director of Primary Care Sport Medicine at the Fowler Kennedy Sport Medicine Clinic in London, Ontario, Canada. "No one knows for sure, but the higher levels of progesterone during this phase may cause a higher body temperature, a higher breathing rate, and higher heart rate. In addition, you retain more fluid in the second phase. All of these factors can make running more difficult."

Does that mean that you won't run as well during the week before your period? Not necessarily. Though running economy may decrease during the second half of the menstrual cycle, your ability to store glycogen and to burn fats increases. "Estrogen increases the uptake of glycogen and shifts your metabolism toward free fatty acids," says Lebrun. "This means that you'll burn more fat during running and hold onto your glycogen stores longer, so you should have better endurance and be able to run longer."

When you consider that your mood and other symptoms of PMS may have a psychological effect on your running, however, it becomes very clear that none of this is clear at all. There's simply no direct answer to the question of how the menstrual cycle affects running. Every woman is different. Lebrun suggests that you keep a log of how you feel during your runs and then study it in relationship to your menstrual cycle to see if you can find any monthly pattern to your performance.

There's really not much you can do about it one way or the other, but knowing how your cycle affects your running can help you understand and accept your body's performance. If you're having a bad run and it happens to be the week before you're due to get your period, it may simply be a matter of hormones and not your ability on that day.

Understanding your body's response to the menstrual cycle may be important in evaluating race performances as well. If you find you race better at certain times of the month than others and performance is important to you, pick your key races to fall on those days that you usually run your best.

Not all women experience noticeable changes in their running before or during menstruation. Experts point out that world records and Olympic medals have been won by women at all phases of the menstrual cycle.

The Effects of Running on Menstruation

Our hormones can be very powerful, but we know, too, that running is a force that affects our minds and bodies. What effects might it have on our menstrual cycles?

Premenstrual Syndrome

If you experience premenstrual symptoms every month—bloating, fatigue, moodiness, cramps—the last thing you feel like doing is going for a run, but give it a try. You might feel better. Many women do.

Studies that have looked at whether exercise alleviates the discomforts of PMS show mixed results. Some have found that, indeed, active women report less discomfort than do inactive women. Other research has recorded roughly equal incidence of PMS among exercisers and sedentary women. All you can do is give it a shot and see if it works for you.

Amenorrhea

Experts estimate that 10 percent to 20 percent of women who exercise vigorously experience amenorrhea. The risks? Infertility and osteoporosis (a decrease in bone mass resulting in bones' becoming porous, thin, and susceptible to fracture). Fortunately, fertility eventually resumes after menstruation becomes regular again, but bone health may not return.

Anytime you miss a period and suspect pregnancy, it's imperative that you see your gynecologist; otherwise, most physicians advise that if you miss three consecutive periods, you should make an appointment. Menstrual dysfunction can have several causes, including a thyroid or pituitary problem. "The only way to determine if exercise is related to the menstrual problem is by excluding other causes," says sports gynecologist Mona Shangold, M.D.

Is running *directly* responsible for loss of menstruation? No. The factors involved in amenorrhea include weight loss, percentage of body fat, a history of menstrual irregularity, psychological stress, and diet, as well as the amount and intensity of exercise. It is the interrelationship of some or several of these factors that affects our menstrual cycles.

For years, the thinking among experts has been that low body weight, and specifically low body fat, causes loss of menstruation among runners. The theory is that a certain level of body fat is

AMENORRHEA DEFINED

You are amenorrheic if you have three or fewer periods a year. Primary amenorrhea is when menstruation has not occurred by the age of 18. Secondary amenorrhea is when menstruation occurs at least once, but then ceases. Oligomenorrhea is when menstruation occurs irregularly every 39 to 90 days, and eumenorrhea refers to regular, consistent menstruation.

necessary for the production of estrogen, but several recent studies have found that among exercising women of equal height, weight, and fat percentages, some are amenorrheic and some are not.

Though amenorrhea occurs more often in thin women than in heavier runners, researchers now believe that it's not low weight or lack of fat that causes problems but a low caloric intake. Very simply, the body requires energy in order to perform all of its many functions, including running and menstruation. If you are expending more energy than you are taking in through food, your body goes to its stores of energy—fat—and begins burning them. The result is weight loss. This is fine if you have lots of fat to burn, but if you don't, your body will also go into an energy conservation mode. Metabolism slows and certain "dispensable" functions—such as menstruation and reproduction—get shut down. It's like having a short supply of fuel to heat your home during a long, cold winter. You warm the rooms you live in and close off the ones that are used least often.

I menstruate regularly, but I'm having trouble getting pregnant. Could my running be affecting my fertility?

It is possible to have regular periods and not ovulate (produce an egg), which clearly makes fertility impossible. Another dysfunction that may be hidden by regular menstruation is luteal-phase defect, in which the second phase of the menstrual cycle after ovulation (the luteal phase) shortens because of a lack of progesterone. The result is that the uterine lining doesn't develop completely, and though fertilization may still be possible, the pregnancy may not take. This condition occurs in nonrunners as well as runners. Experts suspect it may be a precursor to athletic amenorrhea. By charting your menstrual cycle (see Determining Ovulation on page 138) for a few months, you will be able to determine whether you are ovulating or experiencing a shortened luteal phase. If you suspect either, see your gynecologist.

You can burn a lot of calories through running. If you aren't eating enough to fuel both your running and your body's regular functions, something may stop working. For many women, it's their menstrual cycles. This phenomenon is neither new nor specific to exercising women. Historically, there are many instances of women's losing their fertility during times of famine or war.

UNDERSTANDING ATHLETIC AMENORRHEA

Current theory states that when your caloric intake is too low to sustain the energy needs of your body, your menstrual cycle ceases. Research into how this takes place indicates that it starts in the brain at the hypothalamus, which decreases the amount of gonadotropin-releasing hormone (GnRH). Take a look back at the beginning of this chapter and review the chain of hormonal events responsible for normal menstruation. A decrease in GnRH causes a decrease in follicle-stimulating hormone (FSH) and luteinizing hormone (LH) secretions from the pituitary, which results in a reduction of follicles in the ovary, which means very little estrogen and progesterone will be produced. An egg may not develop and ovulation may not occur.

When it comes to running, you can run long and hard and have your periods, too, but you must eat more. How much more? Experts recommend increasing caloric intake by 10 percent to 20 percent. If you consume, for example, an average of 1,800 calories, add 200 to 400 calories a day. Review your diet to ensure that it is well balanced and that you are getting enough protein. Researchers think there may be a link between lack of dietary protein and amenorrhea.

Christy Dueck, Ph.D., of Arizona State University, reports that in working with an amenorrheic runner, she increased the runner's daily caloric intake with a 360-calorie protein-and-carbohydrate drink. In addition, the runner reduced the intensity of one of her weekly workouts. In less than 4 months, menstruation returned to normal.

Running is not our only external energy demand, however. Our jobs, our households, our children, whatever psychological stresses we may experience—all of these become drains on our energy stores. It's easy to create an overload, which might just blow your menstrual fuse in addition to a mental one.

The solution? Balance your energy flow, regularly replenishing what you've spent. Take a good look at your life and ask yourself where your energy is going and where you want it to go. Perhaps you *are* running too much. Maybe you need to find ways to alleviate some emotional stresses. Perhaps you need more help around the office or home. Or maybe you need to make adjustments in several areas of your life.

Then again, maybe you thrive on a full load of activity—loving your long runs, challenging workdays, and busy home life—and simply *do* need to increase your caloric intake. The best solution is a personal one: the right answer is the one that meets your needs for happiness and good health.

Will the pill affect my running performance?

Though some studies show that maximum oxygen consumption ($\dot{V}o_2$ max; a measure of aerobic capacity) decreases in women who use the pill, most research has found that oral contraceptives have no effect—positive or negative—on running performance. Science aside, some runners report that their performance declines when they're on the pill.

For most women considering the pill, the benefits far outweigh any possible decrease in running performance. Oral contraceptives provide the most effective means of birth control. They regulate your cycle, help protect against bone loss, and may decrease your risk of ovarian and uterine cancers. Most women on the pill experience fewer symptoms of premenstrual syndrome (PMS), and because your periods are lighter, you lose less iron.

Keep in mind that several types of birth control pills are available. If you do notice any unpleasant side effects or you feel the pill may be slowing you down, ask your gynecologist about trying a different formulation.

Osteoporosis

Running builds bones. Amenorrhea tears them down.

Solid as they may seem, our skeletons are not static structures. Even after our bodies have reached full development, our bones are constantly producing new cells and absorbing old ones. Estrogen plays a role in this equation by slowing down the resorption or loss of bone tissue. Take estrogen away and bone loss speeds up, faster than it is rebuilt.

This is why women with exercise-induced amenorrhea have lower bone density than do women whose menstrual cycles are normal. In fact, researchers have found that the spines of amenorrheic runners show a decreased bone mass comparable to that of postmenopausal women. The spine isn't the only area affected, however. A 1996 study of amenorrheic athletes performed at the University of Washington Medical Center in Seattle also found low bone mass densities in the femur (thighbone) and tibia (shinbone). It is not surprising, then, that amenorrheic women are more susceptible to stress fractures in the short term and osteoporosis in the long term. Barbara Drinkwater, Ph.D., one of the researchers involved in the University of Washington study, has found that once normal menstruation resumes, bone loss may be regained, but not completely.

Estrogen replacement therapy, through birth control pills or similar prescriptions, has been successfully used to increase bone density in amenorrheic runners, but you have other options, as described earlier. You can concentrate on balancing your energy flow by eating more and/or exercising less to get your menstrual cycle back on track. In fact, some women who followed a program of increased calorie consumption combined with a small decrease in training intensity not only resumed normal menstruation but ran better, too.

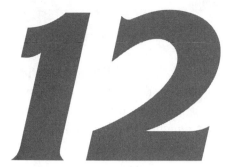

Pregnancy

"I NEVER CONSIDERED NOT RUNNING WHILE pregnant," says Sarah Linstedt, mother of Maggie, 9, and Kitty, 4½. "During my first pregnancy, I ran twenty-five miles a week through thirty-two weeks and probably would have kept going if I had not delivered prematurely at that point. My doctor assured me running had nothing to do with my daughter's early arrival and applauded my efforts to stay aerobically fit. I was able to resume running 10 days after her delivery.

"With my second pregnancy, I ran comfortably through the first six months and then chose to stop. I also took a bike trip to British Columbia when I was five months along. My second daughter arrived just three weeks ahead of schedule and weighed in at a healthy seven pounds eleven ounces. Eight months after she was born, I ran my fastest marathon ever at Chicago.

"In both pregnancies, running lifted my spirits, prevented me from ballooning into a giant couch blob, kept me in shape for two extremely easy deliveries, and helped me stay in touch with my running social life. Granted, my pace naturally slowed as the babies got bigger, but I still felt running contributed to my well-being.

"Now Maggie and Kitty come to the track with me once a week. Maggie times my laps, and Kitty, who loved going out in the running stroller, now likes to run around the track. I think both girls have a very positive outlook on athletics that started even before they had their little legs on the ground."

Like Sarah, many women are discovering that running during pregnancy is a positive and healthful experience for themselves and their babies. Experts now agree not only that running during pregnancy is safe for mom and baby but that it can actually enhance your well-being and maybe even that of your child.

Running and Baby's Well-Being

For years, women were cautious and concerned about running during pregnancy, worrying that it might deprive the fetus of oxygen or nourishment in the form of glucose (blood sugar), that the body might overheat and cause damage to the fetus, or that running might stimulate premature delivery.

Too Little Oxygen?

Pregnancy and running each make high demands on your cardiovascular, respiratory, and thermoregulatory systems. Research has found, however, that a woman's body can handle both—pregnancy and running—at the same time. A pregnant woman's body makes adjustments to accommodate the extra demands of exercise, making sure that the fetus gets the oxygen and nutrients it needs while muscles are burning up oxygen and glucose they use during exercise.

Cardiac output increases 30 percent to 50 percent, and blood volume expands by 35 percent to 45 percent during pregnancy. These increases mean your blood can carry more oxygen, but also, during exercise your body makes adjustments to meet the oxygen needs of the fetus and your working muscles.

Too Much Heat?

Concerns about overheating have been raised by studies with animals that show high temperatures in the first trimester can cause neural tube defects in the fetus. No such studies have been performed on humans, of course, but body temperature has been measured in pregnant women exercising on a treadmill and found to rise only slightly (a degree or less), not exceeding the recommended upper limit of 102° Fahrenheit.

Other research has shown that the body's ability to regulate heat improves during pregnancy and is probably a natural adaptation to help protect the fetus. One aspect of this improved heat regulation is a lower sweating threshhold, meaning that you'll start sweating sooner in the heat than you would if you weren't pregnant. As uncomfortable as sweating might be, it's an important cooling mechanism.

Early Delivery?

As to whether running causes uterine contractions and premature delivery, studies report that women who exercise through their pregnancies show no greater incidence of early delivery than do women who don't exercise.

Small Babies?

Runners' babies generally do weigh less than infants born of nonexercising women; however, the lower birth weights still fall within the normal range. The latest research shows that this lower weight in runner's babies is due to lower body fat—10 percent compared to the usual 15, according to James F. Clapp III, M.D., of the Departments of Reproductive Biology and of Obstetrics and Gynecology at Case Western Reserve University in Cleveland.

Answer: Running Is Safe

Women who run during pregnancy are not compromising the health of their babies. With all the evidence that's been compiled to show this is true, experts around the country, including the American College of Obstetricians and Gynecologists (ACOG), agree that as long as a woman shows no risk factors for a problematic pregnancy, she can continue her exercise program throughout pregnancy.

Running and Your Well-Being

Not only is running during pregnancy *safe* for you and your baby, but it can also offer several health *benefits,* as Sarah described earlier.

Physical Rewards

Women who run experience fewer of the discomforts of pregnancy: nausea, fatigue, leg cramps, and backache. Late in pregnancy, though, many women complain of abdominal and pelvic discomfort during running due to tension on the round ligaments that support the uterus. This may be alleviated by using an elastic abdominal support or by wearing bike shorts.

Regular running seems to improve sleep and appetite while preventing unnecessary weight gain, and it may prevent gestational diabetes. In addition, many (not all) women who exercise during pregnancy have easier and shorter deliveries. Experts believe this is a result of their high level of fitness.

Psychological Pluses

Runners feel better about their bodies during pregnancy than do inactive women. They have a better body image, higher self-esteem, and generally brighter moods.

Aerobic Advantages

If you're wondering what will happen to your fitness as you run through 9 months of pregnancy, getting slower and running fewer miles with every month, you'll be glad to know that you'll probably maintain your aerobic capacity and may even improve it. Experts explain that pregnancy in itself is like exercise. With added weight, you expend more energy standing, walking, running—doing any weight-bearing activity. Plus, during pregnancy, your blood volume and red blood cell count rises. Add regular running, even at a lower intensity than you are used to, and it's easy to see how aerobic fitness is maintained.

A Musculoskeletal Minus

Though for the most part, running during pregnancy is healthful, you may be at a greater risk of injury. Early in pregnancy, the body produces a substance called relaxin, which relaxes the ligaments of the pelvis and softens the cartilage that holds the pelvic bones together. This occurs in other joints as well, which may make a pregnant runner more susceptible to sprains and other injuries.

In the latter months of pregnancy, the extra weight you carry puts additional stress on joints as you run; however, at this point, you will probably have cut back on the intensity and distance of your runs. Also, because you carry the weight of pregnancy in front of you at your abdomen, your center of gravity changes, making balance more difficult; therefore, you want to avoid uneven or potentially slippery surfaces.

Consider running on a track or treadmill during the latter part of pregnancy. Both offer a firm, even surface, which helps prevent undue stress on the muscles of your legs and ankles and protects against sprains. Also, tracks and treadmills are softer than roads, which lessens the impact of running. Many women continue on the road with no problem, however.

Despite this assumed vulnerability that pregnancy puts us at, there are no reports of an increased rate of injury among women who exercise during pregnancy.

Individual Experiences

Every woman's body is unique. Every woman experiences pregnancy differently. Even though the majority of women say that running helped them feel good during their pregnancies, this won't be

IT'S YOUR CHOICE

All the requirements have been met: you're in good health, there are no signs of complications, and the experts have deemed that running during pregnancy is safe. Nevertheless, you just aren't comfortable with the idea of continuing such intense exercise during your pregnancy. Well, that's reason enough not to run. It's most important that you feel good about how you are handling your pregnancy. If you have any concerns about running, take a break from it during your pregnancy. Consider exercise options that you would feel comfortable with—swimming or walking, perhaps. Your pregnancy exercise plan should enhance your well-being, not detract from it by creating stress.

true of everyone. You might be in excellent health going into pregnancy, run comfortably for 9 months, and then experience a difficult delivery. You simply may feel too sick during pregnancy to keep up your running. Ultimately, you will decide for yourself what's best. If you have the permission of your doctor or midwife and you want to run during pregnancy, go ahead and give it a try. You can always stop if it becomes uncomfortable.

Sometimes during a run I have what feels like contractions. Should I be concerned?

"If you experience contractions during running, you should stop and lie down. They will probably subside. If they don't, see your obstetrician right away. In any case, check with your obstetrician to see if it is safe for you to continue running. There is no way for you to tell what these contractions are and whether you should be concerned about them."

—MONA SHANGOLD, M.D., SPORTS GYNECOLOGIST

When Running Is Not Advised

Despite all the good news about running and pregnancy, not every woman will be able to continue her exercise routine while she's pregnant. Certain situations make it unsafe to do so. The ACOG recommends that exercise be limited or discontinued entirely given any of the following circumstances.

Preeclampsia

Some women develop preeclampsia, formerly called toxemia, the symptoms of which are hypertension (high blood pressure), protein in the urine, and fluid retention. Experts think this condition may be linked to a blood vessel problem. Exercise can make toxemia worse.

Vaginal Bleeding

If you notice any vaginal bleeding, stop exercising and see your obstetrician. Some women experience a condition called placenta previa (not induced by running) in which the placenta develops low in the uterus, covering the opening of the cervix and causing heavy bleeding.

Preterm Labor or a History of Preterm Labor

Women who have delivered prematurely in an earlier pregnancy should be conservative in their exercise routines, especially during the second and third trimesters. Consider taking a break from running after a certain point in your pregnancy and taking up walking or some other less intense activity. Discuss your options with your obstetrician.

Poor Growth of the Fetus (Intrauterine Growth Retardation)

At regular intervals, your obstetrician will check the development of your baby using ultrasound. If the growth of the fetus does not meet appropriate standards, it may be a sign that the fetus is not getting enough oxygen. Since exercise draws blood flow away from the uterus, it's wise to stop exercising.

Multiple Fetuses

If you are carrying twins, triplets, quadruplets . . . you are at a higher risk for complications during pregnancy and should not increase that risk with running. Discuss with your obstetrician or midwife a non–weight-bearing exercise routine that would be safe.

Medical Problems

Women with heart disease, high blood pressure, anemia, or thyroid, vascular, or pulmonary disease need to discuss with their health-care providers whether exercise is safe and if so, what type or program would be appropriate.

A Running Program for Pregnancy

Wouldn't it be helpful and reassuring if some obstetrician/coach had developed the perfect running program for pregnant women? Then you could follow a prescription for running that would take all the guesswork out of how far, how fast, and how often to run. Unfortunately, such a schedule doesn't exist. So many factors must be considered—a woman's health, medical history, athletic history, risks of complications, her response to pregnancy—that to devise one plan that's right for every woman is impossible.

As research continues to reassure us of the safety of physical activity for pregnant women, the possibilities for exercise increase.

The 1994 guidelines for exercising through pregnancy drafted by the ACOG states: "An exercise prescription in pregnancy should be individualized and should include a health assessment." That means you need to develop a running program that is appropriate for you. How?

Begin with Your Doctor

Before starting—or continuing—your running program, consult your obstetrician or midwife. Together, you should thoroughly review your medical history, assess your health, and discuss the history and details of your current running program. Taking all this information into account, you can then create an appropriate plan.

Run at Least Three Times a Week

If you get a clean bill of health and if you've been a regular runner, you can probably continue with your usual running program during the early months of your pregnancy. ACOG specifically recommends that exercising at least three times a week is preferable to a sporadic approach.

Determine Intensity and Distance According to Your Ability and How You Feel

ACOG's 1994 guidelines do not put specific limits on the amount or intensity of exercise: "Weight-bearing exercises [running is one] may under some circumstances be continued at intensities similar to those prior to pregnancy throughout pregnancy."

Some women have run incredible amounts during their pregnancies. Sue Olsen, a nationally ranked ultrarunner, ran through her entire first pregnancy at age 38. At 8½ months she completed Grandma's Marathon in Duluth, Minnesota, finishing in 4 hours. A week later, she walked and ran a 24-hour event, covering 63 miles. The next day she delivered a healthy baby boy.

Was Sue endangering herself and her baby? Considering that she can run 134 miles in a 24-hour competition, it's clear that she had cut her intensity by more than half in her 63-mile performance. During the event, she was conscientious about eating and drinking regularly and she stopped to sleep. Also, Sue had the permission of her doctor, who advised that she not get overheated and to stop if she didn't feel well.

Sue is an example of a very fit woman who was able to maintain a rigorous running program throughout pregnancy. Fitness isn't the

PERCEIVED EXERTION

When you become pregnant, your resting heart rate increases, and since we don't know what maximal heart rate is during pregnancy, it becomes an impractical way to determine how hard you should run during pregnancy.

A better approach is to use the Rating of Perceived Exertion developed by a Swedish physiologist named Gunnar Borg, Ph.D. This is a scale of exercise intensity that you apply to your running; you define for yourself, on the basis of your experience, what "very, very light exercise" means and what "very, very hard exercise" means, plus all the levels in between. Applying a technique called rhythmic breathing will help you to gauge the intensity of your running (see pages 39 through 41 in chapter 5 for details).

Using the following scale, the effort of your runs during pregnancy should not exceed a rating of 17, according to James F. Clapp III, M.D., of the Departments of Reproductive Biology and of Obstetrics and Gynecology at Case Western Reserve University in Cleveland.

Exercise Intensity	Rating
	6
Very, very light	7
	8
Very light	9
	10
Fairly light	11
	12
Somewhat hard	13
	14
Hard	15
	16
Very hard	17
	18
Very, very hard	19
	20

only factor in determining what level of running program you should follow, however. Raul Artal, M.D., professor and chairman of the Department of Obstetrics and Gynecology at the Crouse Irving Memorial Hospital in Syracuse, New York, had a patient—an Olympic champion—who not only wasn't able to run during her pregnancy; she couldn't even walk.

We'll never know what the upper limits for exercising during pregnancy are, partly because that would involve subjecting groups of pregnant women to higher and higher intensities of exercise until a problem occurred. The more important issue is that every woman is different. The number of miles we run each week and the paces we keep vary considerably among women who aren't pregnant. Each of us has her own appropriate levels of exercise determined by her individual biomechanics, physiologies, lifestyles, and athletic goals.

You and your doctor should discuss the level of running that seems appropriate, using your current program as a starting point. Then it's up to you to pay attention to your body and adjust the amount and intensity of your running according to how you feel. Here are some guidelines to help you figure out how far and how fast you should run:

- Run at a moderate intensity as determined by how you feel rather than by heart rate (see Perceived Exertion on page 155). You should be able to have a conversation while you are running. If you can't talk, slow down.
- Regarding distance, plan your weekly mileage according to what you think you can do comfortably. If on any particular run you become fatigued, stop running. Do not run to the point of exhaustion.
- As your pregnancy progresses, reduce the amount and intensity of running. You will probably naturally cut back as running becomes more uncomfortable.

Choose Convenient Courses

Map out routes that will allow you several bathroom stops, especially during the first and third trimesters, when urination is most frequent.

Run During Peak Energy Levels

If you're really tired during pregnancy, try to schedule your runs at those times of day that you have the most energy.

Include Stretching

Cool down and stretch at the end of each run. Don't stop running abruptly; walk until your heart rate and breathing have returned to normal and stretch lightly to maintain flexibility and help prevent injury.

Add Exercises to Tone Key Muscles

In addition to running, you should regularly do exercises to improve posture, prevent urinary incontinence, strengthen the muscles that support the breasts, and strengthen the muscles you will use during labor. These include shoulder shrugs and rotations, pelvic tilts and rocks, abdominal curls, and Kegel exercises. (See the section "Cross-Training for Pregnancy" in this chapter.)

Safety Tips

Listening to your body and adjusting your running accordingly is the most important safety measure you can follow. There are a few other precautions you should take, however, to ensure a healthful running program. The following recommendations are a compilation of guidelines from the Melpomene Institute for Women's Health Research in

WHAT TO WEAR?

In the early months of pregnancy, your usual running clothes will fit just fine, but eventually you'll need to change into something more comfortable for your runs. Many women wear cycling shorts, which stretch easily to accommodate an expanding waistline.

In winter, regular running tights should work well, though you may need a larger size than you're used to wearing. For "maternity" running clothes, check out the web site for Fit For Two: **www.snowcrest.net/fitfor2/.**

Here are a few more tips for dressing comfortably during pregnancy:

- Wear two sports bras for extra support and comfort as your breasts enlarge.
- When your belly gets big, try wearing a pregnancy belt.
- Some runners find a unitard comfortable and supportive.
- During summer, wear loose-fitting tops made from CoolMax or any of the other light, breathable fabrics that wick sweat away from your skin to keep you cool and dry. Avoid cotton, which soaks up perspiration and stays wet.
- To help keep feet cool and dry, wear synthetic socks.
- Check that your shoes are in good shape, especially during the later months of pregnancy, when musculoskeletal changes and an altered center of gravity make you more vulnerable to injury.
- Joan Marie Butler, runner and author of *Fit & Pregnant: The Pregnant Woman's Guide to Exercise* (Waverly, New York: Acorn Publishing, 1996), offers this tip: pick up a pair of lace locks, small plastic devices that secure your laces without your having to bend over and retie them.

St. Paul, Minnesota; ACOG; and obstetricians experienced with exercise and pregnancy.

- Run during the cooler parts of the day—early morning or early evening.
- Stay well hydrated to help keep your body cool. You know you are well hydrated when your urine is very pale.
- During warm months, wear loose clothing that provides adequate ventilation.
- In cold weather, wear a hat, since a lot of body heat is lost through your head.
- Make sure your running shoes are in good shape to provide adequate support.
- Avoid running on slippery or very uneven surfaces, especially in the latter months of pregnancy, when balance is poor.
- Stop running when you are fatigued.
- Stop running if you experience any vaginal bleeding.
- Stop running if you experience pain or dizziness.
- Follow a high-carbohydrate diet and make sure you are getting enough calories and an adequate supply of nutrients (see "Eating Right," below, for more information).
- If you can, run with a partner. This is a good safety tip even if you're not pregnant.
- Run in a populated area or in your neighborhood where you can get assistance should you need it.
- After the first trimester, do not do exercises in the supine position (lying on your back). In this position, the uterus compresses a vein (the inferior vena cava), reducing blood flow.

Eating Right

As a health-conscious runner, you probably already follow a nutritious low-fat, high-carbohydrate diet that includes a variety of fruits and vegetables, whole grains, and calcium-rich foods (see chapter 8 for general information on nutrition). Follow this same diet during pregnancy, making just a few adjustments in calories and nutrients.

Calorie Requirements

Pregnant women need 300 more calories a day than do the rest of us, according to ACOG. That's equivalent to a bagel-shop bagel with low-fat cream cheese or a cup of low-fat yogurt and a banana or two slices of bread with 1 tablespoon of peanut butter. Eat according to your appetite and make sure you're getting the calories you need to feed your body, your baby, and your running.

The average weight gain during pregnancy is 30 to 35 pounds, but anything from 20 to 40 pounds may be appropriate, depending on your nonpregnant weight and your level of activity. Your obstetrician or midwife will regularly measure your weight throughout your pregnancy to make sure you are gaining properly.

Nutrient Needs

Several of your vitamin and mineral requirements go up when you're pregnant. Most likely, your doctor or midwife will recommend a multivitamin and/or iron supplement, but you should be conscientious about eating foods rich in protein, calcium, iron, and folate.

Folate, also known as folic acid or folacin, is one of the B vitamins. Studies have shown that deficiencies of this nutrient during pregnancy can result in neural tube defects in your baby. Also commonly called spina bifida, a neural tube defect is when the vertebrae of the spine fail to close in the developing fetus, leaving some of the spinal cord exposed. The result may be as mild as weakness in the legs or as severe as brain damage.

Sports gynecologist Mona Shangold, M.D., recommends that active pregnant women get 1 milligram of folic acid, 1,500 milligrams of calcium, 80 milligrams of iron, and 80 grams of protein daily. (For foods rich in these nutrients, see chapter 8.)

Dietary Don'ts

Don't drink either alcohol or caffeine. The first, of course, can be harmful to your developing baby and the latter can cause premature birth. Also, when you're nursing, caffeine gets into breast milk; and the last thing you need is a baby with a caffeine buzz.

I often feel nauseated and am having trouble keeping food down. I'm concerned I'm not getting enough calories for my baby. What should I do?

On average, women gain 2 to 4 pounds by the end of their first trimester. However, many women lose weight due to morning sickness. So don't be too concerned during those first few months; your baby will get enough nutrition from your body's stores of nutrients. After the first trimester, you should gain about a pound a week.

To help keep calories up early in pregnancy, try frequent small snacks throughout the day rather than large meals, and experiment with different foods to find those that sit comfortably in your stomach.

Cross-Training for Pregnancy

Let's be honest: the joys of pregnancy are accompanied by the pains of pregnancy—backache, poor posture, urinary incontinence, heavy breasts. By regularly practicing certain exercises, you can prevent many of the problems of pregnancy and prepare for an easier childbirth. The following exercise routine will help your posture, strengthen the muscles that support your breasts, help prevent urinary incontinence, and prepare your muscles for delivery. Try to do this program two to three times a week.

• **Shoulder rolls**

Benefit: Strengthens the trapezius muscles of the shoulder, back of the neck, and upper back for better posture.

Technique: Stand with arms straight down at your sides, holding a 2- to 5-pound dumbbell in each hand. Make a circular motion with your shoulders, moving them forward, up, back, and down.

Number of repetitions: Begin with 3 to 5 and gradually build up to 10 to 12.

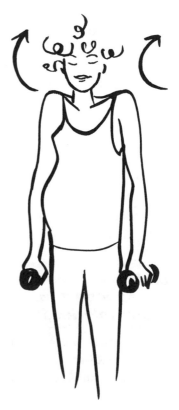

Figure 12-1. Shoulder roll: rotate your arms in a circular motion.

- **Pelvic tilts**

  Benefit: Helps relieve backache.

  Technique: Stand comfortably. As you exhale, pull your buttocks under and forward. Hold for 5 seconds and relax.

  Number of repetitions: Begin with 5 and gradually work up to 10 to 12.

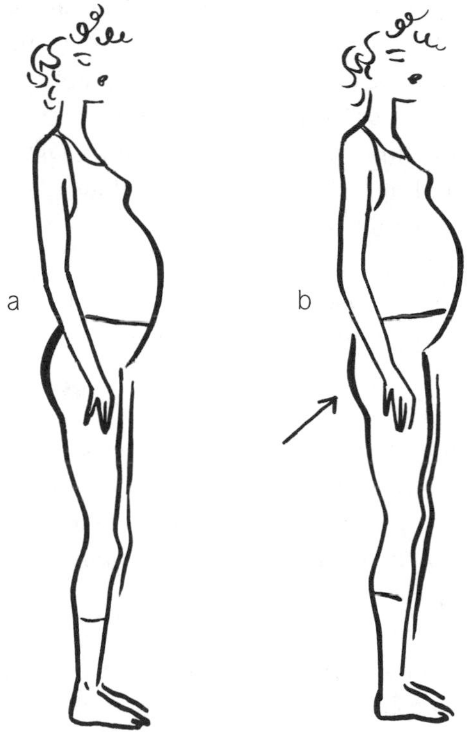

Figure 12-2. Pelvic tilt: stand comfortably (*a*), then exhale and pull your buttocks under and forward (*b*).

- **Pelvic thrust**

  Benefit: Strengthens the lower back.

  Technique: Lie on your back on the floor with your knees bent, feet flat on the floor, and hands at your sides. Raise your pelvis off the floor until you feel a slight arch in your back, then lower your pelvis to the floor.

  Number of repetitions: Start with 5 and work up to 10 to 15.

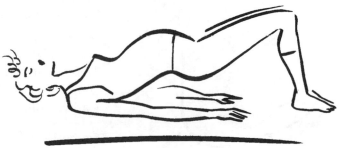

Figure 12-3. Pelvic thrust: raise your pelvis until you feel a slight arch in your back.

- **Kegel exercises**

Benefit: Strengthens the pubococcygeus muscle (PC muscle), which encircles the opening of the urinary tract and the outside walls of the vagina.

Technique: The key to doing Kegel exercises properly is to make sure you are flexing the PC muscle. The exercises were developed by Arnold Kegel, M.D. Sit on a toilet with your legs spread apart and, as you urinate, try to stop the flow of urine midstream without moving your legs. When you can do this, congratulations: you've found your PC muscle. Now that you know how to flex it, you can do Kegels anywhere in any position—standing, sitting, or lying down. Simply tighten the muscle for 3 seconds and relax.

Number of repetitions: Work up to 25.

Tougher Kegels: Tighten your muscles and hold for 10 to 20 seconds. Work up to 10 of these, done throughout the day.

- **The Tupler technique**

Benefit: Strengthens abdominal muscles, prevents back pain during pregnancy, and eases delivery. The Tupler technique was developed by Julie Tupler, R.N., fitness trainer, childbirth educator, and author of *Maternal Fitness: Preparing for the Marathon of Labor* (New York: Simon & Schuster, 1996).

Technique: Sit on the floor, your back against a wall and your legs crossed. With one hand on your abdomen and the other against the small of your back, take a deep breath. Exhale slowly and pull your belly button back toward your spine until you've reached a point that

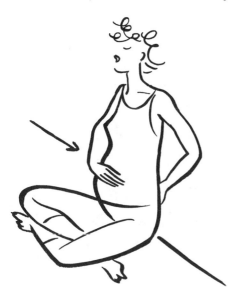

seems midway to your spine. This is the starting position. Now, pull your belly button as far back toward your spine as you can and then release it *just to the starting point.* Repeat this 100 times. That's right, 100 times—and that's only one set. Then relax.

Number of repetitions: Work up to 10 sets of 100 repetitions each for a total of 1,000 contractions. It's tough, but when you're in the delivery room, you'll be glad you did it.

Figure 12-4. The Tupler technique: pull your belly button as far back toward your spine as you can.

Postpartum Running

Some women can begin running again just 2 weeks after giving birth. Others may need to wait 4 to 6 weeks, and still other women find it takes a couple months before they're up to running again. Don't get discouraged. It takes time for all the changes your body has gone through during pregnancy to return to normal.

How quickly you return to running depends on how you feel physically and psychologically, as well as how much help you have at home with child care. When you feel ready to start running again, give it a try. If it becomes very uncomfortable or you get tired after a few minutes, stop running and give yourself a few more days of rest before going out again. You might want to do a combination of running and walking for the first week or so until you feel strong enough to run continuously. Gradually build up your running program as your body, mind, and lifestyle allow.

The Melpomene Institute for Women's Health Research offers these guidelines:

- If you had an episiotomy, wait until all soreness is gone before you exercise vigorously.
- If you exercise and begin to bleed heavily or with bright red blood, give yourself more time to recover. For 1 to 2 weeks after giving birth, your vagina expels lochia, the brownish to dull red blood that comprised the uterine lining during pregnancy.
- Be aware of continuing joint laxity resulting from the hormone relaxin produced during pregnancy; your hormone balance does not stabilize for several weeks.
- Fatigue is a common problem for new mothers, especially those who nurse. If you are tired, consider a nap rather than exercise.
- Drink plenty of fluids if you are a nursing mother.
- Good breast support during exercise is important for nursing mothers.
- You may be incontinent, even for several months, after delivery. Kegel exercises are best to correct this condition.
- Watch your posture. The cumulative effects of pregnancy, labor, milk-filled breasts, and carrying babies can lead to back pain. Do some abdomen-strengthening exercises.
- Warm up before exercise. Cool down, stretch, and relax after your exercise.

- Follow good nutritional habits. Eating properly is difficult with a baby and a busy schedule, but try to find a way. There's no need to rush into weight loss, especially if you are nursing; in fact, nursing itself helps some women lose weight.
- Child-care arrangements and juggling schedules may be difficult as you find time to exercise. Be patient.
- Relax and enjoy yourself. A brisk walk with your baby may be all you can do at first. As you develop a routine and can fit regular exercise into your schedule, you will find it provides important time just for you.

I've heard that running right before breast-feeding can make my milk taste sour to my baby. Is that true?

It was once thought that the lactic acid produced during running crossed into breast milk and made it unpalatable to babies. The most recent studies, however, report that your milk will not be affected in content or volume by running. Nonetheless, your enlarged breasts can become pretty uncomfortable during running. For that reason alone, you might want to feed your baby first. Also, wear a sports bra that offers a lot of support, or try wearing two.

Postpartum Personal Records?

Ingrid Kristiansen, who set world records in many race distances (including the marathon) during her career, ran a marathon personal record (PR) only 5 months after giving birth, and many recreational runners have seen their race times improve after pregnancy, too. As mentioned earlier, pregnancy combined with running can improve your aerobic capacity. In a 1991 study, James F. Clapp III, M.D., measured maximum oxygen capacity ($\dot{V}o_2$max) using a treadmill test, in a group of well-trained women before and after pregnancy and found that $\dot{V}o_2$max was significantly higher 12 to 24 weeks and 36 to 44 weeks postpartum. He also measured $\dot{V}o_2$max in a group of well-trained women who didn't go through pregnancy and found that in the same time period, there was no change in their aerobic capacity. This is not to say that every woman will race faster after giving birth. Performance is individual, and many factors affect how well we run.

What is a PR?

PR stands for *personal record*. It refers to your fastest time at a given distance. European runners use the term *personal best,* or *PB.*

The Birth of New Beliefs

What once we feared might be life-threatening—running during pregnancy—we've learned can be life-enhancing for you and your baby. There are no guarantees, but running may improve your pregnancy experience, and pregnancy may improve your running experience. As we continue to explore the effects of running and other physical activities on our well-being, we learn over and over again that exercise is not a separate piece of our lifestyles—a thing we do—but is a natural and integral aspect of our lives as healthy women.

DO RUNNERS HAVE SMARTER BABIES?

In 1996, James F. Clapp III, M.D., with the Departments of Reproductive Biology and of Obstetrics and Gynecology at Case Western Reserve University in Cleveland, performed a study to look at the effect of exercise during pregnancy on the well-being of a woman's baby at birth and at 5 years of age.

Clapp selected two groups of 20 women each, all of whom were healthy, of similar socioeconomic status and level of education, and who exercised prior to pregnancy. The difference was that one group did not continue to exercise during pregnancy, but the other did. Among the exercisers, 11 were runners and 9 participated in aerobics. Six of them also did cross-country skiing during the winter. Throughout their pregnancies, these women continued to exercise at least three times a week for more than 30 minutes.

Both groups had normal pregnancies, normal deliveries, and healthy babies. The only difference Clapp found was that the babies of exercising women weighed less, owing to lower body fat—an average of 10 percent, versus 15 percent among the offspring of nonexercisers. This was no surprise, as this has been found again and again in other research.

Clapp's study wasn't over, though. Five years, later he measured certain physical and intellectual characteristics in these 40 children. He discovered that at age 5, the children of the women who exercised during pregnancy still had lower body fat percentages, but their height and weight were normal by national standards.

The bigger surprise was that the exercisers' children performed better on tests of general intelligence and oral language skills than did the children of women who did not exercise during pregnancy.

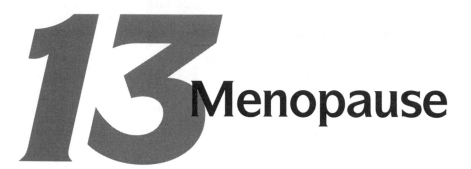

13 Menopause

> *My periods stopped right after I bought a new box of tampons. There is a god; she has a sense of humor.*
>
> —NANCY L. HARLEY, runner

IF THE EBB AND FLOW OF HORMONES we experience each month in our menstrual cycles can be compared to a changing tide, then for some women, menopause is the storm hitting the sea. Great swells and dips in hormones can send emotions rocking, plummet energy levels, and muddy the memory. For others, though, the passage through menopause is so calm and peaceful they hardly notice. Most of us will have an experience that lies somewhere between the two.

If we approach menopause knowing what it can bring and how to handle those events, we can navigate more surely and more comfortably. As runners, we have an advantage over inactive women. Running makes us physically and mentally stronger, better able to withstand whatever ups and downs we might experience. It helps to be braced against the greatest risks—osteoporosis and heart disease.

Menopause—What to Expect

Defined as a woman's final menstrual period, menopause occurs on average at the age of 52. It's the years leading up to menopause, called perimenopause, that can be the most tumultuous: this is when your hormones (estrogen and progesterone) fluctuate before finally settling at low levels. You will still be getting your period, but you'll begin experiencing menopausal symptoms. Perimenopause can last anywhere from 2 to 10 years and can begin in the early forties. After your period stops, you may continue to experience the hormonal effects for 5 to 10 years.

The range of symptoms is wide (see Signs of Menopause on page 168), but most women will first notice a change in their menstrual cycle. Periods may become closer together or farther apart. They may be longer or shorter, heavier or lighter. You may experience moodiness or have trouble concentrating or remembering things. Insomnia is common, and fatigue can at times be almost debilitating. Of course, there are the infamous hot flashes, which may present themselves as moments of hotness or flares of heat and floods of perspiration.

Although 10 percent to 15 percent of women don't even know they're going through menopause, an equal number are, for a time, disabled by it. The rest of us experience some range of manageable symptoms.

If the symptoms vary so much from woman to woman, how can I be sure I'm going through perimenopause?

There is a blood test that measures your levels of follicle-stimulating hormone (FSH), luteinizing hormone (LH), and estrogen. On the basis of these levels, your doctor can tell you what stage of perimenopause you have reached. The glitch here is that during perimenopause, your hormone levels change dramatically, so to get a more accurate picture of what's going on,

SIGNS OF MENOPAUSE

Hot flashes have become synonymous with menopause, but there are many other symptoms. The following list was compiled in January 1996 by Judy Bayliss at Hershey Medical Center in Hershey, Pennsylvania, from a survey she conducted via the internet. Bayliss is the owner and founder of an internet menopause mailing list, which at the time of the survey had 400 subscribers. Don't let the extensiveness of this list scare you. You aren't going to experience all of these symptoms. The first 13 symptoms are the most common. As Bayliss points out, "these signs are not simply a matter of aging. They are seen in young women after the ovaries are removed."

- Hot flashes
- Bouts of rapid heartbeat
- Irritability
- Mood swings, sudden tears
- Trouble sleeping through the night (with or without night sweats)
- Irregular periods; shorter and lighter or heavier
- Loss of libido
- Dry vagina
- Crushing fatigue
- Anxiety, feeling ill at ease
- Feelings of dread, apprehension
- Difficulty concentrating, disorientation, mental confusion
- Disturbing memory lapses
- Incontinence, especially on sneezing or laughing
- Itchy, crawly skin
- Aching and sore joints, muscles, and tendons
- Increased tension in muscles
- Breast tenderness
- Increase or decrease in headaches
- Gastrointestinal distress: indigestion, flatulence, gas pain, nausea
- Sudden bouts of bloating
- Depression
- Exacerbation of existing conditions
- Increase in allergies
- Weight gain, often around waist and thighs
- Hair loss or thinning; increase in facial hair
- Dizziness, lightheadedness
- Changes in body odor
- Electric shock sensation under the skin
- Tingling in the extremities
- Gum problems, increased bleeding
- Burning tongue, burning roof of mouth, bad taste in mouth
- Osteoporosis (after several years)
- Change in fingernails: softer, crack and break more easily

the blood test should be done two or three times over a few weeks. Ask your doctor about a saliva test, which is reported to be even more accurate.

The Two Big-Time Health Risks: Heart Disease and Osteoporosis

Estrogen has many protective effects on our hearts and bones. To lose this hormone as we do in menopause therefore sets us up for possible heart disease and osteoporosis later in life.

Your Heart

Estrogen helps keep total cholesterol levels low and high-density lipoprotein (HDL)—or "good"—cholesterol levels high and prevents the buildup of plaque that can clog arteries. It also affects the walls of your blood vessels, keeping them smooth and relaxed. Take estrogen away and over time, your arteries harden, plaque collects inside them, and your risk of heart attack and stroke rises.

Your Bones

In addition to taking care of your heart, estrogen protects bones from calcium loss primarily by inhibiting the work of bone-eroding cells called osteoclasts. After menopause, when estrogen levels are low, there's little to stop those osteoclasts from tearing down bone

RUNNERS ON MENOPAUSE

"After years of apprehension, anticipating the worst, I can say—at least at this point—hot flashes are more annoying than anything else. For me, they feel like I've walked in front of a pizza oven (minus the aroma) for 15 seconds or so. No night sweats, no flushing red face—and never while running, though who could tell?"

—NANCY L. HARLEY, RUNNER

"I think hot flashes were less bothersome to me than to my friends because as a runner, I'm used to getting all hot and sweaty. It may also be that having a relatively high level of fitness helped keep my menopausal symptoms mild. One effect of menopause is that it is much harder to keep my weight down, which definitely affects my running. Some women have a much greater problem, a real menopause-related weight gain, while in my case, it's more that when I've gained weight (primarily during running layoffs), it's extremely difficult to lose it even when I go back to my normal mileage."

—JANE COLMAN, RUNNER

tissue, so the rate of bone loss increases from 2 percent to 5 percent a year for 5 to 7 years, then slows to 1 percent a year. Eventually, bones become porous, and this is called osteoporosis. Unfortunately, you

WHAT YOU SHOULD KNOW ABOUT OSTEOPOROSIS

Osteoporosis is a porousness of bone caused by a loss of bone tissue, which leaves the bone vulnerable to fractures. Here are some facts compiled from data published by the Melpomene Institute for Women's Health Research in St. Paul, Minnesota, and the National Osteoporosis Foundation in Washington, D.C.

- Osteoporosis affects approximately 20 million American women.
- Approximately 1.5 million osteoporosis-related fractures occur each year: 40% in the spine, 25% in the hip, and 15% at the wrist.
- A 50-year-old Caucasian woman has a 50% chance of developing a fracture sometime in her remaining years.
- Twice as many fractures are reported among Caucasian women as among African American women over the age of 60, but one of every five African American women is at risk of developing osteoporosis in her lifetime.
- The best way to prevent osteoporosis is to build strong bones through exercise and diet *before the age of 35.* You reach your peak bone mass between the ages of 25 and 35; after 35, your bone mass begins to decrease.
- Though osteoporosis occurs primarily in older women, it can develop before menopause.

Risk Factors:
- Being female
- Family history of osteoporosis
- Small frame
- Early onset of menopause
- History of amenorrhea or missed periods
- Northern European ancestry
- No childbirth
- History of eating disorders
- Lack of calcium in diet
- Inactive lifestyle
- Smoking and/or alcohol use
- Use of certain medications, including corticosteroids and anticonvulsants

Drug Treatments:
- Estrogen replacement therapy
- Calcitonin, a naturally occurring hormone that affects calcium regulation and bone metabolism
- Bisphosphonates, compounds that inhibit the breakdown of bone tissue

won't know you have osteoporosis until a fracture occurs. Experts recommend getting a bone density test once you've stopped menstruating, especially if your risk is high (see What You Should Know About Osteoporosis on page 170).

Running to the Rescue

The good news is that as a runner, you probably won't be one of the statistics. You are way ahead of the average woman in preventing heart disease, osteoporosis, and even many of the distressing symptoms of menopause.

Mona Shangold, M.D., director of the Center for Sports Gynecology and Women's Health in Philadelphia, published a report, "An Active Menopause: Using Exercise to Combat Symptoms," in the *Physician and Sportsmedicine* (1996; vol. 24, no. 7, pp. 30–36), explaining the ways exercise relieves some of the problems of menopause. "Those who exercise regularly tend to report fewer menopausal symptoms and problems than sedentary women," she says. Here's what she has found.

Deeper Sleep

Running helps you sleep better through the night, which may help combat the fatigue that comes with menopause. Also, running in itself energizes us.

Merrier Mood

"Regular aerobic exercise improves cognitive function, enhances mood, and promotes daytime alertness," says Shangold.

Better Weight Control

Menopausal women put on pounds easily. Your muscle mass decreases and body fat increases, lowering your metabolism and leading to weight gain. Running is one of the best weight-control exercises around; however, menopausal runners find that it's harder to maintain their weight than it once was. Regular resistance training, which will prevent muscle loss and keep your metabolism high, may help, as will following a low-fat diet.

Stronger Bones

Running is a weight-bearing exercise, which means that as you do it, your musculoskeletal system must bear the weight of your body.

The force causes bone density to increase. Strength training also bolsters the skeleton, another good reason to incorporate it into your weekly routine (see "An Exercise Prescription for Menopause," below). Don't forget your calcium, though. The combination of a calcium-rich diet and exercise reinforces bone density even more.

If you've experienced exercise-induced amenorrhea (cessation of menstruation), which results in a loss of estrogen, your bones may not be as strong as those of a woman who menstruated regularly throughout her life. It depends on the length of the amenorrheic phase and other lifestyle habits. Running will help strengthen your bones and prevent osteoporosis through menopause and beyond, however.

Hardier Heart

Running is an excellent preventive against cardiovascular disease. It strengthens the heart, improves circulation, lowers total cholesterol levels, and raises levels of HDL cholesterol. "In fact, subjects jogging 11 miles per week were found to have significantly higher HDL levels than their sedentary counterparts," reports Kathleen M. Hargarten, M.D., in "Menopause: How Exercise Mitigates Symptoms" (*The Physician and Sportsmedicine,* 1994; 22:49–58). Shangold points out that "many of the adverse effects of aging and menopause on lipids [fats] are *reversed* by aerobic exercise."

An Exercise Prescription for Menopause

Chances are your current physical activities are sufficient to help reduce the symptoms of menopause and lower the risks of heart disease and osteoporosis. Compare your exercise program with the following recommendations based on the advice of Shangold and other experts.

- **One hour of running or some other weight-bearing exercise four to six times a week:** This recommendation comes from the National Osteoporosis Foundation. If running this much each week is too much for you, mix in some brisk walking, stair climbing, or aerobics. Swimming and bicycling are *non*–weight-bearing activities and won't provide the same degree of benefit, but they do improve bone density somewhat.

- **Strength training two or three times a week:** Remember, not only does this help prevent osteoporosis but it also prevents muscle loss. The more muscle you have, the higher your metabolism and the more calories you burn, even when you are not exercising. You can do a program of strength training at home, using free weights, or at your local gym, using resistance machines. See chapter 18 for a complete routine.

- **Daily stretching:** After every run or workout, be sure to cool down, walking until your heart rate has returned to normal, then stretch. This will help you maintain flexibility, another asset that we lose as we age. Good flexibility helps prevent injury. For a thorough stretching program, see chapter 17.

A Nutrition Plan for Menopause

Exercise is only part of a good action plan for a healthy and comfortable menopause. Diet is the other essential piece of the program. What you eat and don't eat can affect weight gain, bone density, and your risk for cardiovascular disease. Here are several important dietary guidelines.

- Make sure you consume plenty of calcium. (See The Calcium Cache on page 91 in chapter 8 for a list of calcium-rich foods.)
- Don't overeat meat, as diets high in protein have been associated with calcium loss.
- Watch your salt intake, since sodium has been linked to calcium loss.
- Avoid alcohol, which inhibits the absorption of calcium.
- Cut back on caffeine, another calcium blocker.
- Avoid eating calcium-rich foods with foods that inhibit calcium absorption, such as spinach, beets, parsley, and tea.
- Make sure you meet your daily requirements of all vitamins and minerals.
- Add soy foods, such as soybeans, tofu, and soy milk, to your diet. Soybeans contain isoflavones, plant estrogens that may help alleviate some of the symptoms of menopause associated with the loss of human estrogen.
- Trim the fat in your diet (particularly saturated fat) to help control weight gain and keep cholesterol under control.

What About Hormone Replacement Therapy?

With running, resistance training, and a healthful diet high in calcium and low in fat, you may prevent many of the symptoms and health risks of menopause. This is all some women need to move through this phase and on to a healthy active postmenopause. Other women may not find enough relief through exercise and diet and may choose hormone replacement therapy (HRT) to help with the discomforts of menopause and for added protection against heart disease and osteoporosis.

What Is It?

HRT is a prescription of estrogen and progestin taken to replace those hormones lost through menopause. The estrogen relieves many of the symptoms of menopause, whereas progestin is prescribed to protect against uterine cancer, the risk of which rises with estrogen therapy. Women who have had a hysterectomy do not need progestin.

The Benefits

Estrogen relieves hot flashes, prevents the drying and shrinking of the vagina, lifts your mood, helps you sleep, and may help maintain your memory and cognitive abilities. Most important, it protects against bone loss and prevents heart disease.

The Risks

HRT has been the topic of much debate among health professionals because of the risks of cancer associated with it. Some studies show that women who take estrogen are at a higher risk for both uterine and breast cancer.

To Take or Not to Take Hormone Replacement Therapy?

The benefits and risks of HRT vary from woman to woman. Whether HRT is right for you depends on your lifestyle, your medical history, family medical history, and what you are comfortable doing. Educate yourself as much as you can about HRT and then have an open, thorough discussion with your doctor about your options.

Beyond Menopause

Our experience of life after menopause is as individual as our experience leading up to it. Some women feel saddened by their loss of fertility and the fact that they are getting older. Others feel relief from the monthly effects of their menstrual cycles and freedom from the possibility of pregnancy. For some women, libido decreases; for others, desire increases.

Many women who've moved beyond their responsibilities to children and career find their postmenopausal years ripe with the possibility of new experiences. Others may be hampered by the caretaking of ill or elderly parents. What's certain is that we all pass through menopause to a new segment of our lives. Running can help us go there in good health.

FOR MORE INFORMATION ON MENOPAUSE

Want to learn more about menopause, treatments, osteoporosis? Check these excellent sources.

BOOKS:

Menopause, Me and You: The Sound of Women Pausing, by Ann M. Voda, R.N., Ph.D. (New York: Harrington Park Press, 1997)
The Pause, by Lonnie Barbach, Ph.D. (New York: Dutton, 1993)

ORGANIZATIONS:

The North American Menopause Society
P.O. Box 94527
Cleveland, OH 44106
(216) 844-8748
web site: www.menopause.org
The Calcium Information Center
phone: (800) 321-2681
3314 S.W. U.S. Veteran's Hospital Road
PP262
Portland, OR 97201
The National Osteoporosis Foundation
phone: (800) 464-6700
1150 17th Street N.W.
Suite 500
Washington, D.C. 20036-4603
web site: www.nof.org

WEB SITES AND INTERNET MAILING LISTS:

Better Health Profiles: Menopause

fbhc.org/patients/betterhealth/menopause/home.html

Doctor's Guide to Menopause Information and Resources

www.psigroup.com/menopause.html

Menopause: Another Change in Life (Planned Parenthood Federation of America)

www.ppfa.org/ppfa/menopub.html

Menopause

www.howdyneighbor.com/menopaus/

You can also join an internet mailing list for women going through menopause. You'll receive e-mail daily from members sharing their experiences and offering their advice. To subscribe, send an e-mail message to **listserv@mailstjohns.edu** with the following content only: Subscribe Menopaus [insert your name here]

"Shuffling" for Balance (and the Occasional Pitcher of Beer)

BY ELIZABETH SHIMER

I WAS 7 YEARS OLD WHEN I GOT MY FIRST PAIR OF REAL RUNNING shoes. They were magenta Nikes, and the only runs I took in them were sprints around the jungle gym to avoid being smooched by my male classmates. I took my first fitness run at about age 13. I attempted a very hilly 2-mile route near my house that left me nauseated, breathless, and discouraged. Nevertheless, I joined the track team my freshman year of high school, and my running hobby left the starting block.

I say "hobby" because I wasn't gifted with speed or a competitive edge. I didn't break records on either the track or the cross-country teams. One of my most memorable running moments occurred as I crossed the finish line of a 3-mile race when my coach patted me on the back and said, "Liz, you're not real speedy, and your shuffling form leaves much to be desired, but I can always count on you to keep on running."

At first I was slightly insulted by my coach's bluntness, but the next day in English class I read the following quote from Shakespeare's *Romeo and Juliet*: "Wisely and slow; they stumble who run fast." I saw the hidden compliment in my coach's sarcasm.

I have not yet stumbled, and I continued running through my senior year of college. My runs provide an escape, a few precious moments to myself. They also teach me discipline and levelheadedness.

As I "shuffle," I write my papers, I contemplate my social dilemmas, or sometimes I just let my mind wander. Some of the most important decisions of my life have been made in the comfort of cushioned running shoes.

When I return red-faced to my roommates, they ask, "Are you tired?" or "Is it cold outside?" I have never been asked, "Did you decide on your thesis statement out there?" Nonrunners see my runs as something tedious and unpleasant. They don't see that I run into my thoughts a few miles down the street.

Physically, my running has helped to counteract what would otherwise be the somewhat unhealthy (yet typical) lifestyle of a college senior. Unlike some of my friends, I have not seen the pizza I consume collecting around my stomach. The pitchers of beer have not inflated my hips to the degree that they have deflated my wallet.

I am not alone in my desire to keep my potentially fattening lifestyle in check with regular exercise; however, most of my fit friends have chosen not to run but to join the gym downtown. As I watch my roommate put on her thong and makeup before going to sweat on the StairMaster, I feel thankful that I am a runner. "Everyone is checking everyone else out" is how my roomate explains her pregym primping session.

Wearing a thong during exercise seems about as close to personal hell as I can imagine. My heaven is being able to throw on sweats and trusty shoes, run around for 40 minutes or so, and have a better, more balanced life. My little run each day has made an enormous difference in my attitude, my self-image, my stress level, and my social life (as I jog by and wave to the guys down the street in my comfortable T-shirt and shorts).

Although I love running, I must admit there are those days when I have trouble getting up 40 minutes early to waddle groggily out the door. I'll either push myself out anyway, hoping that once I get going the run itself will become motivating—which often it does—or I'll leave my shoes under the bed and join my roommates for pancakes, knowing that I'll run again tomorrow.

Running has become an important part of me. Those magenta Nikes of my childhood sent me shuffling down a running path that I will probably never abandon.

Elizabeth Shimer graduated from Pennsylvania State University in spring 1998 with a bachelor of arts degree in psychology.

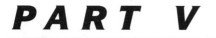

Getting into Gear

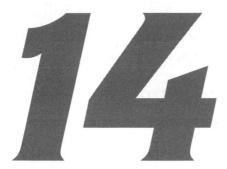

Shoes

IN THE 12 YEARS THAT I'VE BEEN RUNNING, I've never had any serious trouble with my knees. Whenever they do start to bother me, I know, then, that it's not a sign of recurring injury but rather that I've pushed my running shoes past their life span and I'm about to *incur* an injury if I don't replace them fast. As soon as I do replace them, the pain disappears.

When this happens, which isn't too often, it reminds me just how important running shoes are; and not just in terms of their condition. You need to find the best type of shoe for your foot and running style. The right shoe will provide miles of comfortable running and help prevent injury. The wrong shoe can lead to problems that may even stop you from running—for a little while, anyway.

With the myriad running shoes on the market, how do you determine which is best for you? Follow these basic steps:

1. Determine your running profile.
2. Match your profile to one of the four categories of running shoes (see pages 186 and 187).
3. Go a specialty running store, try several pairs, and buy the one that fits best.

Understanding Foot Motion

In figuring out what type of shoe is best for you, it helps to understand the basics of what your foot goes through during running. When you run, you land with a force equal to three times your body weight with every step you take. Most of us take about 180 steps a minute, which comes to 5,400 in a half hour. Clearly, as you run, your body is subjected to a lot of impact. Don't let this scare you, though. Remember, running is a natural activity. Human beings have been running since the beginning of our existence on earth, and the body has the ability to absorb and disperse the impact force of running so that it doesn't cause injury.

Normal and healthy foot motion during running is this: you land on the outside of your heel, then your foot rolls in as it makes full contact with the ground, and finally, your foot flexes forward to the ball and toes as it pushes off the ground. The line of greatest impact is not a direct vertical from heel to toe but more of a diagonal from the outer heel toward your big toe.

Pronation

The inward rolling motion of your foot during contact is called pronation, and it helps disperse the force of impact evenly over the whole foot and up your leg.

Overpronation is when the foot rolls too far inward, which causes extra strain on the muscles of the leg and can result in injury. Knee problems are common among overpronators.

Underpronation is when the foot doesn't roll in far enough—you tend to run more on the outer side of your foot. When this happens, most of the impact of running, rather than being dispersed over the entire foot, is concentrated on the outside of the foot. This increases the impact of running, and it stresses muscles and tendons on the outside of the leg. Iliotibial band syndrome (see chapter 26) is an injury common among those who underpronate.

Female Foot Motion

Women are more likely to overpronate than men are and more likely to overpronate than underpronate, according to Richard Braver, D.D.M., a sports podiatrist who works with the women's running and basketball teams at Montclair State and Fairleigh Dickinson Universities in New Jersey. "Women have naturally wider hips," points out Braver. "There's a greater angle from the hip to the knee, which puts your legs into a more knock-kneed position, with feet wider apart than the knees. This causes feet to collapse and overpronate during running."

Your Running Profile

Whether you are an overpronator, an underpronator, or normal pronator is one of the most important factors in choosing the right shoe. How do you determine your degree of pronation? It's not like you can observe your own foot motion as you run. Following are several indicators of pronation; use them all to help define your running profile.

Do the Wet Test

Whether you have a flat foot, a high-arched foot, or a "normal" foot largely determines how you contact the ground during running. Generally speaking, if you have a flat foot, you will have a tendency to overpronate. Runners with high arches usually underpronate; if you have normal arches, you should pronate properly. How do you tell if you're flat footed or high arched? Not by picking up your foot and looking at it. Do the wet test.

Wet your feet and then stand on a flat, dry surface, one that will show your footprint. You may need to lay a piece of paper on the floor to capture your footprint. Then take a look at your print. If it's full, showing the entire sole of your foot with no curve where your arch should be, you have a flat or low-arched foot. If on the other hand, there's an extreme inward curve between the ball of your foot and the heel, you have a high-arched foot. If the curve, indicating your arch, is moderate, you have a normal foot (see Figure 14-1).

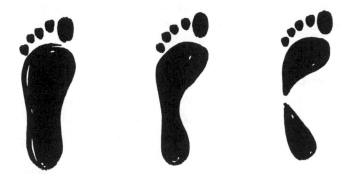

Figure 14-1. Wet your feet, and make a footprint on a flat, dry surface. A full print (*left*) indicates that you have a flat, or low-arched, foot. A curved footprint (*middle*) indicates a normal foot, and an extremely curved print (*right*) means you have a high-arched foot.

Your foot type isn't the only factor to affect the mechanics of your running and the degree to which you pronate. A person might have a normal foot yet still be an overpronator or an underpronator. Here are a few more ways to evaluate the way your foot contacts the ground.

Read Your Worn Old Shoes

Look at the wear pattern on the bottom of your shoes. Forget about the heel; most shoes show wear on the outer edge of the heel, regardless of pronation. Look instead more closely at the ball and toe of the shoe. Wear toward the inner side of the shoe or your big toe indicates that you are an overpronator. Wear on the outer side of the shoe, toward your little toe, indicates that you underpronate, and wear in the middle of the shoe means your foot motion is normal.

Search Your Soles

Calluses occur in areas of greatest pressure. Therefore, an overpronator might have calluses under or around the big toe and an underpronator might have them along the outer edge of the foot.

Look at Your Legs

The more your knees come together (knock-knees) and your feet point outward, the more you will pronate. Bowlegs and feet that point inward result in underpronation.

ANATOMY OF A RUNNING SHOE

Running shoes have become fairly technical pieces of equipment from what they once were, and in trying to determine which shoe is right for you, it helps to have a basic understanding of the components and construction. Let's take one apart and look at all the pieces.

Figure 14-2. An exploded view of a typical running shoe.

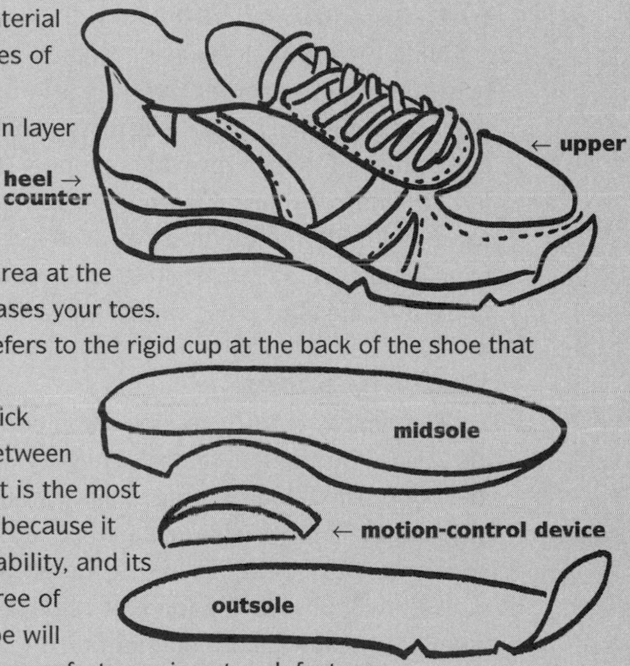

- **The upper:** This is the material that covers the top and sides of your foot.
- **The outsole:** This is the thin layer of material on the bottom of your shoe. It's usually made of a hard rubber.
- **The toe box:** This is the area at the front of your shoe that encases your toes.
- **The heel counter:** This refers to the rigid cup at the back of the shoe that surrounds the heel.
- **The midsole:** This is the thick area of the shoe that lies between your foot and the outsole. It is the most important part of the shoe because it provides cushioning and stability, and its design determines the degree of those qualities that the shoe will offer. The midsole is where manufacturers insert such features as air and gel devices to enhance the cushioning of the shoe.
- **Motion-control devices:** These include medial posts, Footbridges, and the like, which are inserted in the midsole along the inner or arch side of the shoe to help control pronation.
- **The last:** This refers to the shape of the shoe and corresponds to the three basic shapes of the foot. (In truth, a last is the solid mold from which shoes are shaped, but the word has also come to mean the final shape of the shoe itself.) A shoe with a *straight last,* like a flat foot, has very little curve and is essentially straight on both sides. A *semicurved* shoe turns inward some under the arch, like the footprint of a normal foot. The *curved last* has the greatest degree of curve under the arch area and fits most closely the shape of a high-arched foot.

Generally speaking, you should buy a shoe that fits the shape of your footprint. That means that runners with flat feet do best with straight-lasted shoes; those with high arches do best with curved-lasted shoes, and those with normal feet do best with semicurved shoes.

The Shoe Categories

Running shoe manufacturers and running magazines group shoes by the following categories: motion control, stability, cushioned, and lightweight training. (There are also racing shoes and trail shoes, but we'll get to that later in this chapter.)

Motion-Control Shoes

Motion-control shoes are designed to control foot motion (no surprise there) and prevent overpronation. Therefore, they have a rigid construction. Many have a firm midsole and are built on a straight last, both of which provide support and help reduce pronation. Motion-control shoes often have technical devices (a medial post, for example) built into the inner or arch side of the shoe to stop your foot from rolling in too far. Because motion-control shoes are heavier and more durable than most, they are a good choice for heavy runners.

Stability Shoes

The name *stability* creates some confusion as a category of shoes alongside the motion-control category because motion-control shoes are the most stable running shoes you'll find. Stability shoes are also quite stable but provide a bit more cushioning than motion-control shoes do. Cushioning refers to the softness of the midsole. A softer midsole will absorb the force of impact better than a firmer midsole will; it also allows more foot motion.

Stability shoes are usually built on a semicurved last, which allows more foot motion than a straight last does. Several models, however, contain a medial post or an area of dense midsole material along the inner side of the shoe to prevent too much motion.

Cushioned Shoes

Cushioned shoes have the softest midsoles and provide the best shock absorption. Sounds ideal for any runner, doesn't it? Cushioning isn't for everyone, though. Cushioned shoes allow the greatest range of foot motion during running. This is partly due to the softness of the midsole, but in addition, cushioned shoes are built on a semicurved or curved last and most do not contain motion-control devices, allowing your foot to roll inward. Clearly, these are *not* the shoes for overpronators.

Lightweight Training Shoes

Lightweight training shoes are designed for speed training and/or racing or for runners who simply prefer a lighter shoe. They are built on a semicurved or curved last and weigh less than most training shoes do. Offering less stability and motion control than most other running shoes do, lightweight trainers should not be worn by over-pronators, heavy runners, or runners who seem prone to injury. Some shoes in this category are more stable than others.

The Matchup: Runner to Shoe

Having read about all the categories of shoes, you probably have a pretty good idea which type of shoe you should consider.

Overpronators: Motion-Control Shoes

If you overpronate, especially if you do so severely, you should look at shoes in the motion-control category. Most runners with flat feet or low arches overpronate.

Underpronators: Cushioned Shoes

Underpronators need good shock absorption and a shoe that promotes foot motion. Most runners with high-arched feet are under-pronators.

Normal Pronators: Stability Shoes

Runners with normal arches and no pronation problems are best suited for stability shoes, which provide a good blend of cushioning and stability.

Quick, Light, Efficient Runners: Lightweight Trainers

Runners with no pronation problems who rarely experience injury and who enjoy the feel of a light shoe on their foot can consider lightweight training shoes.

The Perfect Match

The recommendations above provide a *starting point* to your search for the perfect running shoe. Neither shoes nor runners can be categorized or cross-matched exactly. Within each category of shoes you'll find a range of features and cushioning and stability properties, and among runners there exists a whole spectrum of degrees of pronation and biomechanics. One runner who over-pronates severely may do best in a motion-control shoe, whereas another runner who shows a small degree of overpronation might be fine in a stability shoe.

You need to take what you know about shoes and your running style to your local running shop, talk with the experts there, and try some training shoes on for size. Keep in mind there is no best shoe or shoe company. The perfect shoe for you is the one that fits best and feels most comfortable.

Shopping for Shoes

The best place to buy running shoes is at a store that specializes in them. There you'll find the best selection plus salespeople (usually runners themselves) who know running shoes and how to fit them to your foot.

SHOES FOR WOMEN

When you pick up the women's model of a particular shoe, are you really getting a shoe designed for a woman's foot, or is it simply a smaller version of a men's shoe? "Companies do have different men's and women's lasts [the last is the form on which shoes are built] but generally only in overall width. Men's shoes are made on a D width and women's on a B," says Paul Carrozza, *Runner's World* shoe consultant and owner of the Run-Tex running store in Austin, Texas.

This may explain why many women have a hard time finding shoes that fit well, especially in the heel. Kate Bednarski, president of Ryka, Inc., which makes running and other athletic footwear for women, has done thorough research on the structure of women's feet. What she's found is that women's feet are dimensionally different than men's. Specifically, a woman's heel is narrower relative to the girth measurement or circumference of her forefoot. In other words, if you look at a man and a woman who have the same girth measurement in the forefoot, the woman's heel will be narrower. In general, women need shoes that have enough room in the forefoot to accommodate the girth of their feet yet are small enough at the back to fit their narrower heels.

Ryka and Saucony, where Bednarski also worked, both make women's shoes on lasts built for the special dimensions of a woman's foot. As the numbers of female runners continue to increase, we're likely to see more shoes designed specifically to fit our feet.

Talk to the salesperson about how much running you do, the type of surface you run on most often (roads or grass and other soft surfaces), whether you do lots of hill work or speed training, whether you overpronate or underpronate, what types of injuries you've had, and whether you use orthotics. Take an old pair of running shoes or athletic shoes to show the wear pattern. Some running shops have treadmills that you can run on so a salesperson can observe your running style. All of these factors will help the salesperson help you fine-tune your selection.

Next, try on several pairs. Check the fit, and take each pair for a test run; most running shops will allow you to go for a spin around the block. The deciding factor in choosing a shoe should be fit. Again, if you're an overpronator, that doesn't mean you have to buy a shoe from the motion-control category; if a stability shoe fits best and feels most comfortable on the run, that's the shoe for you.

Tips for a Good Fit

Pay special attention to how a shoe fits in the heel and the toe box. Many women have a hard time finding shoes that fit snugly around the heel, and slippage can cause friction and blisters. (I used to wear holes in the back of my socks where my heel slid up and down against the shoe.) If a shoe doesn't fit in the forefoot, the result could be bunions, neuromas, or hammertoes, says podiatrist Richard Braver. Here are several other tips for making sure your shoes fit well.

- Try on shoes late in the day when your feet are somewhat swollen, because your feet swell during running.
- Wear the same type of socks that you wear running.
- If you use orthotics, be sure you've brought them along.
- Check that there's about a thumb-width of space between the top of your longest toe and the top of the shoe. Do this with both shoes, since one foot is likely to be larger than the other; the larger foot should be your measure.
- The shoes should feel snug but not tight.
- When going for a test run, your foot should not slide around in the shoes, your heel should not slip, and your toes should not bang against the front end. If you notice any of these problems, try another pair.

LACE 'EM UP TIGHT

If even the best-fitting shoe needs to be a little snugger around your heel, this lacing technique should help. Lace your shoes as usual, stopping at the next-to-the-last eyelet. Then, rather than cross the lace over to the other side, thread it down through the remaining eyelet closest to you. This will create a little loop. Do the same on the other side. Next take each lace and thread it through the loop on the opposite side. Your shoe should now tie a little tighter, for a snugger fit at the heel.

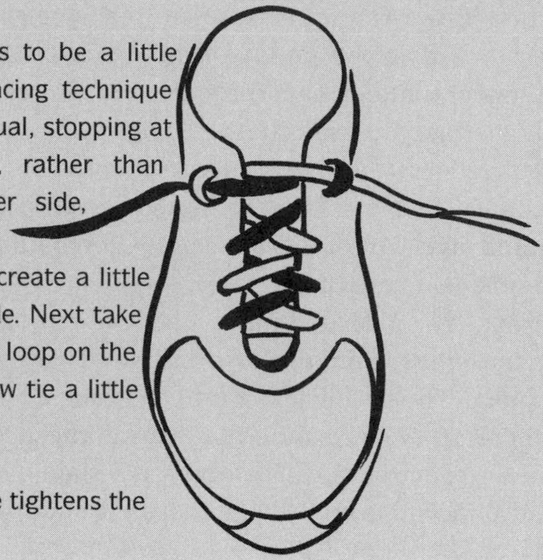

Figure 14-3. This lacing technique tightens the heel of the shoe for a snugger fit.

Go for Quality

If you're new to running and not sure whether you'll like it, it's okay to buy a less-expensive, lower-end shoe to start, but definitely buy a running shoe, not a cross-trainer or tennis shoe. If running is an important part of your life, however, don't skimp when it comes to buying a pair of training shoes. This isn't to say that the more a shoe costs, the better it is. You don't have to buy the most expensive shoe on the market to get the best shoe for your foot, but you should expect to pay at least $75. Do it—you're worth it.

The Life of Running Shoes

How will you know when your running shoes need to be replaced? Don't do what I've done and let pain be the signal. Still, it's not always easy to tell by looking at your shoes. On the surface, they may appear to be in good shape, yet inside, the midsole may be broken down. The best advice experts give is to replace your shoes after about 500 miles of running. In the meantime, take good care of them so they'll be their best in providing cushioning and stability for your feet.

Keep your shoes in top shape with these tips:

- When they get wet, don't put them in the dryer. The high heat will damage them. Place them on shoe trees and let them dry at room temperature or dry them with a fan.
- Don't throw them in the washer, either. The harsh chemicals in detergents can shorten the life of your shoes. Simply clean them with a brush and a little mild soap and water.
- After your run, take the time to take them off by hand rather than prying them off with your feet. The latter can ruin the heel of your shoe.
- Wear them only for running, not as casual footwear.

I've heard it's best to buy two pairs of shoes and alternate them. Is this true?

Yes, "rest days" can be as beneficial to your shoes as they are to your legs. The extra time between wear allows shoes to fully bounce back from the compression that running causes, and you'll benefit by wearing shoes that are fresher than if you were to wear the same pair every day.

Trail Shoes

Are you a wild woman, preferring rocky, root-strewn trails that snake through woods and up mountains to the smooth asphalt of the streets? Then you should consider owning a pair of trail running shoes—that is, if you don't already.

Trail shoes have a tougher construction than regular training shoes do. The uppers are reinforced to take a beating from rocky terrain, and many are water resistant for those times when the trail takes you skipping across a stream. Some shoes have a toe bumper, which protects your forefoot and the front of the shoe from scrapes and hits. The outsoles are firm and have treads that provide good traction over rugged surfaces, and the midsoles are designed to allow your foot to sit low in the shoe for better stability. Trail shoes range in design from those that have enough flexibility and cushioning to wear on the roads to seriously rugged models that are really suitable only for off-road running and will feel rough and uncomfortable on asphalt.

You'll find the best selection at your local running store. Talk with the salesperson about the kind of trail running you plan to do—whether you'll be mostly traveling down dirt paths and tame trails or scrambling over wild and woolly passages. Try on the appropriate pairs and go with the one that fits best.

Racing Shoes

Many of the runners I know—both women and men—think they'd look foolish to buy a pair of racing flats. "It's ridiculous. I'm not fast enough to wear racing shoes," they say. If you like to race and you think you'd enjoy wearing a shoe that's light, fits like a glove, feels fast, and *is* fast, then go ahead and get a pair.

I've had a few pairs of racing shoes in my day, and I've loved them. My feet feel free, unencumbered, and quick. Racing flats are the final touch to race readiness. Psychologically, they give me a lift: wearing them helps me believe I'm fast, boosts my confidence, makes me want to run my very best.

Mental boosts aside, racing shoes can help you pick your feet up faster when you run. Experts say that you will save 1 second per ounce of reduced shoe weight per mile. Let's say your usual training shoes weigh 11 ounces and your racing flats weigh 7 ounces. That's a savings of 4 ounces, or 4 seconds. Wearing those racing flats over a 5-K (3.1 miles), you'll run 4 seconds faster per mile, for a total of 12.4 seconds. Doesn't sound like much, does it? It can make the difference, though, in whether you achieve that hoped-for personal record (PR). How many times have you come close to the finish line of a race, struggling to get there in under a certain time, and then fallen short by just a few seconds?

Racing shoes are *not* for everyone, though. Some people *don't* feel comfortable in them, finding them too skimpy and unprotective. Many stability and cushioning features must be sacrificed to hone these shoes into the featherweight footwear they are. Severe pronators and heavy runners would be wise to wear a pair of lightweight training shoes to race in; they offer more support and protection.

Can I wear my racing shoes during a marathon?

Unless you are a very experienced runner and run free of injury most of the time, you should save your racing flats for the 5-K and 10-K or maybe the half-marathon. If you really want to wear a lighter shoe for longer races, go with a lightweight training shoe, which offers more cushioning, support, and stability.

Finding the Right Pair

Follow the same principles in buying racing shoes that you do when choosing a daily trainer. If you train in shoes built for stability and motion control, you should look for racing flats that offer some stability as well.

Most racing shoes come in unisex sizes, although there are a few models made specifically for women. When trying on a pair, begin with a shoe that's 1½ sizes smaller than your training shoes. Try a few different models, give them a test run, and choose the one that fits best and feels most comfortable. Keep your feet happy and healthy and you'll be happy and healthy, too.

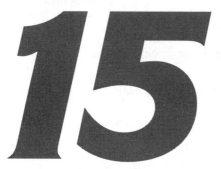

Clothing

A cotton shirt can more than double in weight when it gets wet, and it retains 80 percent more moisture than most synthetic shirts do.

—EILEEN PORTZ-SHOVLIN, apparel editor for *Runner's World*

WHEN YOU'RE LOOKING FOR RUNNING clothes, remember one word: *breathable.* Whether it's hot and humid or cold and snowing, you'll be most comfortable running in breathable fabrics for every piece of clothing, right down to your sports bra. Why? Because they allow perspiration to evaporate from your skin. This cools you off in the heat and keeps you dry—which means warm—when it's cold out.

The average runner sweats a quart or more of fluid every hour during running, and this can double or triple in hot and humid conditions. The faster this sweat evaporates off your skin, the cooler you'll be. Breathable fabrics make the evaporation process quick and easy. They are woven from polyester fibers that suck moisture off your skin and transport it to the outer surface of the garment, where it evaporates easily. The best known of these materials is CoolMax. Other brands include Supplex, Dri-F.I.T., and Ultrasensor.

Cotton, as light, natural, and ecologically desirable as it may be, is just about the worst fabric you can wear. In the summer, it soaks up sweat, sticks to your skin, and keeps you hot and drippy. In winter, it soaks up sweat, sticks to your skin, and chills your body to the bone. Save your cotton tees for spring and fall days when temperatures are moderate.

AVOID INFECTION

If you're prone to yeast infections, you want to be especially careful to buy running shorts and tights made with a breathable fabric like CoolMax and to change out of your sweaty clothing as soon as you're done running. The same goes for sweaty socks. The fungus that causes athlete's foot loves moist conditions.

Sports Bras

The sports bra is your most important piece of running apparel for both comfort and health. Our breasts are supported by weak ligaments that stretch easily. Running bounces breasts up and down, which isn't particularly comfortable, but more important, it stretches ligaments and can lead to premature sagging. Who needs it?!

Even small-breasted runners are more comfortable wearing sports bras, and though they don't need as much sag prevention as large-breasted women do, they still need support.

BLACK TOPS?

Wear dark-colored clothing rather than light colors when running under a strong sun. Dermatologist Rodney Basler, M.D., did a study that showed that light-colored clothing lets ultraviolet (UV) light pass through to your skin, whereas dark colors absorb UV rays, preventing their penetration through fabric. "I got the idea for this study one day after my little girl had come back from spending a day at the beach in a striped bathing suit."

BEST BRAS FOR WELL-ENDOWED WOMEN

I often hear complaints from larger-breasted runners that they have a difficult time finding a sports bra that offers them enough support. Some have had to resort to wearing two bras, one on top of the other. Fortunately, manufacturers have finally realized that not all female runners have chests as flat as pancakes, and some excellent sports bras are now available for larger-breasted women.

In 1997, Moving Comfort (manufacturer of women's sports apparel) introduced the Athena Bra for women with a C, D, or DD cup who participate in such high-impact sports as running. Its design separates and supports the breasts with two form-fitting cups. It provides good coverage and is made from a nylon/Lycra mesh lined with breathable fabric that provides good motion control and doesn't chafe.

Champion offers an underwire sport bra in sizes 32 to 42 and cups C to DD for women who need maximum support, and Title Nine Sports has created the Frog Bra "so you can leap without bouncing." It's made with a woven fabric that provides better control than do the knits used in many sports bras; plus, it contains 32% Lycra for excellent compression.

If you can't find these bras in your local running shop, call Moving Comfort at (800) 763-6000, Champion at (800) 621-3582, and Title Nine Sports (for their catalog) at (800) 609-0092.

Design

Bras come in two basic designs: the compression type, in which the fabric stretches across both breasts and presses them into your chest, and the encapsulation design, which has cups to hold and support each breast separately. Compression bras are best for small- to medium-breasted women. Large-breasted women will find more support in encapsulation-type bras.

Fit

Good fit is crucial to comfort and support so be sure to try a few on before you buy. The bra should feel snug but not tight. Run in place with it on to test its support, and check for any seams or places where the bra might rub against your skin and cause chafing.

Outerwear for Women

When you're looking at them on the rack, running shorts look pretty much the same whether they're men's or women's, but they're not equal. "A man's short is cut more like a rectangle, and a woman's like a box," explains Ellen Wessel, cofounder of Moving Comfort, manufacturer of sports apparel for women. "Women's shorts are broader in the hips and narrower in the waist and have a longer rise," she says, meaning that they come up higher onto your waist than men's shorts would. "They're more contoured than men's shorts, and longer, for better coverage of the thighs and butt."

Don't let a salesperson talk you into buying a pair of men's running tights as once happened to me. There, too, the rise is different— shorter in men's, as I found out when I couldn't pull the tights up far enough over my hips for a comfortable fit. Then again, that's me. I know women who actually prefer men's shorts and running tights. Try them on before you buy.

As for shirts, "those made specifically for women are narrower in the back and shoulders, shorter in the torso and arms and fuller in the chest," says Wessel. Even singlets vary: men's have those long, looping armholes that expose more chest for quicker evaporation of sweat. Women's singlets have smaller armholes and provide more coverage.

THE START OF SOMETHING

In 1976, Ellen Wessel and her training partners were running 70 miles a week and competing in races, but nobody was making women's running clothing, so they wore men's shorts. "I spent a long time thinking that if I were skinnier, they would fit right," says Wessel.

She and running friend Valerie Nye spent a long time searching for clothes that would fit better. Finally, they got tired of looking, so they decided to make some. They were living in Washington, D.C. At about that same time, Henley Gabeau, currently executive director of the Road Runners Club of America (RRCA), organized the women's running club RunHers in their area. "We were just going to make clothes for the club," recalls Wessel.

Then in the spring of 1977, a friend of Wessel's wrote an article about their effort, which appeared with an ad for Moving Comfort clothing in *Running Times* magazine. "We got five letters from retailers asking for our catalog," says Wessel. "We hustled together our first catalog—one sheet of paper, photos on both sides, folded over." With that, Moving Comfort was launched into the retail world.

Wessel eventually took up partnership with Elizabeth Goeke, and they've made the company into one of the largest and most successful manufacturers of women's sports apparel in the country. Though born from the needs of female runners, Moving Comfort now offers clothing suitable for a variety of activities.

Designs for Bigger Women

Big doesn't mean fat. Many women have a large frame with big bones and thick muscles but are not overweight. Though they may be very fine runners, they don't fit the stereotypical thin-bodied physique, nor do they fit into the typical tiny-waisted running shorts that you find in most stores. They look down the rack of running shorts to the "large" sizes, turn around, and run out of the store. What about the woman who *is* overweight, who needs to drop several pounds for her health and would succeed best with running but has trouble finding decent clothes to run in? It's not easy for larger women to find comfortable and attractive athletic wear. You need to know where to look.

I have trouble with chafing between my thighs when I run. Are there any shorts that might help?

Many women find that bike shorts offer protection. Also, you might try the dual-layer shorts by Junonia, which combine a cycling type of short under a free-flowing layer; call (800) 671-0175 for more information.

One place is Junonia, a manufacturer of activewear for women size 14 and up. The name derives from the Junonia shell named after the Roman goddess Juno, protector of women, who is depicted as having majestic size and beauty. The founder of Junonia, Anne Kelly, herself doesn't have a typically athletic figure. "I'm a 16 petite," says Anne. "Looking around in my aerobics class one day, I realized there are more women like me than there are very thin women. In fact, depending on what statistics you look at, 30 percent to 50 percent of American women are a size 14 or larger." With that realization, Anne started designing sports clothing for such women. Call (800) 671-0175 for a free catalog.

Danskin has also recognized the need for larger sizes in athletic wear and offers a line of apparel called Danskin Plus. And Champion introduced a line of plus-size sports apparel in 1998 called Champion Woman, which includes sports bras, T-shirts, shorts, and leggings.

Winter Running Wear

Understandably, a run may not seem too appealing when the thermometer reads freezing or below, but manufacturers of sports apparel have become *so* good at making warm, lightweight running clothes that you can stay cozy during some of the cruelest winter weather. When you're warm, bounding down a snow-covered lane can be exhilarating.

The best way to dress comfortably for cold weather is in layers. A few light layers of clothing keep you warmer than one thick garment does because air gets caught between layers, acting as extra insulation as it warms with the heat of your body. The other advantage to dressing in layers is that if you've put on too many and get too warm, you can take one off, tie it around your waist, and keep on running comfortably.

The tricky part is figuring out how many layers you need. It depends, of course, on the temperature and conditions (wind, rain, snow) and on your personal cold tolerance. Also, the faster you intend to run, the more heat you will generate and the lighter you can dress. Here's a basic guide to progressive layering.

- **Cool (40° to 50° Fahrenheit):** Long-sleeved crewneck top or turtleneck, shorts or running tights; gloves are optional
- **Cold (30° to 40° Fahrenheit):** Long-sleeved crewneck top or turtleneck, vest or light jacket, running tights, gloves or mittens, hat
- **Colder (10° to 30° Fahrenheit):** Heavy long-sleeved turtleneck, jacket, thick running tights, mittens, hat
- **Really cold (0° to 10° Fahrenheit):** Long-sleeved turtleneck, jacket, thick running tights, wind pants, mittens (maybe thin gloves and mittens), hat
- **Coldest (below 0° Fahrenheit):** Long-sleeved turtleneck, vest or second top, jacket, heavy running tights, wind pants, gloves and mittens, hat and/or knit face mask

For these systems to work effectively, each layer must be—yes—breathable. Mix a cotton shirt in there, and you've created major interference in the moisture management of your outfit.

Special Circumstances

Every now and then, your usual running clothes just won't suffice.

MATERNITY CLOTHES

If you run throughout your pregnancy, you'll eventually expand out of your regular running clothes. Some women find bike shorts comfortable in the latter months of pregnancy, or you can buy roomier running shorts. Title Nine Sports carries shorts for active pregnant women; call (800) 609-0092. Also, check out the web site for Fit For Two at **www.snowcrest.net/fitfor2/** Fit Maternity at **www.fitmaternity. com** for their selection of maternity running apparel.

Raincoats

You can head out in the rain in only a shirt and shorts or tights. When it's warm out, that's exactly what you should do—it feels great. When the air is cool, though, you'll be more comfortable with a jacket.

Gore-Tex is still the only water*proof* material you'll find. It's still fairly heavy and fairly expensive, but if you live in a wet climate, it may be worth owning a Gore-Tex jacket and pants. It'll last for years of running.

All other running outerwear is made from water-*resistant* material, which can keep you fairly dry on a short run and at least prevents your getting drenched and chilled. Activent is a fabric made by the Gore company that is highly water resistant and is lighter and more breathable than most other outerwear fabrics used in jackets.

Night Lights

If you have to run in the darkness of evening or early morning, wear something reflective so you can be seen by oncoming cars. Many running jackets and pants—and even shoes—have reflective strips, or you can wear a reflective vest. Illuminite is a material that is used by several clothing manufacturers in their outerwear. It has excellent reflective properties, making you very visible in the night.

Accessories

You can't forget your extremities. What you wear on your feet, hands, and head can seriously affect the comfort of your run.

Socks

Your socks are the only thing that come between your feet and your running shoes, and if yours rub the wrong way, you'll end up with blisters and maybe even a ruined run. They seem like simple things, socks, but there are several considerations that go into choosing the right type. First of all is fit—they need to fit your foot *and* your shoe. A sock that's too big for your foot will bunch up inside your shoe and cause blisters; too small, and it'll just feel uncomfortable. A sock that's too thin for your shoe will allow your foot to slide around (blisters); too thick, and your shoe will fit too tightly around your foot, which over time can lead to bunions, neuromas, or other problems. Always try on running socks and shoes together before purchasing either.

The fabric of your socks can make a big difference in whether you develop a blister. Synthetics, such as acrylic and CoolMax, are preferable to cotton because they disperse perspiration more effectively, and it's the friction caused between a moist foot and a shoe that most often leads to blisters. Also, check to make sure there are no seams in the toe area that might cause you trouble. If you are particularly prone to blisters, try socks that offer extra padding in areas of high impact—the heel and forefoot. Thorlo brand running socks are supercomfy, but make sure they'll fit your shoe, because they are thicker than most.

Gloves

Even when the weather's just beginning to turn cold, you might want to wear a light pair of knit gloves. As the days get colder, switch to heavier gloves or mittens. Choose ones made from a breathable fabric. In frigid temperatures, double up: wear a knit glove or mitten under a water- and wind-resistant shell.

GLOVELESS?

Can't find your winter running gloves? Wear a pair of running socks over your hands instead. They act like mittens—without the thumb, of course—and some runners actually prefer them.

Hats

Every runner's closet should have an assortment of running hats. You need at least two types: baseball caps and knit hats. A baseball cap is a must when you run in the rain because it keeps the water out of your eyes so you can see where you're going. You may also want to wear one during the summer to keep the sun out of your face and off your head. Secure your cap with hairpins so it doesn't blow off in a wind.

A knit hat is essential if you run in cold weather. You lose 90 percent of your body's heat from your head, so a hat can be the most important piece of clothing for keeping you warm when it's cold out. Check out the offerings at your local running shop. They usually carry winter running hats made of polypropylene or another synthetic material that's light but warm.

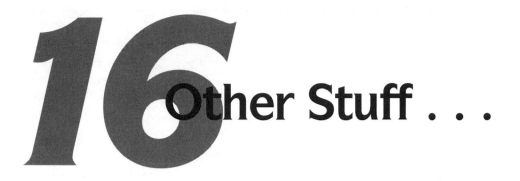

16 Other Stuff . . .

RUNNING IS SIMPLE, AND THAT'S ONE OF ITS joys—spontaneous, unencumbered movement. There are a few accessories you'll find very useful, though—in addition to, of course, shoes, a bra, a shirt, and a pair of shorts.

Sunscreen

Sunscreen is a must. You should cover all areas of exposed skin whenever you go for a run, not only to prevent premature wrinkling and sun damage but also to protect you from malignant melanoma—skin cancer—which, if not caught early, can kill you. "The effects of sunlight on the skin have to be taken seriously. There is no question that overexposure to the sun causes wrinkles, precancerous growth, and malignant melanoma," says Rodney Basler, M.D., a dermatologist from Lincoln, Nebraska, who is past chairman of the task force on sports medicine for the American Academy of Dermatology. "And the incidence of skin cancer is going up. Part of the reason is that the population is aging, but I believe it's also a result of depletion of the ozone layer and that there is greater damage to skin per given amount of time spent in the sun than ever before."

How do I know if a spot is suspicious and should be checked for malignancy?

"If a spot is changing in size or shape and part of it is coal-black in color, you should have it checked by a dermatologist. If a malignant melanoma is caught early—at less than a centimeter in size—the survival rate is excellent."

—RODNEY BASLER, M.D., DERMATOLOGIST

Basler recommends running early in the morning or late in the day to avoid the sun at its highest intensity. "Early morning is best. The damaging effects of the sun persist even beyond four P.M." Here's Basler's advice on sunscreen:

- Use it!
- Apply sunscreen 20 minutes before you go out so that it binds with the upper layer of your skin.
- Cover all exposed areas.
- Reapply sunscreen every 4 hours.

Does wearing sunscreen prevent the absorption of light necessary for my body to manufacture vitamin D?

"It does to a certain level, but plenty of sunlight reaches your skin even with a sunscreen of SPF (solar protection factor) 15. And the truth of the matter is, you don't need very much sunlight to make all the vitamin D you need."

—RODNEY BASLER, M.D., DERMATOLOGIST

A side benefit to wearing sunscreen is that it may keep you cooler in hot weather. A study done at Oregon State University found that people who wore sunscreen during 45 minutes of stationary cycling in a room heated to 90° Fahrenheit had skin temperatures 15 percent to 20 percent lower than those who wore none.

You should wear sunscreen year round and even on days that are overcast: cloud cover does not block harmful ultraviolet (UV) rays.

When you buy sunscreen, look for

- An SPF (solar protection factor) of 15 or higher
- Protection against ultraviolet A (UVA) *and* ultraviolet B (UVB) rays
- A waterproof formula that won't drip off your skin with sweat
- One that won't burn if it drips into your eyes

Is it true that an SPF (solar protection factor) of 15 is all you need for good sun protection and that to spend more for sunscreens with a higher SPF is a waste of money?

An SPF of 15 is sufficient for most occasions, but sunscreens with higher SPFs do offer more protection and should be used if you'll be in the hot sun for a long time or if you're visiting or living in an area that's closer to the equator or at altitude where the effects of the sun's rays are much stronger. "The incidence of skin cancer is twice as high in Tucson, Arizona, as it is in Chicago," says dermatologist Rodney Basler, M.D. He cautions, however, that sunscreens with high SPFs have added ingredients that can cause skin irritation in active people, particularly runners.

Sunglasses

Some runners feel a little self-conscious wearing sports sunglasses, as if they're trying to be too cool. After all, sports sunglasses are kind of flashy, but put your inhibitions aside and put on a pair of shades: wearing sunglasses protects your eyes from damage, such as cataracts that result from long-term exposure to intense sunlight and UV radiation. They also shield your eyes from wind, dust, bugs, and other small flying objects. As for vanity, it's a good thing in this case: wearing sunglasses prevents you from squinting, which can lead to early wrinkling of the sensitive skin around your eyes. If you live in a climate where it snows in the winter, sports shades protect your eyes from the sun and the glare of bright light that reflects off a snowy landscape.

When you buy sports sunglasses, look for

- 100 percent protection from UV rays
- A lens color that is appropriate to the light conditions in which you run most often. If you run often on trails or shady streets, you'll want a lens that lets in more light so you can see where you're going. If you usually run in bright light and open areas, you should wear a lens that blocks more light. Some companies, such as Oakley, sell glasses with interchangeable lenses so you can alter them, depending on the light conditions.
- Wide lenses. The more the lenses wrap around your face, the more light they block.
- If you sweat heavily, glasses that have foam strips above the brow and/or along the nose bridge to absorb moisture
- Glasses that fit snugly enough that they won't feel like they'll fall off during running, yet that are light and comfortable on your ears and nose

Sports Watches

If you've never owned a sports watch, try one. Before long, you won't be caught running without it. Not only can you use one to time your run, but you can program it to beep at regular intervals if you're doing a timed *fartlek* run or to keep track of your times when you're doing speed work or to record your mile splits (the time it takes you to run each mile) during a race. Plus, most have a built-in alarm, and many have a light that you can press on when you need to see what time it is when you're running in the dark—or even when you're in a movie theater.

When you buy a sports watch, look for

- A stopwatch function, also called a chronograph, which you can use to time your runs
- Lap memory. An 8-lap memory is sufficient for most runners who want to be able to record timed intervals during speed work or who want to be able to record their pace for each mile of a race (5 kilometers [3.1 miles] to 8 miles in distance). You can buy watches

that have a memory of up to 100 laps if you like to keep track of all your miles during a marathon or ultrarun.

- Ease of use. All sports watches are a bit confusing at first, but test the various functions of a few brands before you buy.
- A beeper function. This is useful if you like to do runs in which you change your paces at certain timed intervals.

KNOW YOUR WATCH

Take the time to read the instructions for and learn and practice all the functions of your sports watch. Many runners buy watches, use them to time their runs, and neglect the other possibilities, thinking them too complicated and not worth the bother, but it's really easy to program your watch, and it *is* worth it. Have you ever found yourself, at the end of a race, wishing you knew exactly how fast you ran each mile? Well, with the press of a button, you can bring up your mile times, one after another, on your watch.

Water Carriers

As long as you're conscientious about drinking plenty of fluids during the day, you probably won't need water during a run of an hour or less, but go much longer and you should plan a route that takes you past a few water sources (water fountains, friends' homes, convenience stores . . .), or you should take some water with you. Experts recommend that you drink about 8 ounces of water or sports beverages roughly every 15 minutes to stay well hydrated during a run. (For more information on fluid consumption, see chapter 8.)

If you regularly run long distances, especially on trails, wear a water carrier. It may seem cumbersome to do so at first, but staying well hydrated helps you run better and prevents heat problems during the summer. You'll enjoy your long, hot runs more, and it'll be worth the little bit of extra weight and bulk.

There are two basic types of water carriers: those that hold water bottles, which you simply remove when you need a drink, and the pouch type, which holds water in a bladder and has a long plastic tube that you sip from as you run.

When you buy a water carrier, look for

- A comfortable and convenient fit. Try both carrier and pouch styles to see which feels as though it will work best for you. Ask the salesperson if you can fill them with water before trying them on.

- A fluid capacity that fits your needs. The longer you run, the more water you'll want to take with you. Options include single-bottle carriers that hold about 21 ounces of water, double-bottle belts that allow you to take along 40 ounces of water, and bladder-type carriers that can hold 50 ounces or more.
- The water bottle should open and close readily, or in the case of the bladder design, the tube should be easy to access.
- Comfort. Those made with mesh material or some other coolness feature will make them more comfortable to wear.

Heart Rate Monitors

A heart rate monitor may sound like a complicated technical device to be used only by the most serious runners, but in fact, it can be most helpful to a new runner who isn't yet very familiar with the pace she should run. Using a monitor can prevent you from running too hard, a common mistake among beginners. Monitors are, of course, also useful to competitive runners for measuring the effort of speed-training sessions. You can design an entire training program based on heart rate (see Training with a Heart Rate Monitor on page 209).

When you buy a heart rate monitor, look for

- Chest and wrist bands. The chest band picks up the signal from your heart and sends it to the watchlike monitor on your wrist.
- An easy-to-read digital display
- Ease of operation

Duffle Bag

Now you need something to carry all this running stuff in, right? Every runner needs a duffle bag. Even if you usually run from your home every day, there will come a time when you don't start out your front door but rather meet your running partners at a friend's house, or perhaps you'll drive to a nearby park for a trail run or will need to take a change of clothes to a race. If you run from the office, a good sports bag is essential—and there is a difference between a good duffle bag and a bad one.

TRAINING WITH A HEART RATE MONITOR

All training programs combine workouts of different efforts or paces: long, slow runs to build endurance, fast intervals or up-tempo runs to develop speed, and easy runs to promote recovery. One way to determine how fast to run during these different workouts is heart rate. Easy runs are done at 60%–70% of your maximum heart rate, long runs at 60%–75%, tempo runs at 80%–85%, and fast intervals at 90%–95% of maximum heart rate.

Obviously, the first thing you need to know is your maximum heart rate. The method you see recommended most often is the traditional formula—220 minus your age—but this can be off by as much as 25 beats per minute. A better way, though more inconvenient, is to go to a track or treadmill. After warming up with some slow running, run 800 meters (2 laps around a typical 400-meter track or ½ mile on the treadmill) at what feels like close to top speed. Jog or walk for 1 minute and then run a second 800 meters very fast. As soon as you stop, find your pulse (the neck is easiest) and take your heart rate. This is your maximum.

Now you can use this number to determine what your heart rate should be when doing the different types of workouts described above. Before a run, program your monitor with the appropriate heart rate range for the workout, and then as you run, adjust your pace to stay within that heart rate. The monitor will help you by beeping when you've gone too high or too low.

There are three things to keep in mind:

- The chest band must be wet and snug to ensure a good reading of your heart rate.
- Power lines and motorized exercise machines, such as treadmills and stair climbers, emit electrical energy that can interfere with the function of a monitor.
- Heart monitors are inappropriate during pregnancy because your maximum heart rate is higher than usual, and pregnancy is no time to be trying to determine what your max is.

The information here is a simplified explanation of how to train with a heart monitor. It's a fine place to start, but if you are serious about this, purchase a copy of *Precision Running* by Roy Benson, who has many years of experience using heart rate monitors to coach runners. This booklet is available in running supply stores and comes free with a Polar Heart Rate Monitor.

The worst sports bag you can buy is the kind with a zipper at the top and only one compartment into which you toss your running shoes, sports bra, shirt, shorts, deodorant, sports sunglasses, sunscreen, water bottle, snacks . . . You only hope the water bottle and the sunscreen don't leak all over your clothes and that there's not too much dirt on your shoes from yesterday's run.

When you buy a duffle bag, look for

- Lots of compartments so you can separate shoes from clothes from lotions from water bottles from cosmetics . . .
- Mesh pockets on the outside of the bag for storing shoes and sweaty clothes after you run so they can dry out
- A size appropriate to your needs
- Sturdy material and well-sewn seams
- Comfortable shoulder strap or handles

The duffle bag—a symbol of running's simplicity. It holds all the gear you'll ever need for a good run.

Thank You, Mr. Sidelines

BY MEG WALDRON

OUT OF A NEED TO ESCAPE THE TEASING AND CHASING OF A
younger brother, I began to run, first through the hallways of my
Victorian home, then around its porch, hydrangeas, and large yard. Tear-
stained and muddy, the joy of a day in nursery school now tarnished, I'd
run to my mother's skirts, only to be caught again by my brother, his
energy unflagging, while my mother busily pressed and folded, pressed
and folded, high above my frail little arms.

It was natural, then, that when the opportunity arose—a classmate
slid the flier to me announcing a running league—I took up racing. By
the age of 13, I was beating the boys and traveling to races out of town,
always attended by my father.

Regardless of chores, weather, and the needs of eight other children,
this big-hearted man would take the only car we owned and accompany
me to the scary urban championship courses of Garret Mountain and
Van Cortland Park.

I'd pour heart and soul into each race, with my father often running
alongside to cheer me on. I was naive and tentative, my biggest fear
being that I'd give in to the desire to stop and walk. My father told me
I'd be disqualified if I did so. "That means you won't be counted when
you cross the finish line," he would say. Whether he believed this to be
true or simply used it as a means of building my character, I do not
know. It did, however, work—I never quit a race.

At the midpoint of a hill, my father would appear, gangly and tall
with shirttails flying, cheering with such distraction that inevitably his
glasses would fly out of one pocket while his pipe escaped another. We'd
spend the hour after the race touring the course together, trying to
track down these objects that more often than not also included his
wallet and car keys. In the process, my father would make friends with

the officials and, to my horror, the parents of my rivals and manage to happily engage them all in this game of lost and found.

Too soon into my early successes, his big heart gave out. The train platform in Orange, New Jersey, became an oddly poetic resting place for this hard-working son of Newark, Catholic father of nine, and mayor of our town. In his final moments, as his long legs buckled, I imagine his glasses folded tightly in their case, the pipe sinking deeper into his overcoat pocket, his wallet in a safer place, and the casual strangers he had befriended on the commute suddenly and inexorably becoming bound to his life.

Long after the town honored him with a memorial race, my running continued. A successful high-school career, fueled by a passion to be somebody other than just another skinny kid, led to higher honors, bigger races, a college scholarship.

Somehow along the way, I have maintained a certain healthy kinesis. Running has remained a guiding and steady force, defining me as much as it does my career rebuilding and training injured athletes. At 33, the Olympic bug has bitten, and I find myself compelled to gather what's been lost. Somewhere from some sideline, my father is calling to me: "Don't stop now or you won't be counted."

Meg Waldron is a neuromuscular massage therapist and owner of Megafit, a massage therapy and fitness clinic in Bernardsville, New Jersey. She is training to qualify for the 1999 Olympic Trials Marathon.

PART VI

Running
Enhancements

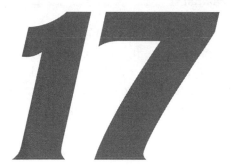

Stretching

Those of us who stretch seem to have a pleasure center accessible by no other route; firing its nerve endings becomes a necessity for sustaining mobility, if not life itself.

—JOHN JEROME, author of *The Elements of Effort*

SOME RUNNERS WOULDN'T DREAM OF starting or finishing a run without stretching, whereas others would never even bother to try to touch their toes. Who's better off? No one knows for sure. Sports science has fallen short on finding the answer to whether stretching improves performance, as some have espoused, or prevents injuries, which is the more common reason for exercising your flexibility.

At a meeting of the American College of Sports Medicine, editors from *Runner's World*

215

magazine asked a group of sports scientists whether they would recommend stretching to runners. Despite agreeing that there is little research to prove its benefits, most did recommend stretching to help prevent injury. Perhaps more important, as exercise physiologist David Martin, Ph.D., points out, "Stretching is part of the fitness continuum."

Styles of Stretching

First we bounced, then we s-t-r-e-t-c-h-e-d, and now we have a method that's a cross between the two—sort of a stretched bounce. Here are the three methods.

Ballistic Stretching

Ballistic stretching sounds dangerous, and it can be, which is why this method is no longer used. With ballistic stretching, you bounce while in the stretch position. The quick movements can cause soreness and even muscle tears.

Static Stretching

With static stretching, you slowly move into the stretch position and hold it for at least 12 seconds. It's the most common form of stretching used by runners today, but some experts argue that holding a stretch for many seconds can also cause muscle soreness and tears.

Active Isolated Stretching

Remember that old principle, "every action has an equal and opposite reaction"? It applies to your tendons, which exhibit what's called a stretch reflex—when you stretch a tendon, it reacts by contracting. (Anatomy note: tendons and muscles are not the same; tendons are the thicker tissue at the ends of muscles that attach muscle to bone.)

With rapid movement (like that in ballistic stretching), the reflex occurs immediately. During a slow static stretch of several seconds, it occurs after 2 seconds. Either way, you and your tendon end up pulling in opposite directions.

The principle behind active isolated (AI) stretching is that you ease into a stretch and hold the position for only 2 seconds so as not to elicit the tendon contraction.

Another aspect of AI stretching is that the positions used force the muscle group opposite the area you're stretching to contract. What's the advantage? The contraction of one muscle group automatically causes the opposite muscle group to relax, which facilitates stretching. You can do this with static stretches also, but depending on the position, you may have to consciously contract the muscles opposite those you stretch; for example, when stretching your hamstrings (back of the thigh), you would contract your quadriceps (front of the thigh). Finally, when performing an AI stretch, you use a rope, towel, or your hands to further enhance the stretch.

Clearly, it's a bit more complicated than static stretching. Is it worth it? The answer is still under debate. Many runners prefer AI stretching to static stretching, saying that the latter leaves their muscles sore. Other runners find that static stretching works well. Experts, too, are divided. Some physical therapists argue that 2 seconds doesn't stretch the *muscle* significantly. Others point out that with numerous repetitions, muscles are sufficiently stretched with the AI technique.

Which Should You Use?

"Both static stretching and active isolated stretching are effective," says Budd Coates, coach, runner, and corporate fitness director. "The decision often comes down to a matter of how much time you have. AI stretching takes more time than static stretching does."

Is yoga a good form of stretching for runners?

"I don't recommend it," says Budd Coates, coach and marathoner. "You need some tension in your muscles to perform well during running. It gives a little 'spring' to your muscles. If you are too supple, you won't run your best." None of the top runners do yoga, he adds.

Stretching Do's and Don'ts

One thing we do know about stretching is that you should do it after your run or in the middle of your run, not before it. "It isn't wise to stretch tight muscles," warns Martin. "The best time is after running when you are metabolically warmed up and a little loose."

How often should you stretch? After every run would be ideal, but it's most important to stretch after a long run, a hard run, or a race—

the most stressful running you do. "This is when your muscles are more likely to tie up and get tight," says Coates. "Stretching will help you maintain flexibility and limit discomfort."

The key underlying principle to stretching is that it should complement your running, says Coates, who suggested the routine in this chapter, which includes stretches for the major muscle groups used in running: the lower back, quadriceps, hamstrings, and calves. The program provides a basic foundation to which you can add and subtract stretches as you need them.

Focus on those areas that are tight and don't bother muscles that are flexible. You'll know what's tight and what's not when you stretch. For example, when you do the standing toe touch described below, if you feel tension in your lower back and hamstrings and you can reach only down to your knees, well, you know what that means . . . this is one stretch you should do regularly in addition to others that isolate the lower back and hamstrings. On the other hand, if you can place the palms of your hands flat on the floor, you're loose enough.

Certain aches, pains, and minor injuries can be helped by stretching. If your shins are troubling you, add a shin stretch to your routine. Pain along the outside of your knee may indicate the iliotibial band (ITB) stretch.

How do you know when to add a new stretch and which one to do? "If you've been experiencing a nagging soreness or pain, you can call an orthopedic surgeon," says Coates. "Most work with athletic trainers who can recommend a stretch to try."

Keep your stretching program flexible, tailoring it to your needs as they change with running.

STRETCHING MATERIAL

If you're looking for more stretches or more information on active isolated stretching, here's where to go:

- **Static stretching:** Read *Stretching* by Bob Anderson (Bolinas, California: Shelter Publications, 1987). This classic book on stretching provides easy-to-understand instructions and crystal-clear illustrations for just about every stretch you'd ever need. It includes routines for cyclists, swimmers, golfers, and tennis players, as well as runners.
- **Active isolated (AI) stretching:** For a book or video on AI stretching or for information on clinics, call Maximum Performance International at (800) 240-9805.

A Basic Stretching Program

The following routine uses static stretching (for an AI stretching program, see Stretching Material on page 218). As you do each stretch, ease into position and hold it for 12 to 20 seconds, counting each time you breathe so you go slowly and because as you exhale, your muscles relax even more. Repeat each stretch three times, taking it a little farther each time. Do not stretch to the point of pain—just until you feel tension in the muscle you are working.

Standing toe touch

The target muscles: Lower back, hips, groin, and hamstrings (backs of the thighs)

The purpose: Helps prevent hamstring pulls and back pain

The procedure:

- Stand with your feet about shoulder width apart, knees slightly bent.
- Bend over slowly at the waist, letting your arms drop straight down in front of you.
- Stretch toward your toes until you feel tension in your hamstrings and hold (most people cannot touch their toes).
- Relax, slowly return to the starting position, and repeat.

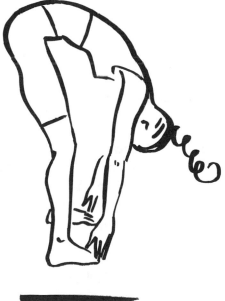

Figure 17-1. Standing toe touch: stretch toward your toes until you feel tension in your hamstrings.

Straight leg stretch

The target muscles: The gastrocnemius, one of the two muscles that make up the calf

The purpose: Helps prevent calf pulls and shinsplints; relieves soreness in the calves and Achilles tendons and along the heels and arches of the feet

The procedure:

- Stand 2 to 3 feet away from a wall or other immovable object and

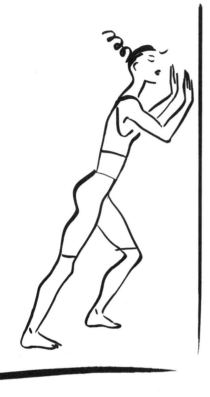

lean forward, placing your palms against the wall.
• Relax your left leg, bending it at the knee.
• Keep the right leg straight, heel on the ground, and lean into the wall until you feel tension in the calf; hold.
• Relax and then stretch the other leg the same way.

Figure 17-2. Straight leg stretch: lean into the wall until you feel tension in the calf of your outstretched leg.

Bent leg stretch

The muscles: The soleus, one of the two major muscles of the calf, and the Achilles tendon

The purpose: To prevent strains and pulls to the calf and Achilles tendon and help relieve soreness

The procedure:

• Stand facing a wall at a distance that allows you to place your arms straight out in front of you with palms against the wall.
• Relax and bend your left leg at the knee just to lift your heel off the ground.
• Keep your right foot and heel flat on the ground and bend your right knee, lowering your body until you feel tension in the lower calf and Achilles tendon, then hold.
• Relax and stretch the other leg.

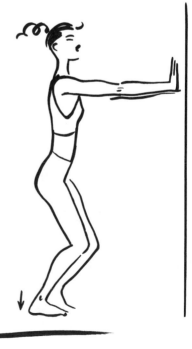

Figure 17-3. Bent leg stretch: lower your body until you feel tension in the lower calf and Achilles tendon.

Spinal twist

The muscles: Stretches a large area of the body including the neck, rib cage, back, and hips

The purpose: Helps prevent back and neck pain; relieves tension in those areas; can help prevent "stitches," those sharp pains we all get sometimes in our stomach and sides

The procedure:

- Sit on the floor with your right leg straight out in front of you.
- Bend your left leg, cross it over your right leg, and place your foot on the floor up against the knee of your right leg.
- Turn your upper body to the left and place your left hand behind you on the floor for support. Cross your right arm over your bent knee, placing your elbow against the outside of that knee.
- Slowly turn your upper body and neck to the left to look back over your left shoulder. Press your arm against your bent knee to help you stretch. You will feel the tension in your neck, back, and hips. Hold this position for 12 to 20 seconds.
- Relax and repeat on the other side.

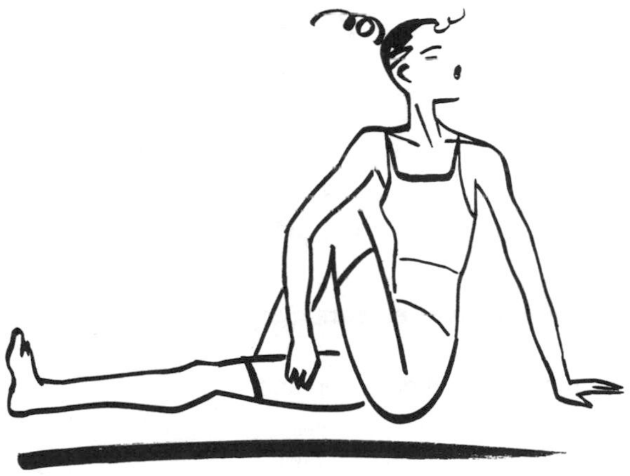

Figure 17-4. Spinal twist: slowly turn your upper body to look back over your shoulder. You'll feel tension in your neck, back, and hips.

Legs overhead and seated hamstring stretch

The muscles: Hamstrings (back thigh) and muscles of the back

The purpose: To loosen tight muscles in the back and along the spine and to relieve back pain; helps prevent hamstring pulls and alleviates soreness

The procedure:

- Sit on a carpeted floor or mat with legs together and knees bent.
- Slowly roll backward, bringing your legs and feet over your head as far as you can go without straining any muscles in your back or legs. Some people will be able to touch their toes to the floor behind their head; others will not.
- Use your hands to support your hips and hold this position.

- Slowly roll forward and into a sitting position.
- Place your right leg straight out in front of you.
- Lean forward from your hips toward the ankle of your straight leg until you feel tension in your hamstrings (you may also feel this stretch at the side of your lower back opposite the leg you are stretching). Hold.
- Relax and stretch the opposite hamstring.
- Relax and then slowly roll back into the leg-overhead stretch and repeat the sequence.

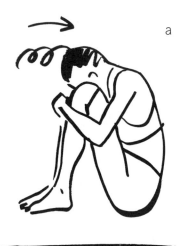
a

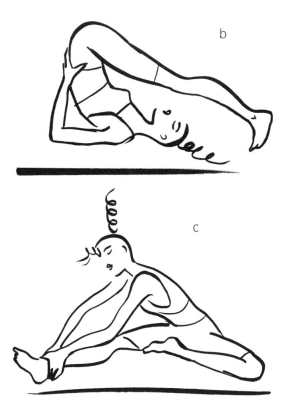
b

c

Figure 17-5. Legs overhead and seated hamstring stretch: Begin from a sitting position (*a*); slowly roll backward, bringing your legs over your head (*b*); roll forward and into the hamstring stretch (*c*).

The ankle pull

The muscles: Quadriceps (front thigh)

The purpose: Helps prevent quadriceps pulls and relieves soreness

The procedure:

- Lie on your stomach with one leg straight and the other bent toward your buttocks.
- Loop a towel around the ankle of your bent leg, holding the ends of the towel in your hands.
- Lift your bent leg and try to straighten it against the towel until you feel tension in your quadriceps muscle; hold.
- Relax and repeat; then switch to the other leg.

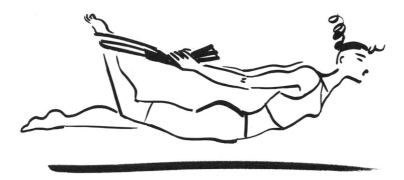

Figure 17-6. Ankle pull: try to straighten your leg against the towel until you feel tension in your quadriceps muscle.

Groin stretch

The muscles: Those of the groin
The purpose: Helps prevent groin pulls
The procedure:

- Sit on the floor, put the soles of your feet together, and pull them in toward your groin.
- Place your elbows on your knees and push your knees down until you feel tension in your groin; hold.
- Relax and then push up with your knees while at the same time pushing down with your elbows. Hold this for 4 seconds, relax, and then repeat the groin stretch.

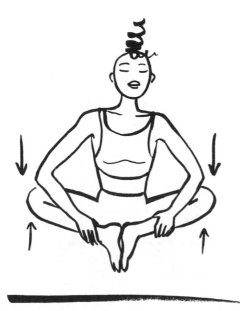

Figure 17-7. Groin stretch: push your knees down with your elbows until you feel tension in your groin, and hold. Relax, and then push up with your knees while pushing down with your elbows.

For Women Especially

Because our hips tend to be wide and angled sharply relative to the position of our knees, we women tend to pronate more than men do and are more susceptible to shin problems and ITB syndrome than they are. The ITB is a ligament that runs from your hip along the outside of your thigh and attaches at the knee. It can become inflamed and painful at the knee or hip.

Here are stretches for the shin and ITB in case you should develop tightness or soreness in these areas. If you have recurring problems with your shins or ITB, add the following stretches to your regular stretching routine.

Shin stretch

The muscles: Those along the front of the shin

The purpose: Helps prevent shinsplints and relieve the pain of them

The procedure:

- Kneel on a mat or carpeted floor, legs and feet together and toes pointed directly back.
- Slowly sit down onto your calves and heels, pushing your ankles into the floor until you feel tension in the muscles of your shins. Hold.
- Relax by moving forward off your heels, and then repeat.

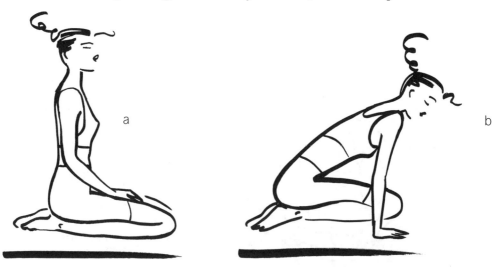

Figure 17-8. Shin stretch: slowly sit down onto your calves and heels (*a*), then relax by moving forward (*b*).

Iliotibial band stretches

Following are two stretches for the ITB. You may not feel much of a stretch in the standing position. If not, try the seated stretch.

The muscles: The ITB from the hip along the outside of the thigh to the knee

The purpose: Helps prevent ITB syndrome and relieve pain at the knee or hip

The procedure for the standing stretch:
- Stand sideways 2 to 3 feet from a wall or other unmovable structure and cross the outside leg over the inside leg.
- Extend your arm and place your hand on the wall.
- Put your other hand on your hip and push your hip toward the wall until you feel tension along the outside of your outside thigh; hold.
- Relax and repeat; then turn around and stretch the other side.

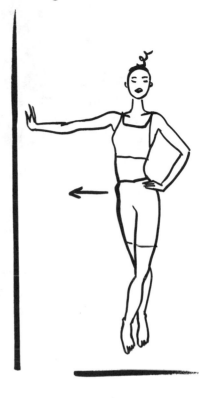

Figure 17-9. Standing iliotibial band stretch: push your hip toward the wall until you feel tension along the outer side of your outside thigh.

The procedure for the seated stretch:
- Sit on the ground with your knees bent and feet flat on the floor and slightly more than shoulder width apart; place your hands behind you for support.
- Place your left leg over your right knee and push your right knee toward the floor, keeping your right foot and hip flat on the floor. When you feel tension along the outer thigh of your right leg, hold the position.
- Relax and repeat; then stretch your left leg.

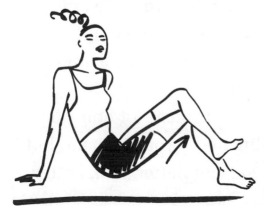

Figure 17-10. Seated iliotibial band stretch: use your left leg to push your right knee toward the floor, keeping your right foot and hip flat on the floor. You should feel tension along the outer thigh of your right leg.

18 Strength Training

The musculature is a suit of power draped over our otherwise helpless bones . . .

—JOHN JEROME, author of *The Elements of Effort*

FOR YEARS, WOMEN HAVE SHIED AWAY from the weight room at the gym, feeling intimidated by all the testosterone-pumped, muscle-busting men grunting and grimacing and heaving heavy barbells above their chests—but no longer. In increasing numbers, women are lifting dumbbells and pushing barbells right alongside those strapping male bodybuilders.

And with good reasons. Not only does strength training make you stronger, but it can also help you run better, look better, feel better, and keep you young. Whether you are 17 or 70, a competitive racer or recreational runner, short or tall, thin or well endowed, you should make strength training an integral part of your running program.

Won't strength training make me bulky? I don't want to look like those female bodybuilders on the covers of muscle magazines.

You practically have to make a career out of strength training to achieve that rippled look. Building muscle mass is difficult for women because we have very little testosterone, a key ingredient in muscle development. Strength training will give you a firm, smooth muscle tone, and it will tighten your jiggly spots. You'll look fit and feminine.

The Benefits

What exactly can strength training do for you?

Strengthen Your Total Body

Running makes your legs strong, but it doesn't do a whole lot for the rest of your body. Strength training develops total body fitness. Plus, a strong upper body helps you maintain good form during running, which allows for better breathing and helps you finish strong at the end of a run or race.

Prevent Injury to Muscles and Bones

Resistance training builds not only muscle but also bone. With a strong musculoskeletal system, you'll have better balance, and you'll be more resistant to overuse injuries—strains, joint problems, and fractures that occur when bones and ligaments are not strong enough to handle high mileage or high intensity.

You can use strength training to help compensate for a biomechanical weakness. Say you are somewhat knock-kneed and have a tendency toward knee trouble: the right strength exercises can build up the muscles around your knees to make them more resistant to injury.

Prevent Osteoporosis

Running, which is a weight-bearing activity, builds strong bones in your legs and on up your spine. With resistance training, you can build up the bones in your arms and shoulders, which are not affected by running. The way it works it this: the muscle contraction required to lift weight against the forces of gravity stresses the bone, and where stress occurs, bone cells are deposited.

Though considered an older woman's disease, osteoporosis is a health concern we should address in our youth because bone density achieves its peak between the ages of 25 and 35. After that, we begin to lose bone tissue at a rate of approximately 1 percent a year until menopause, when loss accelerates to 3 percent to 5 percent. (For more information on osteoporosis, see chapter 13.) Ideally, women should begin resistance training in their twenties and continue throughout their lives to keep this loss to a minimum, but weight lifting can also help rebuild bone that has deteriorated because of age or poor nutrition and can prevent further loss.

Runners who are amenorrheic, those who are approaching menopause, and those who are postmenopausal should be especially conscientious about lifting weights two or three times a week, since lack of estrogen speeds the deterioration of bone tissue.

Improve Body Composition

Regular strength training won't produce bulging biceps, but it does increase muscle mass, producing a higher muscle-to-fat ratio. Body composition is a better indicator of health and fitness than body weight is and may have some effect on your running performance. Muscle works for you when you run; fat just comes along for the ride. One of the reasons men run faster than we do is that most have a higher percentage of muscle and lower percentage of fat, so they're carrying less "extra baggage," so to speak.

PUMP IRON, NOT PILLS

Feeling a little depressed? Lift your spirits by lifting weights at the gym. At Tufts University in Medford, Massachusetts, a few years ago, researchers assembled 32 volunteers (20 women and 12 men) who had been diagnosed with mild to moderate depression. Seventeen were put on a 10-week strength-training regimen using weight machines 3 days a week. The other 15 did not exercise during those 10 weeks but were asked to participate in a health education program (lectures and videos on health and nutrition). At the end of the study, 14 of the 17 weight lifters were free of the symptoms of depression, an improvement equivalent to that produced by antidepressants. Only 6 of the 15 volunteers who went through the education program felt better at the end of the 10 weeks.

Speed Up Your Metabolism

Even when you're not running, muscle is busy burning calories. The more muscle you have, the faster your resting metabolism runs and the more calories you'll burn.

Tone Your Muscles and Firm Flab

Want to get rid of that extra jiggle under your arms? Pick up some weights on a regular basis. Strength training tones muscles, giving them some shape and firmness.

Improve Your Body Image

You'll like your body more for its muscle tone, leanness, strength, and its ability to run more powerfully. The strength you gain with resistance training makes you fitter and healthier. Plus, your friends will be really impressed when you help haul around the heavy furniture during their next move.

Improve Your Self-Image

Building strength through weight lifting is an accomplishment. It strikes another blow against the old but not dead image of woman as weak, frail thing. It builds our self-image as athletes and as strong, capable women.

Keep Yourself Young

After the age of 40, women start to lose muscle mass and bone density, both of which contribute to the frailty and lack of balance that can come with old age. "We lose about a third of a pound of muscle every year after age 40, and we're also losing bone," says Miriam Nelson, an assistant professor of nutrition at Tufts University in Medford, Massachusetts, and the author of *Strong Women Stay Young* (New York: Bantam, 1997). However, we can prevent that decline with regular strength training and preserve our muscle strength well into our seventies.

The Basics

Convinced? Good. Before we look at specific strength exercises, let's review the basic principles of a good strength program for runners. First, as with stretching, it's important that your strength-training program complement your running. It should work the muscle groups of the upper body and lower body that are used in running, but it shouldn't work those muscles too strenuously. If your athletic priority is running, that's where you want to put most of your effort and attention. Strength training should enhance your running, not detract from it.

How Much and How Often?

Two or three strength sessions a week is all you need. Any more would be detrimental to getting the maximum benefit from your program. Research has shown that 1 or 2 days of rest between weight-lifting workouts is necessary for your muscles to recover and rebuild to maximum strength before they're stressed again. Research has also shown that one round of resistance exercises per session is just as effective as two or three sets for building strength—good news for those of us pressed for time.

Schedule your weight lifting on days on which you don't run or on which you run easy. If you do both on the same day, lift first and then run in order to achieve maximum strength gains from weight lifting. Better yet, combine the two into one session (see The Strength Sandwich on page 231).

Free Weights Versus Machines

You can get an effective workout whether you use dumbbells and barbells or strength-training machines such as Nautilus or Cybex equipment. One reason to use dumbbells is that you work one arm or leg at a time, whereas with machines you use both arms or legs at the same time to lift the weight, which allows the stronger limb to compensate for the weaker one. When you use dumbbells, every muscle gets equal exercise.

Use Good Technique

Whether you choose machines or free weights, get instruction from someone qualified to teach you how to use them properly. Not only will good technique allow you to get the most benefit from your strength training program but it can also prevent injury. If you belong to a gym or health club, arrange with the trainer to go over your routine with you and teach you proper form for each exercise. If you have equipment at home, call your local YWCA or health club and make an appointment with one of the athletic trainers for a weight-lifting lesson.

Here are a few basic points of technique:

- Go slowly, using a smooth, steady motion as you lift and release the weight.
- Make sure you complete a full range of motion for each lift. Your movements should not be short and rapid but long and smooth.
- Maintain good form throughout each repetition of each lift—if you can't, you're lifting too heavy a weight.

THE STRENGTH SANDWICH

It can be hard enough to find time to run, let alone try to get in some strength training, too, even if it is only two sessions a week. And given a choice between running and weight lifting, I know I'd rather run.

The solution? Combine running and weight lifting into one session. The advantages are that you don't have to do two separate workouts in the same day, it offers a nice variation to the usual 4-mile run, and it's easier to get psyched to go for a run and then do some strength training in the middle of it rather than to try to get motivated just to lift weights.

Here's how it works: Run for 1 mile—2 max—and then do the strength-training routine described on pages 233–242. Top that off with another mile or two of running. It's ideal if you live close to a gym and can run there, lift, and then run home, but you can make it work with a home gym, too. Another option is to run on the treadmill at the fitness center before and after lifting.

A performance benefit to this run-lift-run routine is that after lifting, your upper body will be fatigued when you go back out and run. Although this does detract somewhat from the enjoyment of that final mile or two, it's good practice because this is how you feel at the end of a race. By practicing it in training, you'll get stronger and you'll run stronger to the finish line.

Step it up: To turn up the difficulty of this workout, add 30 seconds to 1 minute of aerobic activity between lifts during the strength portion. Jump rope, run in place, or do some stair stepping. Prepare to sweat.

A Strength-Training Program

The following routine was developed by Budd Coates, marathoner, corporate fitness director, and the coach who designed the training schedules that appear in part VII of this book. This program will give you balanced strength throughout your body. It will help you maintain good posture and form throughout a race or long run and will help prevent injury.

It is not designed specifically to make you faster. There are exercises that can help runners develop more explosive power in their legs. These are often used by sprinters and track athletes but are not covered here. "Distance runners get faster by doing speed workouts—intervals and tempo runs," explains Coates. It's a matter of training specificity: if you want to run faster in a race, the best thing you can do is run faster in training.

Nonetheless, the strength-training program included here will help you maintain a good pace. If you have a weak upper body, your arms, shoulders, and back will tire in the later miles of a race; your form will begin to fail; and you'll slow down. With a strong body, you'll be able to power right through the finish line of a 5-K or hold up well in the last couple miles of a marathon.

I have run all my best races when I've been consistent with strength training. One year, I let myself fall out of the habit of lifting weights for several months, and I noticed that at the end of all my races, even 5-Ks, my arms would become very tired and sore. I'm convinced I would have run faster in those races if I had just stuck to my strength workout, which, by the way, is the one presented here.

The Logistics

You can do the program below in your home with a set of dumbbells (5 to 20 pounds should cover your needs to start) and a weight bench. (Important: buy a weight bench that includes a leg extension/curl apparatus). Do the exercises in the order presented.

For the upper body, start with an amount of weight that you can lift at least 8 times in good form; for the lower body, lift 12 times.

Do 8 to 12 repetitions for each upper-body lift and 12 to 18 repeti-

MUSCLE GROUPS

What's a trapezius? Here's a list of the muscle groups discussed in this chapter and their general location on your body:

- **Biceps:** Front of the upper arm
- **Deltoids:** Shoulders
- **Hamstrings:** Back of the thigh
- **Latissimus dorsi:** Sides of the back
- **Pectorals:** Chest
- **Quadriceps:** Front of the thigh
- **Trapezius:** Top of the shoulder and middle of the back
- **Triceps:** Back of the upper arm

tions for each leg exercise. When you can do the maximum repetitions comfortably, move up to a heavier weight.

One set is sufficient and should take about 20 minutes, unless, that is, you decide to go the superaerobic route and jump rope for 30 seconds between lifts. (If you plan to lift at the gym, see The Weight Room on page 243 for an adaptation of this program.)

Bench press

Muscles trained: Pectorals, deltoids, triceps
The procedure:
- Lie on a weight bench with your feet flat on the floor.
- Hold a dumbbell in each hand at the sides of your chest, arms next to your body and palms facing forward or inward.
- Push the dumbbells directly upward until your arms are fully extended.
- Slowly bring the dumbbells back to the starting position and repeat.

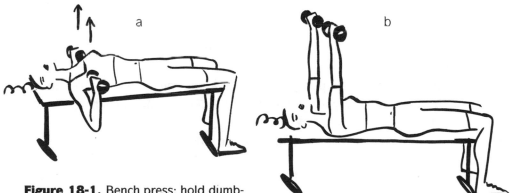

Figure 18-1. Bench press: hold dumbbells at the sides of your chest (*a*), then push them directly upward (*b*).

Dumbbell fly

Muscles trained: Pectorals
The procedure:
- Lie on a weight bench with your feet flat on the floor.
- Hold a dumbbell in each hand at the sides of your chest, near your ears, palms facing forward or inward.
- Push the dumbbells up and together over your chest in a somewhat semicircular motion, extending your arms fully.
- Slowly lower the dumbbells back to the starting position and repeat.

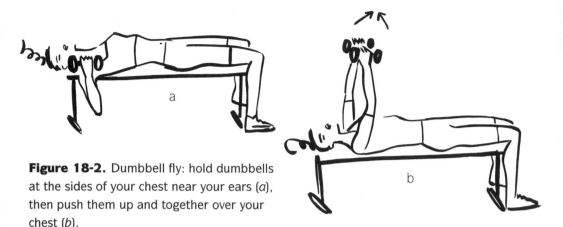

Figure 18-2. Dumbbell fly: hold dumbbells at the sides of your chest near your ears (*a*), then push them up and together over your chest (*b*).

One-arm dumbbell row

Muscles trained: latissimus dorsi (lats), biceps

The procedure:

- Grab one dumbbell for this exercise.
- Kneel on the end of your weight bench with your right leg, keeping your left leg on the floor.
- Use your right arm to support your body in a bent position over the bench.
- Hold the dumbbell in your left arm and extend that arm straight down alongside the bench.
- Lift the dumbbell in a straight line up to the side of your chest.
- Lower the dumbbell and repeat.
- After 8 to 12 repetitions, switch sides.

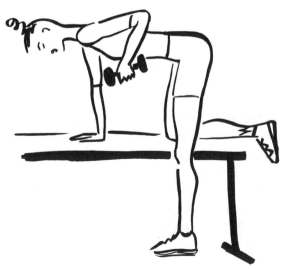

Figure 18-3. One-arm dumbbell row: lift the dumbbell in a straight line up to the side of your chest.

Leg extension

Muscles trained: Quadriceps

Reasons to do it: In general, the hamstrings get used more during running than the quads. This exercise, done in conjunction with the hamstring curl (page 236), develops an appropriate balance of strength between these two major muscle groups, which helps prevent injury. Developing stronger quadriceps also helps prevent knee injuries, which are common among women runners.

Notes: You can do this exercise with ankle weights if your bench does not have a leg extension apparatus. To get the right balance between your quadriceps and hamstrings, you must lift a weight ratio of 3 to 2, quadriceps to hamstrings, meaning if you can lift 30 pounds doing leg extensions, lift only 20 pounds for leg curls.

The procedure:

- Sit at the end of the bench and place both your legs under the padded weight bar. The pads should rest on your shins, just above your ankles.
- Grasp the bench behind you for support.
- Raise both legs until they are straight out in front of you and then drop one leg back to the floor.
- With the other leg, slowly lower the weight about 45 degrees and then lift it to the starting position.
- After 12 to 18 repetitions, switch legs.

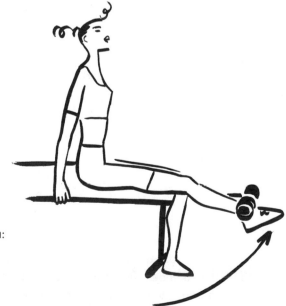

Figure 18-4. Leg extension: lift the weight until your leg is horizontal.

Leg curl

Muscles trained: Hamstrings

The procedure:

- Lie facedown on the bench with your legs under the weight bar. The pads of the bar should rest at the bottom of your calf muscles.
- Hold on to the bench for support.
- Slowly lift the weight, with one leg, up and toward you as far as you can, then lower the leg.
- After 12 to 18 repetitions, switch legs.

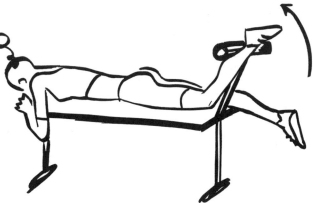

Figure 18-5. Leg curl: slowly lift the weight with your leg as far as you can toward your buttocks.

Dumbbell press

Muscles trained: Deltoids, triceps

The procedure:

- Stand with your feet shoulder width apart.
- Hold a dumbbell in each hand at your shoulders, palms facing forward.
- Slowly push the dumbbells up and bring them together over your head.
- Lower the dumbbells back to the starting position and repeat.

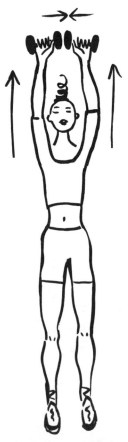

Figure 18-6. Dumbbell press: push the dumbbells up from shoulder height and bring them together over your head.

Lateral raise

Muscles trained: Latissimus dorsi (lats)
The procedure:

- Stand with your feet shoulder width apart and a dumbbell in each hand.
- With your arms bent at 90 degrees, hold the dumbbells in a vertical position out in front of you.
- Keeping your arms in this 90-degree position, raise them to the sides so that your elbows come up to shoulder height.
- Lower your arms to the starting position and repeat.

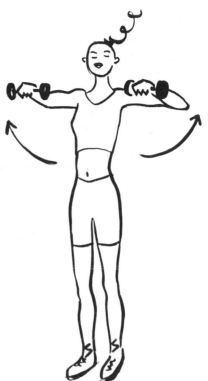

Figure 18-7. Lateral raise: keeping your arms bent at a 90° angle, raise them to the side until your elbows come up to shoulder height.

Shoulder roll

Muscles trained: Trapezius
The procedure:

- Stand with your feet shoulder width apart.
- Hold a dumbbell in each hand, your arms straight down at your sides.
- Move your shoulders in a fluid circular motion forward, up, back, and down.

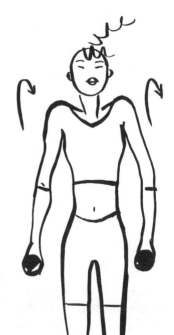

Figure 18-8. Shoulder roll: rotate your shoulders in a circular motion.

Upright row

Muscles trained: Deltoids, biceps, trapezius

The procedure:

- Stand with your feet shoulder width apart and hold one dumbbell straight down in front of you with both hands.
- Slowly lift the dumbbell straight up to your chin, keeping it close to your body.
- Lower the dumbbell to the starting position and repeat.

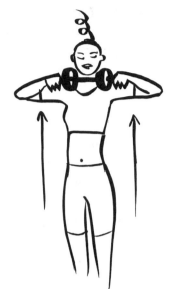

Figure 18-9. Upright row: holding a dumbbell at each end, lift it straight up to your chin, keeping it close to your body.

Triceps press

Muscles trained: Triceps

The procedure:

- Standing with your feet shoulder width apart, hold a dumbbell in your right hand and extend your arm fully overhead, keeping your arm close to your head.
- Lower the dumbbell in a semicircular motion behind your head until your elbow is bent about 90 degrees.
- Raise the dumbbell to the starting position and repeat 8 to 12 times.
- Repeat with your left arm.

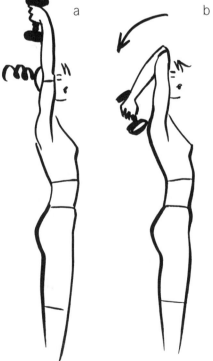

Figure 18-10. Triceps press: hold a dumbbell overhead in one hand (*a*), then lower it in a semicircular motion behind your head (*b*).

Dumbbell curl

Muscles trained: Biceps

The procedure:

- Stand with your feet shoulder width apart and a dumbbell in each hand, arms straight down at your sides.
- Keeping your arms next to your sides, lift one dumbell up toward your chest, bending your arm at the elbow.
- Slowly lower the dumbbell to the starting position and then lift the dumbbell in your opposite arm.
- Curl alternately with your right arm and then your left until you complete 8 to 12 repetitions for each arm.

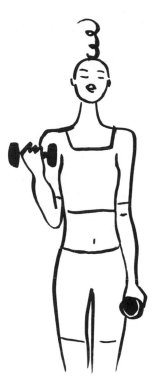

Figure 18-11. Dumbbell curl: lift one dumbbell at a time toward your chest, keeping your arm next to your side.

Dumbbell pull-over

Muscles trained: Pectorals and muscles of the rib cage

The procedure:

- Use one dumbbell.
- Lie on a weight bench, your feet flat on the floor.
- Hold the dumbbell with both hands straight above your chest.
- Slowly lower the dumbbell over your head and back as far as you can without causing pain.
- Lift the dumbbell to the starting position and repeat.

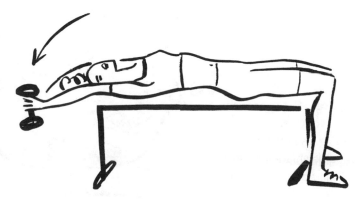

Figure 18-12. Dumbbell pullover: beginning with the dumbbell straight above your chest, slowly lower it over your head and back as far as you can without causing pain.

Abdominal Addendum

Strengthening your abdominal muscles (abs) and lower back can enhance your running posture further and help prevent back problems. The first thing that comes to mind when most people think about strengthening the abs is crunches, but they are only part of the solution. The abdomen is composed of four muscles. The rectus abdominis runs vertically up and down the center of your abdomen from your pubic area to just beneath your breasts. This is the outermost abdominal muscle—the "washboard abs" of well-trained body-builders. The external and internal obliques run diagonally out to the sides of your hips and waist. The transversus abdominis runs horizontally across your lower abdomen, is the deepest of the four abdominal muscles, and is used in breathing.

Crunches, the most popular of the ab exercises, work only the rectus abdominis—more specifically, the upper region of it. To fully strengthen your abdomen for better posture and back support, you need to exercise the upper and lower part of your abdomen and the sides—the oblique muscles.

Here's a routine designed for your abs and lower back. This is a supplement to the strength-training routine presented above. It's not necessary, but it develops good core body strength and helps offer extra back support.

Crunch

Muscles trained: Upper rectus abdominis

The procedure:

- Lie down on the floor with your legs bent 90 degrees and your calves resting on top of your weight bench.
- Cross your arms over your chest.
- Raise your head and shoulders just until your shoulder blades have come off the floor. Do not bend your head forward or pull with your neck muscles; you should feel all the effort in your upper abdomen.
- Slowly lower your body to the starting position.
- Begin with 10 repetitions and increase the number gradually each week.

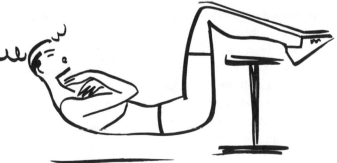

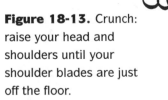

Figure 18-13. Crunch: raise your head and shoulders until your shoulder blades are just off the floor.

Reverse sit-up

Muscles trained: Lower rectus abdominis

The procedure:

- Lie on the floor on your back, with your legs bent and your feet flat on the floor and your arms straight down at your sides and palms facedown.
- Raise your legs so that your thighs are perpendicular to the floor. This is the starting position.
- Slowly bring your legs back and your knees into your chest. Your pelvis should come up off the floor.
- Slowly lower your legs to the starting position.
- Begin with 10 repetitions and increase the number gradually each week.

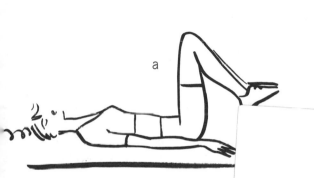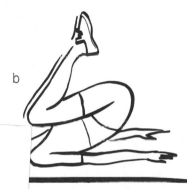

Figure 18-14. Reverse sit-up: s[...]endicular to the floor (*a*); slowly bring your knees into your [...] the starting position (*a*).

Reverse trunk twist

Muscles trained: Internal and external obliques

The procedure:

- Lie on the floor on your back, with your arms straight out to the side, palms facedown on the floor.
- Put your legs together and bring them straight up into the air from your hips so that your body makes a 90-degree angle.
- Keeping your head, back, and arms in position, lower your legs to one side until they touch the floor, then slowly raise them to the starting position.
- Repeat, lowering your legs to the other side.
- Begin with 10 repetitions on each side and increase the number gradually each week.
- If the exercise is too difficult with your legs fully extended, bend them at your knees.

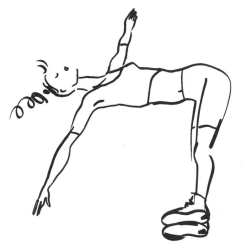

Figure 18-15. Reverse trunk twist: keeping your back and arms flat on the floor, lower your legs from the vertical starting position until they touch the floor.

Cat Cow

Muscles trained: The spinalis, longissimus, and iliocostalis muscles of the back, collectively known as the erector spinae

Note: If you do your strength training at the gym, you can substitute the back raise, done on a glute-ham machine (gluteals–hamstrings), for this exercise.

The procedure:

- Kneel on the floor with your hands directly under your shoulders and your knees directly beneath your hips. Looking at the floor, tuck your chin slightly toward your chest.
- Slowly arch your back upward, pulling your abs up and into your rib cage. You should feel a stretch through the length of your back.
- Slowly arch your back downward, letting your stomach drop toward the floor, and hold this position until you feel a stretch across your abdomen.
- Repeat, moving up and down.
- Begin with 10 total repetitions (1 repetition = arch up, arch down), and gradually increase the number.

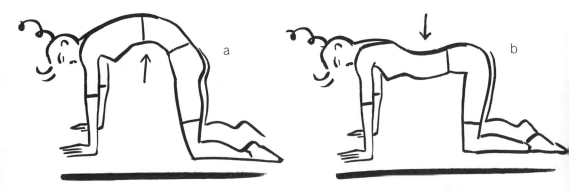

Figure 18-16. Cat cow: slowly arch your back upward until you feel the stretch in your back (*a*), then slowly arch downward until you feel a stretch across your abdomen (*b*).

THE WEIGHT ROOM

The key to successful weight training is consistency. Some runners prefer to lift weights in the privacy and convenience of their homes; others are more motivated to get out of the house and pump iron at the gym. The routine in this chapter can be done at your health club or local YWCA using free weights as described or a combination of free weights and resistance machines. Work with a trainer to learn proper technique and use of equipment. Here's a list of the exercises, in order, with one addition—the lateral pull-down, which requires a resistance machine.

- Bench press
- Dumbbell fly
- Lateral pull-down
- One-arm dumbbell row
- Leg extension
- Leg curl
- Dumbbell press
- Lateral raise
- Shoulder roll
- Upright row
- Triceps push-down
- Dumbbell curl
- Dumbbell pull-over

19 Cross-Training

RUNNING IS YOUR FIRST LOVE, certainly, but there may be times when you'll want or need to do something different. Injury can force you off your feet for a while; a long period of high mileage can leave you wanting a physical and mental break from running; or maybe you just don't want to run every day but crave daily physical activity. These are the times to consider cross-training—taking up another activity in addition to or temporarily in place of your running.

Experts will tell you that certain methods of cross-training will improve your running performance, but if you're healthy and your goal is to become a better runner, cross-training isn't the best means. If you want to get faster, you need to run faster (speed work). If you want to go farther, you have to run farther (long runs). If you want to get stronger, you need to run harder (hill runs). It's all about specificity of training: you become a better runner by running. Of course, there are exceptions.

How quickly will I lose fitness if I stop running?

Studies have shown that after 10 days of complete rest, declines in fitness begin to appear in many athletes. However, you can cut back on running quite a bit and maintain fitness for several weeks. Jim Bledsoe, Ph.D., writing in the September 1997 issue of *Running Research News,* states that "a typical athlete can reduce either the frequency (number of workouts per week) or volume (number of miles covered per week) of training by up to 67 percent for 10 to 15 weeks without losing any fitness at all, as long as the remaining workouts are fairly high quality."

What does he mean by high quality? Bledsoe recommends running three to five 1-mile repeats at a hard pace, with 4 minutes of easy running between each hard mile. Do this only twice a week, says Bledsoe, and you'll be in great shape after 10 weeks even if you do no other running.

Bledsoe goes on to say that runners who have overtrained for a period of time—are tired, sore, irritable, lackluster in their performance—can take 3 weeks off completely and actually show fitness improvements at the end of this period. It appears that rest gives their bodies the opportunity to recover and rebuild to a level higher of cardiorespiratory strength.

Some of us just aren't meant to run every day even though we'd like to. We're prone to injury and fall prey to it after too many consecutive runs on the road. What cross-training can do is provide a means of "active recovery." It allows you to get off your legs and recover from a hard run while maintaining fitness through cardiovascular activity. If this is your situation, plan to cross-train on those days that you would run relaxed, and do a workout similar in terms of intensity and duration to what you would do on the roads. Don't use cross-training to go hard in between days of hard running. You'll become overtrained and possibly injured and your running performance will suffer.

The five best reasons to cross-train are these:

- To maintain your fitness when you're injured
- For variety in your running schedule
- Because you enjoy sports other than running
- To give your body and mind a rest after months of running
- To help prevent injury if you are vulnerable to it

Cross-Training for Fun

Whether you've just finished a period of intense running and want to take some time off or you simply like the variety of cross-training, consider choosing an activity that uses muscles you don't use very much during running. This gives your running muscles a better rest and enhances your overall fitness. The best cross-training activity, though, is the one you most enjoy. After all, if your goal isn't to maintain or achieve a high level of fitness but to stay active and reasonably fit, cross-training should be fun. Following are several options.

Cross-Country Skiing

A great alternative to running during the winter months if you live in a snowy climate, cross-country skiing is an excellent all-around sport. It builds total body strength, raises your heart rate for an extended period of time, and produces very little impact on your body. Plus, it gets you outdoors in the winter and can take you through some spectacular landscapes. The indoor version provides a great workout, too.

Cycling

A common second sport among runners, cycling can be quite a leg burner but without the impact stresses of running. As you'll see later, it is one of the better cross-training activities for runners who want to stay in shape when they're injured, but relaxed cycling makes for an excellent form of active rest. In fact, light cycling is sometimes recommended the day after a marathon to help loosen up your muscles without impact. This is one activity that doesn't do a whole lot for your upper body, but it can cut a mean pair of quads. By riding your bike in a standing position, you use your muscles more as you would in running.

Technique tip: Make sure the bike seat is adjusted so there is only a slight bend in your knee when your leg is extended. Use pedal clips, which allow you to pull and push as you spin.

Elliptical Trainers

One of the newest pieces of indoor exercise equipment, the elliptical trainer is sort of a cross between a stair climber and a treadmill. While in a standing position, you move your feet on the pedals in an elliptical motion. You can get an excellent aerobic workout that's not too distant from running but without the pounding, and it's easy to do.

Technique tip: Maintain an upright position and keep your weight over your feet to replicate running motion as closely as possible.

In-line Skating

Put some speed on your feet with a pair of in-line skates. Though it's not as heart pounding as running, skating can deliver a good aerobic workout, especially if you power up a few hills. Plus, it doesn't deliver the impact stress—at least not unless you fall down. It's fun and fast and enhances the strength of your lower body, particularly your quadriceps.

Rowing

Rowing is most enjoyable with a few friends and a picnic basket on a river or lake, but the indoor version has its benefits, too—it'll probably make you exercise a little harder. Rowing is an excellent upper-body activity, and if you are careful to use good technique and row through a complete range of motion, you'll work your legs, too. Rowing can be as aerobic as you want it to be. It produces minimal stress to your musculoskeletal system, although the monotony might produce some psychological stress.

Technique tip: Poor form can strain your back and knees. While rowing, keep your back straight throughout the movement and don't bend your knees excessively. Keep your elbows close to your body.

Stair Climbing

Though stair climbing is a weight-bearing activity, it doesn't create high impact unless you've chosen as your venue the solid concrete steps outside the Capitol Building, art museum, or baseball stadium. With a quick aerobic pace, you can produce quite a burn in your butt and thighs, but your upper body doesn't see a lot of action.

A 1993 study done by researchers at California State University that compared the effects of stair climbing versus running in groups of women over a period of 9 weeks found that stair climbing produced a comparable level of fitness to running. Hitting the stepper can be a good way to maintain a high level of fitness if running is hard on your body.

Technique tip: You can hold onto the arm rails when you use a stair climber, but don't use them to support your weight. Stand erect and push on the pedal with your whole foot, not just your toes.

Swimming

The water bears your weight as you swim, making swimming the lowest-impact activity of all. Most of the effort of swimming comes from the stroke, so it's a great upper-body builder. To elevate their heart rate significantly, good swimmers have to stroke rather swiftly, but if you're a novice, a few laps can have you gasping for air, and not because you've been holding your breath.

Walking

When you don't feel like running, walk. You use the same muscles as you do in running, but with less force and of course with less aerobic effect. Walking does offer a healthful rest from running, though, and it allows a better view of the scenery.

Cross-Training Through Injury

Most running injuries heal rather quickly if you catch them early and treat them properly. You might need to take a few days off from running, but not enough to cause any loss of speed or fitness. A severe knee injury or a stress fracture, however, can keep you off the roads for several weeks. If you're in the middle of marathon training or building toward a great 5-K or 10-K, you can lose essential fitness if you can't run. Fortunately there are a few activities that can keep you in decent shape through the mending period.

Deep-Water Running

Deep-water running is the cross-training activity of choice among top runners who don't want to lose any fitness because of injury. The reason? It uses the same muscles as running in the same ways, and it's aerobically equivalent as well. Studies have confirmed what runners have long known—that aquarunning produces cardiorespiratory fitness nearly equivalent to that from dry-land running and that it is an excellent way to continue training when you can't run.

You can train in the pool just as you would on the roads, but without the impact; all you need is a flotation belt so you can keep your head above water. It'll seem a little strange at first, but put yourself in the deep end of the pool and move exactly as if you were running, using the same form—arms bent at 90 degrees, swinging straight forward and back, and good posture.

Of course, there aren't mile markers to guide you; the parameters of pool running are time and effort. If your schedule calls for a relaxed 5 miles, you should water run at an effort level that feels the same as the effort of a typical 5-mile road run and for the same amount of time.

Trying to get into race shape? Here are a couple "fast-paced" workouts for the pool.

TEMPO WATER RUN

Warm up with 10 to 15 minutes of relaxed deep-water running. Increase the difficulty to an effort comparable to what you would feel in a tempo run on dry land—the exertion should feel hard but manageable. Keep up this pace for 10 to 20 minutes and then slow down to a relaxed effort for a 10-minute cool-down.

DEEP-WATER *FARTLEK*

Warm up with 10 to 15 minutes of easy deep-water running. Then run for 1 minute hard—an exertion comparable to what you would feel during fast intervals on the track (hard but not an all-out sprint). Then relax for 1 minute. Repeat, alternating hard and easy minutes until you've run 10 hard. Cool down with 10 minutes of easy pool running. If this isn't tough enough for you, alternate 2 minutes of hard running with 2 minutes easy.

Cycling

Cycling puts your legs through a motion similar to that of running; to increase the similarity and get the most benefit, ride in a standing position. Cycling is also an excellent quad-strengthening activity, which can boost your power on hills. Pedal at a rate of 90 to 95 revolutions per minute, which is equivalent to optimal stride rate during running, and change the resistance of the bike according to how hard an effort level you want to achieve.

As with deep-water running, you can transfer your running workouts to the bike according to effort and time. Because cycling is a nonimpact activity, it can help you get through most injuries, but check with your sports physician or an athletic trainer to make sure it's appropriate for you.

You could transfer either of the speed sessions described for the pool to the bicycle or try the following workout.

400s ON THE BIKE

Recall how you run 400-meter repeats on the track or road. How long does it take to run just one? What does the effort feel like? Now, warm up with 10 to 15 minutes of easy cycling, then spin hard at your 400-meter effort for the same amount of time it would take to run it. (Remember, you always want to pedal at 90 to 95 revolutions per minute, so you'll need to raise and lower the resistance of the bike to achieve hard and easy effort levels.) Cycle slowly for the same amount of time and then pick up the pace again. Do as many 400s on the bike as you would on the track—6, 8, 10. Cool down with 10 minutes of easy spinning.

20 Treadmill Running

The treadmill can do anything you want it to.

—KIM JONES, top American marathoner

A TREADMILL CAN BE A WOMAN RUNNER'S most valuable piece of equipment next to good shoes and a sports bra. True, there's nothing better than running outdoors in fresh air and sunlight, exploring landscapes or sharing miles of conversation with friends. Even running in rain on a warm day or down snowy roads in the winter can be exhilarating, but it's not always possible or very wise to go out for a run.

Dark mornings and black nights aren't the safest times for women to be running, especially if you live where streets are lonely, poorly lit, and uneven. Icy roads in winter can slip you up and cause a pulled muscle or a bruised knee, and running on a summer day that soars in temperature and humidity can lead quickly to dehydration, possibly even heat exhaustion. If you have a family or demanding career or both, finding time to run can be a challenge no matter what the conditions outside.

With a treadmill at home, you'll have a much easier time being consistent with your running and sticking to a running program, whether for fitness or performance. At night, when it's dark and snowy, after the kids are in bed, or after you've finished that report due on your supervisor's desk tomorrow morning, you can hop on the treadmill for a quick 20 or 30 minutes to vanquish the day's stress and do something good for your body.

Plus, treadmills offer a few training advantages over the roads. They are softer, making the impact force lower and easier on your legs. If you are prone to stress fractures, an injury more common in women than men, you might want to consider alternating road running with time on the treadmill.

With motorized treadmills, the belt maintains a steady speed, forcing you to keep an even pace. This can be especially helpful for speed workouts: it's easier to slow down running under your own power on the track than when you're keeping up with the movement of your treadmill. Though you can slow the speed of your treadmill at the press of a button, it's a more conscious decision and effort, and you'll be inclined to postpone that decision as long as possible so as not to feel too much like a sissy.

But running on a treadmill is *so boring,* you say. There's no denying that it can be very tedious. The first 10 minutes go by pretty quickly, but each minute after that can feel like an hour if you don't figure out some distraction. With a little creativity, however, you can make treadmill running an enjoyable experience.

Running on a treadmill at my usual 9-minute pace feels so much harder than when I'm running outside. Why is that?

It's a matter of perception, according to exercise physiologist and runner Ken Sparks, who does all his speed training on the treadmill. Nothing is moving around you; your brain notices that you're working really hard to go nowhere.

The perception principle works in reverse during evening runs outdoors. In semidarkness, the landscape appears to be moving by you so quickly that you feel like you're running faster than usual without any additional effort. It just goes to show you the powerful influence the mind can have on the body.

Finding Fun in Treadmill Running

First, if you can, buy a treadmill with enough bells and whistles to give you some interesting workout options. Ideally, you want a machine that includes a variety of preset "courses" to choose from in addition to allowing you to program your own. It should offer a wide range of speeds and inclines and have a monitor that displays pace, time expended, miles run, and calories burned and that shows you an elevation diagram of the course you are running, along with your progress on that course as you run.

Regardless of the type of treadmill you buy, here are some suggested workouts to make your run more fun. Because most of them will require you to change your pace or the incline at which you run, they can help make you a better runner, too.

FINESSE YOUR FORM

One valuable aspect of treadmill running is that you can use it to develop better form. Set a full-length mirror in front of your treadmill so that you can see yourself from head to toe. While running, check your form and make corrections. Look for these points:

- You should have an erect posture—no slumping or curved shoulders.
- Your arms should be close to your sides and bent at roughly 90 degrees.
- Your arms should move directly back and forth, passing your hips and coming up near shoulder height; they should not cross from side to side over your chest.
- Your shoulders should be relaxed, not tight up around your neck.
- Your hands should be relaxed, as if you are holding an egg in each one; your palms should be facing inward, not up or down.
- Don't worry about your legs; they'll automatically coordinate themselves with the movements of your arms.

When you think you're running in good form, pick up the pace and see how well you maintain it.

Movin' to the Music

The *only* place to use headphones and a portable tape player during running is when you're on the treadmill. Here's a way to use music to motivate your run and erase the monotony.

THE PREPARATION

First, you need to record a running tape—30 minutes, 45 minutes, an hour, whatever you need. Pick songs of varied tempos—slow, medium, and fast—which will correspond to the different speeds you will run during this workout. Record about 10 minutes of easy-tempo music at the beginning of the tape, then add songs in whatever order you like, varying the tempos. Finish with 10 minutes of relaxing music; a few soothing instrumental pieces might be nice here.

THE WORKOUT

You've probably figured it out already. As you're listening to the tape, change your treadmill running pace to suit the tempo of the music. Warm up with an easy pace to the first 10 minutes of slow-tempo music, and at the start of the first up-tempo piece, punch up the speed of your treadmill. At the next song, speed up again or slow down, depending on the music. Keep on running and changing paces with each song, finishing your treadmill run with a 10-minute cooldown to the final soothing sounds of your recording.

Listening to music not only makes the run more interesting, but studies have shown that different types of music elicit different physical responses. The up-tempo tunes will actually help you run faster.

VARIATIONS

Do a hill run. Instead of changing the speed, change the incline of the treadmill with the music so that you are running flat or downhill when the tempo is slow, then use the up-tempo pieces to pump you up the inclines.

Do a nature run. Record a tape of different environmental sounds: the beach, the rain forest, a rainstorm. Rather than focusing on changing your pace, imagine yourself running through each environment. Picture the waves crashing on the shore, feel the sand under your bare feet, smell the salt air, notice the seagull gliding. Then make your way through the lush rain forest with its greenery and high trees, exotic birds and flowers, soft ground, moist air . . .

TV Tempo

You're no couch potato if you're getting in a good run while watching your favorite sitcom.

THE PREPARATION

You'll need a television in front of your treadmill for this one. Choose a favorite 30-minute show with commercials.

THE WORKOUT

Depending on how long you want to run, you can do an easy 10-minute warmup on the treadmill before the show starts or at the beginning of the program. Then whenever the show is on, increase the treadmill speed to a pace that requires effort but that you can maintain for several minutes. When the ads come on, take a commercial break, slowing to an easy pace. Run hard again when the program returns. Continue changing paces until 10 minutes to go or the end of the program, and then cool down with easy running.

The idea is to run hard when you are mentally involved in the show and to relax during the less-interesting TV ads. The changing paces and the show break the monotony of this 30- to 50-minute treadmill run.

VARIATIONS

Instead of changing the treadmill speed, you can change the incline for a good hill workout.

Two-in-One Workout

Here's a superefficient treadmill workout—combining running and toning exercises in one session. Watch the evening news and you'll triple the value of this treadmill run.

THE PREPARATION

No preparation is required.

THE WORKOUT

Warm up with 10 minutes of easy running. Then stop running and do 5 to 10 push-ups. Get back on the treadmill and run for 5 minutes. Stop and do 10 to 20 abdominal crunches. Run for 5 minutes. Stop and do 10 to 20 reverse sit-ups. Run for 5 minutes. Stop and do 10 to 20 reverse trunk twists. Run for 5 minutes. Stop and do

5 to 10 push-ups. Finish with 10 minutes of easy running. (See chapter 18 for specifics on abdominal crunches, reverse sit-ups, and reverse trunk twists.)

VARIATIONS

You can do this workout any way you like, using any combination of exercises, and you can shorten or lengthen the treadmill intervals to your preference.

Sixty-Second Switch

The workout described below uses changes in incline to make things interesting, but you can also vary treadmill speed.

THE PREPARATION

No preparation is required.

THE WORKOUT

At zero incline, run for 10 minutes at a comfortable pace. Set the incline to 1 percent and run at the same speed for 1 minute. Drop the incline to –1 percent and run for 1 minute. Raise it to 2 percent for a minute, then down to 0 percent for a minute. Go up to 3 percent for 1 minute, then down to 1 percent; up to 4 percent, down to 2 percent; up to 5 percent, down to 3 percent. Then work your way back down: 4, 2, 3, 1, 2, 0, 1, –1, and finish with 10 minutes of comfortable running at "sea level." The total time of this workout is 38 minutes, with 14 minutes running "uphill."

VARIATIONS

The idea behind this workout is to use changes in incline to break up the monotony of treadmill running. You can alter the above workout any way you like. It's not an easy workout, because even though you are alternating higher inclines with lower inclines through the middle of the run, you are still running "uphill" for several consecutive minutes. If this is too difficult, alternate running 1 minute at 3 percent, 4 percent, or 5 percent incline with 1 minute at 0 percent incline or 1 minute "downhill."

You can also do this workout by changing the speed of the treadmill, rather than the incline, with every minute.

Mount Everest

You won't want to do this workout all in one day. Attack it the way climbers would attempt a mountain: climb a certain distance, take a break, climb, take a break, and so on, until you reach the peak.

THE PREPARATION

Hang a big picture of Mount Everest on the wall in front of your treadmill for inspiration. Off to the side, draw a vertical line from the base to the top. Mount Everest is 29,028 feet high—5 1/2 miles. Divide the vertical line into 11 equal sections, each representing a half-mile. Now, you are ready to begin climbing.

THE WORKOUT

Go at your own pace and according to your own ability on this one. As always, warm up with 10 minutes of easy running at zero incline. Then increase the incline to 1 percent and note the mileage point on the monitor; this is where your climb begins. Run at this incline until you need a break; then note how far you've climbed, drop the treadmill to zero and go easy until you are ready to climb again at 1 percent.

Continue, always noting the distance of the climbing intervals, until you don't feel like climbing anymore. Cool down with 10 minutes of easy running at "sea level." Add up the distance you ran "uphill" for that workout and mark it on the vertical scale next to your picture of Mount Everest.

The next time you do this workout, climb at an incline of 2 percent—after all, the higher up the mountain you go, the harder the climb. Mark your progress on the scale. Each time you come back to this workout, run at a higher incline and mark your mileage. See how many workouts it takes to scale Mount Everest. (Don't do these treadmill climbs on successive days—they can be comparable to hill runs. If you are running them hard, one a week is plenty.)

Once you've reached the peak, consider descending the mountain, using the same principles as you did for the climb, but you'll be alternating zero inclines with negative inclines on the treadmill. Remember, the steepest part of the descent is at the top of the mountain.

Race Practice

Do you have an important race coming up? Give it a test run on your treadmill. Visualizing yourself running a race ahead of time is a technique recommended by sports psychologists to help you mentally prepare for a good performance. The following workout allows you to run both a mental and a physical simulation of the race course.

THE PREPARATION

Obviously, to do this, you need a programmable treadmill and an elevation map of the race you'll be running (sometimes given on the entry form, or you can contact race organizers). Program the course into your treadmill.

THE WORKOUT

Warm up and then run the race, not at race pace but at your usual training pace; save your speed for the real event. As you're running, imagine yourself in the race, moving strongly and smoothly from start to finish. This provides excellent preparation for body and mind.

How to Buy a Good Treadmill

What defines a good treadmill? One that you will use. It should have a design that makes it comfortable to run on, a running surface that's not too soft or too hard, a smooth action, and features that make it interesting to operate. No, you don't *need* all the flashing lights, a dozen different courses to choose from, a wide range of speeds and inclines, and a monitor that displays every increment of height, pace, and mileage in vivid color, but they sure make the treadmill experience much more enjoyable. I say go for as many "bells and whistles" as you can afford.

How much do you have to spend for a good treadmill? Most experts say at least $1,500, and the more you spend, the longer your treadmill will last, the more comfortable it will feel, the more features it will have, and the more you will enjoy running on it. Grab your credit card and head for a store that specializes in selling indoor exercise machines, preferably one that has several models of treadmills that you can try and compare. Don't let a salesperson talk you into his or her favorite brand. A treadmill is a personal piece of equipment; each has its own particular "feel" and design. Shop around, try several, and buy the one that fits your body, stride, and running style.

The Feel

Your treadmill should feel comfortable for running. What does that mean?

- The belt should be wide enough and long enough that you won't feel like you'll easily run off the edge or fall off the back.
- The running surface should be not too hard or too soft. The softer—the greater the cushioning—the more your foot "sinks" into the surface. The harder it is, the faster your foot will push off the surface and the greater the impact will be as you run. The amount of cushioning you choose depends on personal preference. Just remember that there is a difference from treadmill to treadmill.
- The belt should move smoothly. It shouldn't slip or hesitate when you change speed or incline.
- The design of the console and handrails should feel comfortable. Some treadmills don't have side rails. Would that make you uneasy or give you a pleasant sense of space? The console should be a comfortable height and reach.
- The monitor should be very readable with buttons that are easy to press so that you can adjust speed and incline quickly.

The Mechanical Aspects

The feel of the treadmill depends on the quality of construction. So does durability. Put the following points on your treadmill shopping checklist.

- The treadmill should have structural integrity. It shouldn't wiggle or wobble or feel flimsy underfoot.
- Ask the salesperson about the construction of the deck or bed, which is the heart of the treadmill, lying just beneath the belt. High-quality decks are made from layers of laminated wood and then coated with a lubricant to reduce friction between the deck and belt. Some decks are reversible, which doubles their life span.
- The console should be sturdy and appear durable.
- Listen to the motor as you run. Treadmills vary in how loudly they operate. Quieter is better.
- The motor's horsepower (hp) should be 1.5 or higher "continuous duty," meaning that the treadmill runs continuously at that horsepower regardless of load or time. If you see the horsepower listed

as "peak performance," it means that is the maximum horse-power the treadmill can reach; it will not run at that level of power consistently.

The Features

Every treadmill should come with a monitor that displays pace, miles run, time elapsed, and calories burned, but there are so many more options. When selecting features, be honest about what you'd like your treadmill to have; don't go overboard, but don't skimp.

- Treadmills vary in how fast they'll go. Make sure you buy one that will go at least as fast as you do, but faster is better because the treadmill will accommodate your needs as you improve.
- Check that the speed of the treadmill changes in small increments and consistently over the whole range of speeds. You don't want to have to jump from, say, a 9-minute pace immediately to an 8:30 pace.
- The range of incline should suit your purposes, and buy a machine that allows you to run "downhill," too.
- Having several automatic courses programmed into the treadmill gives you variety in your runs, and a display that shows the course and your progress can give you something to focus your attention on every now and then.
- A treadmill that allows you to program your own courses gives

FINE TREADS

Who makes a good treadmill? Many companies do. Here are several excellent treadmill manufacturers. Call to find a dealer near you.

- **Aerobics, Inc.:** call (201) 256-9700
- **Cybex International:** call (800) 228-6635
- **Icon (Pro Form):** call (800) 999-6750; see their web site at **www.iconfitness.com**
- **Landice:** call (800) 526-3423; see their web site at **www.landice.com**
- **Life Fitness:** call (800) 877-3867; see their web site at **www.lifefitness.com**
- **Precor:** call (800) 477-3267; see their web site at **www.precor.com**
- **True Fitness:** call (800) 426-6570; see their web site at **www.truefitness.com**

you infinite variety in the types of runs you do and allows you to practice your upcoming race.

- A cup holder that'll take your water bottle comes in handy for longer, harder runs.

Putting It to the Test

Don't buy a treadmill you haven't tried. Put on your running clothes and shoes and take this book to the shop with you. Test out several models. Run on each of them for about 10 minutes, paying attention to all the feel factors listed above. Go as high as you can on speed and then incline, noting how smoothly the machine shifts from one pace or height to the next and how stable it feels.

Visit a few different stores, test a variety of treadmills that have the features you're looking for, and then choose the one that feels good and fits you comfortably. It's a lot like buying a running shoe. In the end, it comes down to personal preference and what fits you best.

Hurt So Good

BY VIDA MORKUNAS

THE SUN IS SETTING. THE CLOUDS ARE PARTING. THERE WILL BE
no more rain. The track is dark, dirt soaked with water. On the far curve,
large puddles sit right at the bend.

We have gathered for our weekly speed workout, runners of all
abilities from the area. Tonight's workout is 10 400-meter repeats with
200-meter recoveries. We're split into four groups according to speed.
Coach John assigns a 2:10 pace for Ab and me.

I am a little cautious about going out too fast on the first round. Not
so Ab—he pulls me along. I push my legs, take long strides, relax my
upper body, and let the legs do all the work. We cross the 200-meter
mark in 55 seconds. Suddenly, striding becomes more difficult, but I
need to keep Ab in check. I struggle to keep up and succeed in finishing
at the same time as he—1:56.

We recover for 200 meters, then line up again. Ab screams, "*Go!*" I
think, *hunh?* And he's off again.

I'm striding, having fun, running through the puddles. Gosh, that
feels so good . . . just like being a little kid again, under ominous skies,
running to my heart's content, pushing, pushing, pushing . . .

If I am to post a good time, if I am to run like Ab, then I have to
concentrate. I have to banish all thoughts, especially the negative ones,
from my mind. And I have to want it. I have to want to run, to run fast,
to give it all I've got, to push till it hurts, to push till I'm almost out of
breath but not quite, till the legs burn, till I know that this is the best
that I possibly can give at this exact moment. I have to tap into the
absolute desire, the unwavering determination to finish what I started,
to get to the goal, to do what I set out to do. To finish the distance and
give it my best. And not think about it at all because thinking and
running at once don't bring results.

So there I am, at 200 meters again, running a 56, and I am thinking that I'd better speed up 'cause I am about to post a slower time than the first lap, and gee, it's gonna be hard 'cause there are puddles around the bend, and they are deep, and I wonder if I'm gonna lose a shoe in there eventually . . . and—of course—soon enough, Ab is gaining ground.

Then it's push, push, push to the end line, and I give it all I've got, and we cross the line in the same time, at the same time.

Eight more left!

I relax, think positively. I remind myself to be smooth, to flow, and to switch on that will, to push the body past the edge, to blank the thoughts. I concentrate only on form. Relax the legs. Pump the arms. Drop the shoulders. Keep breathing. Don't mind the squishy shoes.

There are two kids playing with a football in the center of the field. As I recover, I watch them play with a friendly retriever who's also trying to go for the ball. The dog is fast. The kids are simply tossing the ball to each other, but the dog really gives his all just for the ball.

I think of the dog as I bound out of the starting line. Our clothes are getting dirtier and dirtier. I run right through the puddles, the mud softening under my feet, becoming deeper and deeper with each lap. I feel the water flick on my back as I kick to push faster.

Ab refuses to tire. I refuse to let go. We run our last lap fast. I push all I can, till I see fireworks just outside my field of vision, till my legs cramp a little, till my throat burns from labored breathing.

And then it's over. Over. Over. Over. I feel joy. I pushed. I did my best. And it was good.

Vida Morkunas has written about her running experiences in *Ultrarunning* magazine and other publications. She currently lives in Vancouver, British Columbia, Canada, where she divides her time between her career in marketing, writing, and running.

PART VII

Racing

21 The Joy of Racing

Racing teaches us to challenge ourselves. It teaches us to push beyond where we thought we could go. It helps us to find out what we are made of.

—PattiSue Plumer, two-time Olympic 3,000-meter runner

"I'M AFRAID I'LL COME IN LAST."

"I'm too slow."

"I'm not competitive."

These are the reasons many women give for why they choose not to race. Although it's true that *someone* has to finish last, chances are it won't be you. Many women go to their first race with this fear, only to cross the finish line well ahead of other runners.

Too slow? No one is too slow to run a race. Many of today's races welcome walkers as well as runners of all abilities, and everyone is lauded for her participation.

FINISHING LAST

"I've come in last plenty of times. Once, the pickup car at the back of the race came up to me and the driver asked if I needed a ride back to the finish. I said no and kept on running.

"I don't race for speed or trophies but for social reasons. I like the excitement and the people cheering, and it's something my husband and I can do together. This isn't to say I'm not competitive. I always play a game to win, but with running I realize I have this one speed, and I'm not going to get much faster. In a race, I just take the attitude that I'll get there when I get there. My outlook is that I'm faster than the people who are there watching."

—SUE GETZ, RUNNER

Not competitive? Really? That's more often a cover for lack of confidence and fear of competition than it is the truth. Give racing a try or join in with a group of women who do speed training; you may be surprised at your desire to pass the person ahead of you—and then your excitement when you do. Even if you truly don't want to test your racing prowess against others, though, you can compete with yourself, striving to beat your best race times. As you do, you'll become fitter, mentally tougher, and you'll feel great about your accomplishment.

Reasons to Race

So you have no reason not to race, but why *should* you race? For sport, motivation, achievement, for a cause, but most of all for fun.

Good Times

It used to be that racing meant seeing who could run the fastest between two points, and races were pretty stark affairs. The gun fired; runners in dull-colored shorts charged down the road, crossed the finish line; some collected medals and all promptly went home. All that has changed, thanks to women (see chapter 30 to learn about women's influence on racing).

Races have now become "events." Hundreds, sometimes thousands, of runners of all ages and abilities, along with their friends and families, gather to walk or run 5-Ks, 10-Ks, and marathons. The courses are often very scenic. There's usually music at the start and the finish and maybe even a band or two along the way. Some events draw throngs of spectators cheering from the sidelines. Then there's the party afterward: food, drink, and general merriment. You choose the role you want: serious competitor, which includes anyone who puts forth her strongest and fastest effort, regardless of pace, or race reveler, who basks in the sights and sounds and the active spirit of hundreds of women and men running together.

Motivation and Improvement

Trainer Bob Greene used races as goals to help keep Oprah Winfrey on her running program, and it worked: she completed a marathon and lost 72 pounds. In my first couple of years as a runner, before running became a daily habit, I often found that when I didn't have a race planned, it was much easier to take a couple days off or allow my runs to get shorter.

If you have trouble getting out the door regularly, commit to doing a race even if you don't want to run it competitively. Any race will do—a 5-K, 10-K, 10-miler, marathon. Of course, the greater the distance, the longer your preparation will need to be. Write down a training schedule that takes you up to the date of that race. You'll need to follow that plan just to be able to run the race comfortably, so you're likely to stick to it.

WOMEN AND COMPETITION

In our male-dominated society, competition takes on a very aggressive meaning, says sports psychologist Jerry Lynch, Ph.D. "The male instinct is that of the warrior, and the traditional male competitor strives to beat his opponent into the ground," says Lynch. "It's no wonder that many women are turned off by the idea of competing." According to Lynch, the feminine nature approaches competition in a very different way, truer to the real definition of the word.

Compete comes from the Latin *competere,* meaning to strive together for (*com-,* together; *petere,* to seek). The feminine way of competition is to strive together toward the same end. Rather than annihilation of the opponent, it uses the collective strength of competitors to push individuals to their best performance.

Lynch points to the competitive relationship between Joan Benoit Samuelson and Grete Waitz in marathons as an example. Joan always welcomed Grete's presence because it helped her to race her very best. "Your competitor is a gift," says Lynch. "She gives you the opportunity to do your best."

Racing can further motivate you by providing athletic challenge. Finishing a race is exciting. Finishing your second race faster than your first is even more exhilarating. It's very easy to get caught up in the ecstasy of achievement, and as long as you set realistic goals for your races, you can continue to improve for a long time.

To Be an Athlete

Maybe you were never encouraged to play sports in high school or college or you didn't have the opportunity. One of the beauties of racing is that it embraces athletes of all abilities. You line up at the start right along with the very best in the sport, and you don't need speed to race competitively—just desire. Serious racers are those who follow a training plan geared to produce improved performances, and when they race, they do so to the very best of their ability. It doesn't matter if your best time for a 5-K is 27 minutes or 17 minutes; if you have trained well and raced hard, that is what makes you an athlete. The difference between running for fitness and running for athleticism is only a couple of "hard" runs a week, as you'll see in the following chapters.

A Stronger Self

Being an athlete enhances self-esteem. There is accomplishment, certainly, in simply running. When you take up racing as a sport and you train hard and challenge yourself every time to go faster, you feel an even greater sense of accomplishment. It's been only in recent history that women have had the freedom to express their full physical strength and stamina. That, too, makes our athletic achievements even more meaningful.

The Thrill of Victory

Victory occurs at many points in a race and for many runners, not just those who cross the finish line first.

Imagine this: You always run 25-something for 5-Ks. Your best and most recent time was 25:05. You're determined to break 25 minutes and you train diligently toward that goal. When race day arrives, you're a little nervous. You know you need to run at about an 8-minute pace. You run the first in 7:55—A little quick. You pass the second mile in 16:00. You're on pace, but you slowed down during that second mile. You pick it up just a bit, but can you hold on? You focus. Finally, around the corner onto the last stretch of road, you can see the finish line. You're breathing hard and it hurts, but you keep pushing. You see the clock: 24:51. You grit your teeth and push: 24:52, 24:53, 24:54, 24:55—you cross the finish line. You did it! You broke the 25-minute barrier.

Perhaps your goal is simply to run a strategic race—to go easy in the beginning and see if you can run faster in the second half. You do exactly that, running the early miles with effort but comfortably. Of course, it seems like everyone is passing you and you're at the back of the pack. With half the race to go, though, your pace starts getting faster and you feel good. You look to the runner just ahead of you and realize you're getting closer. You pass him, and then you look to the next runner. You reach her, and then she picks up the pace, not wanting you to pass. You stay right on her shoulder and eventually move ahead. With a mile to go, you pass runner after runner after runner who started the race too fast. You feel strong, and it inspires you to run even faster. A hundred yards from the finish, you kick it in, crossing the line in a good time, having run a perfect race and coming in first in your age group.

Improving your race times, using your strength and speed to pass other runners on the course, winning age-group awards—these are the victories that every runner can experience.

Women-Only Races

If you've never run a race before and the whole idea of it is a bit intimidating, start with an all-women event. You may feel more comfortable. The greatest aspect to these races, however, is the unique experience of sisterhood they offer. When you are running among thousands of women, you feel a special connection, a collective strength, a pride and significance in being a woman.

I recall feeling all of this at my very first women's race in 1986, what was then called the L'eggs Mini Marathon in New York's Central Park. This was just any other race, I thought. Then halfway into the first mile, I looked around at all the women running and was overcome with emotion. Besides the connection I felt to every other runner, there was the feeling that by running en masse through that park, we were asserting our significance in a world in which we are often made to feel insignificant. Together, that day, we had stepped out of the shadow of men.

I had a similar experience running the Idaho Women's Fitness Celebration in Boise in September 1997. There, over 17,000 women had come out to run or walk the 5-K. They hadn't come to raise money and awareness for a cause, as is the case at many women's races (causes are another good reason to participate in women-only events); they had come for themselves. Women of all ages, all sizes, and all abilities were there, to celebrate their fitness and good health.

We become so immersed in taking care of others—our children, our partners, our parents when they become less able, and our friends—that we readily put our needs second to the needs of others. For a day, at the Idaho Women's Fitness Celebration, 17,200 women affirmed their well-being, making a statement to themselves and to others about the significance of their health and fitness. No one there could help being affected by it.

WOMEN'S RACES

The number of women's races increases every year, especially as Race for the Cure spreads from city to city across the country. Here's a list of the country's best all-women events and race series.

Avon Running New York Mini Marathon

Formerly sponsored by L'eggs and then by Advil, this 10-K has become part of the Avon Running Global Women's Circuit (see below). It draws women of all abilities and showcases a front-running lineup of some of the fastest female distance runners in the world. With a beautiful course and a festive atmosphere, this is one fun race.

When: June

Where: New York, New York

For more information, contact:

New York Road Runners Club
9 E. 89th Street
New York, NY 10128
phone: (212) 860-4455

Avon Running Global Women's Circuit

New in 1998 but patterned after a running circuit Avon sponsored from 1978 to 1986, this series includes 11 events across the country and several overseas, culminating in a championship race to be held every November. Each event includes a 10-K run and 5-K walk. Women of all abilities are invited. Top women compete for points to qualify for a free trip to the championship race.

When: Races are held from April through November

Where: Atlanta, Baltimore, Chicago, Cincinnati, Dallas, Denver, Hartford (Connecticut), Kansas City, New York, Sacramento, Portland (Oregon)

For more information, contact:

Avon Running
1345 Avenue of the Americas, 27th floor
New York, NY 10105
phone: (212)-282-5350
web site: **www.avon.com/running/**

Freihofer's Run for Women

This 5-K is limited to 3,000 runners and welcomes everyone from first-timers to world-class athletes. Kids' races and a community walk make this an event for the whole family. The cite of the 5-K USA National Championships, Freihofer's draws the best female runners in the country.

When: May, usually

Where: Albany, New York

For more information, contact:

Freihofer's Run for Women
P.O. Box 1200
233 Fourth Street
Troy, NY 12180
phone: (518) 273-0267
web site: **www.freihofersrun.com**

Idaho Women's Fitness Celebration

One of the biggest women's running/walking events in the country, this 5-K event drew more than 19,000 women in only its sixth year in 1998. There are bands along the course, men in tuxedos cheering at every mile mark, and a huge celebration party at the finish in Ann Memorial Park.

When: September

Where: Boise, Idaho

For more information, contact:

Idaho Women's Fitness Celebration
511 W. Main Street
Boise, ID 83702
phone: 208-331-2221
web site: **www.celebrateall.org**

Race for the Cure

This series of mostly all-women run/walk 5-Ks was founded in 1983 in Dallas by Nancy Brinker, whose sister, Susan G. Komen, died of breast cancer. The goal of this series is to increase awareness about breast cancer and to raise funds for research, education, and screening. Many of the participants run in memory of a loved one or are themselves survivors of breast cancer. You can't run a Race for the Cure without being deeply touched by the cause and moved by the incredible stories of the participants.

When: Throughout the year

Where: In over 80 cities around the country as of 1998, with more added annually

For more information, contact:

    Susan G. Komen Breast Cancer Foundation

    Race for the Cure

    5005 LBJ Freeway, suite 370

    Dallas, TX 75244

    phone: (800) 653-5355

Tufts Health Plan 10-K for Women

This is another outstanding all-women race, attracting the country's best each year.

When: October

Where: Boston, Massachusetts

For more information, contact:

    Tufts Health Plan 10-K for Women

    250 Summer Street

    Boston, MA 02210

    phone: (617) 439-7700

Women's Distance Festival 5-K

Every year, under the supervision of the Road Runners Club of America (RRCA), this series of nearly 90 races takes place around the country.

When: Throughout the year

Where: Cities around the country

For more information, contact:

    Road Runners Club of America

    1150 S. Washington Street, suite 250

    Alexandria, VA 22314

    phone: (703) 836-0558

Mixed Races

A women's race offers a unique and very special experience, but this doesn't mean you won't have a great time racing in a mixed event. Running with men is fun, and though you will come across a few who can't stand it if you pass them, most men are very supportive of women runners.

Running is the least sexist sport there is. In very few sports do women and men compete one on one, equally, against each other— but to be a bit sexist and travel down the feminist road again, it feels great to beat out that guy who hates to be passed by a woman.

You'll find community in mixed races, too. Perhaps because it is so mentally and physically demanding, running breaks down barriers between people and between sexes. It is a great equalizer because everyone who races hard is stripped down to his or her essential athleticism. The struggle is equal no matter what the level of talent or ability, man or woman. We *all* suffer the fatigue of exertion, the pains of pounding, the labor of breathing. Each of us struggles to squeeze out every bit of strength, speed, and endurance in our push for high performance. In the race to be our best, we are all the same. We share in each other's pain and glory regardless of sex, race, religion, or nationality.

22 Training to Race

RACING CAN BE INFECTIOUS. YOU RUN one, it's fun. You do another and run faster, that's even more exciting. Before you know it, you're looking to see just how fast you can run a 5-K or a 10-K or a marathon. At first you get faster just by running regularly and increasing your mileage, but eventually, if you want to continue to improve, you'll need to do some specific training other than runs at your usual pace.

The Principles of Training

You've heard it said that when you break a bone, it heals to become stronger than it was in the first place. That's the way training works. You stress your body, and it responds by becoming stronger and faster. Training to improve is a constant process of tearing down and rebuilding.

When you push your body to run harder than it's used to, you're causing extra stress to the muscles. In fact, you're breaking them down to a slight degree; this is why you feel sore after a race or after your first few speed workouts, a long run, or hills. During recovery, your muscles rebuild and become stronger in such a way that they'll be better able to handle that stress next time it comes around.

Hard–Easy

Of course, this cycle of breaking down and building up is why you need to alternate hard and easy days in your training. You must give your body time to recover from the stress of speed workouts or long runs or hills. If you don't, you will continue to break down even further until you are injured and can't run at all. Called overtraining, this is the primary cause of injury among runners.

Think about a house that gets hit by a hurricane. If you don't have time to repair it before another storm hits, more damage will occur. The structure will become even weaker, and it'll take you longer to rebuild it. Imagine if storm after storm after storm hit: eventually, the house would be a shambles. This is what happens to your body if you run hard every day. Without time to recover, you won't get stronger—you'll become weaker, and the damage to your body will increase until you are injured.

Specificity

Training isn't just a building process; it's also a learning process. When you run faster, longer, or hard up hills, your body learns what's required of those situations. All the chemical, nerve, and muscular reactions that take place will occur more readily as you repeat them over and over through training. This is the principle behind specificity of training. If you want to run fast, you need to do some speed workouts. If you want to run a marathon, you need to do long runs. If you are going to race on a hilly course, you need to practice running on hills. This is also why cross-training isn't necessarily going to make you a better runner. Though cycling, for example, requires many of the same muscular actions and reactions that running does, it isn't an exact match. Cross-training is effective, however, for those who become injured easily if they run every day.

It's like building a home. The house you would construct in southern Florida, where it's hot and humid, wouldn't perform very well through the winters of Minnesota. Your body is your house; you need to develop it in the ways that will allow it to perform its best under the conditions it will encounter. Think about what you want to do with your running—short races, long races, hilly races, hot races—then you can design a training plan that will help you achieve your goals.

The Biology of Training

To understand how different types of training can improve your running ability, it's helpful to know some basic physiology. Very simply, muscles contract to move your body down the street, up the trail, around the track, and over the hill, and those muscles need energy to perform. Your body produces energy in a variety of ways, the most prominent being a chemical reaction called oxidative metabolism, and the two main ingredients of that chemical reaction are glucose (blood sugar) and oxygen. Glucose circulates in your blood and is also stored as glycogen in your liver and muscles. Oxygen comes from your lungs. Both glucose and oxygen are delivered to your muscles through your bloodstream.

As oxygen and glucose are used by your muscles, they need to be replaced so that your muscles can continue to work. The harder your muscles work, such as when you run fast or uphill, the faster they use oxygen and glucose and the quicker these substances need to be replaced. To speed up delivery of oxygen and glucose, your heart pumps faster to move blood more quickly to working muscles. Now you can see why the harder you run, the higher your heart and breathing rates become.

The ability of your muscles to use oxygen and glucose for energy doesn't depend just on how quickly those substances get to your muscles, however. Once they get there, your body has to be able to process them quickly to produce energy. Just as you have a top running speed, your body has a maximum speed at which it can use oxygen. The scientific term for this is $\dot{V}O_2max$. It has absolutely nothing to do with your breathing rate or the size of your lungs. It refers to the ability of your muscles to make use of the oxygen that's delivered to them. Training at high intensity forces your body to use oxygen at a high rate, and eventually, you become more efficient at doing so.

Aerobic and Anaerobic Activity

You run, you need oxygen, your heart pumps oxygenated blood to your muscles, and your muscles use that oxygen to produce energy. You are running aerobically.

The faster you run, the faster your heart beats to get oxygen to your muscles. There comes a point, however, when your muscles simply can't process oxygen fast enough to produce the energy you need. Fortunately, your body has a backup system.

Your muscles also produce energy through a different metabolic process that burns the glycogen in your muscle without using oxygen. This is called anaerobic metabolism, and it creates several by-products, including lactic acid. These by-products are removed from the muscle, but generally not as fast as they are produced, so if you continue to exercise at a high intensity, they will accumulate. The point at which lactic acid and these other chemicals start collecting in your muscles is called the lactate threshold, or anaerobic threshold, and is an indication that you are running anaerobically.

Many runners mistakenly think that lactic acid brings on muscle fatigue, but this isn't true. It's other by-products of anaerobic metabolism that eventually cause your muscles to shut down if levels get too high. In fact, lactic acid can be used to produce energy. By training at high intensity, you teach your muscles to maintain intensity despite the accumulation of these metabolic by-products, plus your body becomes better at removing these fatigue-causing chemicals more quickly. The bottom line is that you can run faster without fatigue.

Running Economy

Probably the most important factor in how fast you run or race is efficiency. The higher your running efficiency, the less energy you will expend running at a given pace. The more you practice running, the more efficient you become at it. Through training, you develop better form, the chemical processes of energy metabolism speed up, and the transmission of signals from nerves to muscles that initiates contractions and movement occurs more quickly and smoothly. Running becomes easier and faster.

All types of training will improve your running economy, but one of the best ways is with very fast, short intervals (described on page 281). By running as fast as you can for 100 or 200 meters, you demand quick reactions from nerves and muscles and immediate production of energy to propel you forward. Do this over and over again, and your body will learn how to become more efficient.

Rhythmic Breathing

One of the most important aspects of training and racing is effort or pace. Different types of training require different paces: long runs—slow; intervals—fast. How do you know if you are running the right pace? You can find all kinds of charts and methods for figuring out what your pace should be for every kind of workout, and there's one in the appendix of this book on page 416. To use such a chart, you must first figure out your level of fitness by running a race or doing a timed mile at your best effort and then calculating what your pace per mile should be. Then ideally, you'd do all your training on measured and marked courses so you could check your watch along the way to make sure you're maintaining a 9-, 8-, or 7-minute-per-mile pace. Fortunately, there's a more convenient way to gauge your running pace—by paying attention to your breathing. It makes perfect sense: the quicker and harder you run, the quicker and harder you breathe.

Rhythmic breathing is a specific method of gauging running effort. It involves coordinating your breathing with your stride cadence such that you inhale and exhale over an odd number of foot strikes. We discussed it in chapter 5, but here again is how it works.

For Relaxed Running

With all of your runs, except speed workouts, your effort and breathing should be comfortable so that you can inhale for three steps and exhale for two steps (a 3:2 ratio).

Footstrike	Breathing Pattern
Left	Inhale
Right	Inhale
Left	Inhale
Right	*Exhale*
Left	*Exhale*
Right	Inhale
Left	Inhale
Right	Inhale
Left	*Exhale*
Right	*Exhale*

For Fast-Paced Running

When you are running intervals or a race, your breathing rate is much faster, so you will be inhaling for only two steps and exhaling on one (a 2:1 ratio).

Footstrike	Breathing Pattern
Left	Inhale
Right	Inhale
Left	*Exhale*
Right	Inhale
Left	Inhale
Right	*Exhale*

To Monitor Your Pace

At first, learning to breath using the 3:2 pattern may be difficult, unless this is your natural rhythm, but within a week, it will become second nature. Then when you run hard, such as during a speed-training session, you will automatically shift into a 2:1 breathing pattern.

This doesn't mean you have only two speeds, slow and fast. You have a whole range of paces. The most significant point to remember, though, is that once your breathing has shifted into a 2:1 pattern, it means you are running anaerobically, and this is the effort you want to maintain when you are doing speed training or when you are racing a 5-K.

If you are running hard but are able to maintain a 3:2 breathing pattern, it means you are very close to your anaerobic threshold. This is the effort you want to maintain during tempo runs, described on page 286. By paying attention to your breathing when you run, you will learn how to correlate different intensities of breathing with different intensities of effort, and you won't need to rely on a heart monitor or your watch to tell you that you are running the right pace.

Furthermore, gauging your effort through rhythmic breathing means that you are running according to your body, not to some predetermined pace that may be appropriate one day but not the next. Some days you feel energetic, and you run faster because running (and breathing) feel easier. When you're tired, you'll run more slowly, which is what you should do. Though improvement in running requires that you push yourself into an uncomfortable zone during certain workouts, you should still always be running at an effort that's appropriate for you. By practicing rhythmic breathing, you will become finely attuned to your body and you will know instinctively whether you are pushing too hard or not hard enough.

Now that you have a better understanding of what training is all about, let's look at the different types of training and workouts and how each can help your performance.

Endurance

Endurance is the ability to run at a given pace for an extended period of time. The most obvious example in racing is the marathon, in which you set out to run at a particular pace for 26.2 miles. What many people may not realize is that endurance is essential even in the mile, where your goal is to maintain a very fast pace for a relatively long time. It's one thing to run fast for 100, 200, or 300 meters, but to keep running fast for 1,600 meters (approximately 1 mile) requires stamina.

You can improve your endurance by increasing your weekly mileage, but the more efficient and effective way is with a weekly long run. Runners who complete marathons on low mileage do so by making sure they include long runs in their training, but more on that in chapter 24. Whether or not you're training for a marathon, it's always good to go a little longer 1 day a week.

What defines a long run? It's simply the longest run you do each week. The length depends on your goals. If you're training for a 5-K, you may run no more than 4 to 8 miles on your long run. Those who have more time to train and want to improve their endurance for stronger 5-K performances might choose to run 12 to 15 miles for their long run. Marathoners will run 15 to 22 miles once a week in preparation for their event. Regardless of the distance, long runs tax your body. Limit them to once a week and follow up with 1 or 2 days of rest, which might be short, slow runs; a day off; or cross-training. Run them at a relaxed pace that allows you to chat with a friend. Your breathing should feel easy.

I've heard the terms warmup and cool-down. What do they mean?

A warmup is the 10–15 minutes of easy running you do before running hard and fast in training or in a race. It loosens up your muscles and brings your heart rate and metabolism up in preparation for the high intensity of running you are about to do. Not only can a warmup improve your performance by getting your body ready to run, but it prevents injury that might occur with the shock of sudden fast running.

A cool-down is the relaxed 10–15 minutes of running you do at the end of a quality run or race. It eases your heart rate and metabolism gradually back toward a resting rate and decreases the pooling of blood in your legs. Also, after your muscles have been working hard, they respond by tightening up. Add some stretching here and your legs will feel refreshed.

Speed

When most runners think about speed training, what comes to mind are intervals, also called pace workouts, and this is the best form of training if you want to get faster. There are other ways to work on your speed, however, including running up hills, and each has its benefit.

Fartlek

Swedish for "speed play," *fartlek* really is fun because it is so random and spontaneous. You head out on one of your favorite training runs, preferably one with few hills or this won't be so enjoyable. After you've warmed up with 10 to 15 minutes of relaxed running, pick a point in the distance—a tree, a mailbox, a street sign—and then run fast (hard but comfortably) to that point. Slow down, and then when you're ready to run hard again, pick another landmark and go. Continue in this way, alternating fast and slow running as many times as you desire, and finish with 10 to 15 minutes at a slow pace. You can double the fun by doing a *fartlek* run with a friend, taking turns calling out a landmark and leading to that point.

Fartlek is a great way to introduce yourself to speed training if you've never done any before, or if you haven't done any in a while—it's more relaxed than other types of workouts are and you're less likely to overdo it. On the other hand, if you've been doing intense pace workouts on the track week after week, *fartlek* provides a great mental break and can be a way to motivate yourself to do some speed training when thoughts of repeat quarter-miles make you moan. Even those who don't want to race can use *fartlek* to put a little variety into their running.

PARTNER POWER

The beauty of running is that you can do it on your own; you're not dependent on finding a friend or group to train with. When it comes to long runs, hill runs, or speed sessions, however, running with someone helps with motivation and effort. Time flies on a long run when you're flying along with a friend, and the conversation prevents you from dwelling on any discomfort.

You won't be talking too much during a speed session, but doing it with friends allows you to tap into the group energy, which helps you maintain your fast pace more easily than if you were on your own. Also, by planning to meet friends for pace workouts, you're more likely to do them week after week. It's not easy to find the motivation to go to the track and run your butt off by yourself. If your friends don't run, join a running club. Most organize group speed workouts and long runs for members. You might also ask at your local specialty running shop if the store offers group runs.

You can always start a local women's running group, as a friend of mine, Jane Serues, has done in my hometown. Every Tuesday night at 5:30 P.M., anywhere from 20 to 40 women of all ages and levels of ability gather in the local park to run speed workouts. We've discovered faster legs and new friends.

Pickups

Pickups are a more structured form of *fartlek*. Rather than randomly switching paces, you'll go by time, using your watch. For example, if you were to do 1-minute pickups, you'd pick up your pace (hard but comfortable effort) for 1 minute, then slow down for 1 minute, then pick it up for 1 minute, and so on. As always, finish off your workout with a cool-down.

You can structure pickups in any number of ways. Here are a few examples:

- Halve the recovery. Run 8 to 10 pickups of 2 minutes each with 1 minute of recovery between each.
- Repeat a set of pickups. Run 1 minute hard, 1 minute easy; 2 minutes hard, 2 minutes easy; 3 minutes hard, 3 minutes easy. Repeat this set once or twice.
- Do a "ladder." Run pickups of 1, 2, 3, 4, and 5 minutes, following each pickup with an equal amount of slow running, and then come back down the ladder with pickups of 4, 3, and 2 minutes and 1 minute.

Like *fartlek,* pickups are a good way to begin speed training if you're new to speed work or haven't done it in a while. For runners who are more advanced in their training and want to do two speed sessions a week, use either pickups or *fartlek* for a good second session, as they are less intense than tempo runs or pace workouts, described below.

Pace Workouts (Intervals)

When most runners think about speed training, pace workouts (also called intervals) come to mind. They make up the heart of your speed training as you prepare to race. Intervals teach you to run fast, and they raise your anaerobic threshold and $\dot{V}o_2$max.

A pace workout involves running several measured distances at a fast pace with slow recoveries in between. For example, if you were going to run six "quarters," you'd run 400 meters (quarter-mile) fast, then recover by running 200 meters very slowly, and repeat this sequence five more times. All the fast running in these workouts should be done at your anaerobic pace, the effort that forces you into a 2:1 breathing pattern. This pace is also roughly equivalent to your 5-K pace. It should be hard but not so hard that you are totally out of breath after each fast effort. Also, you should be able to maintain the same pace for each of the fast segments. If you slow down, it means you've been running too hard. Run the recoveries very slowly. This allows your muscles to "catch their breath" before you run hard again. As with any other form of speed training, warm up to prepare your legs for the intensity of fast running and cool down to prevent muscles from tightening.

Usually, intervals are done on a track, where you can easily figure the distance. Most outdoor tracks measure 400 meters (approximately a quarter-mile) around. Obviously, 2 laps would be 800 meters or a half-mile; 3 laps, three quarters of a mile; and 4 laps, a mile. Another advantage to the track is that the surface is flat and even, which allows you to run at a consistent pace. You don't have to go to a track, though, if you know of a bike path or cinder trail where distances are marked. Check with your local running club to find out where they run intervals, and then consider joining them so you'll have some company.

Do pace workouts during the weeks of preparation leading up to a race. If you plan to run several races over a period of 6 or 7 months, doing intervals once a week will keep you race ready. You'll find specific pace workouts in the next two chapters.

Fast-Paced Intervals

Fast-paced intervals improve running economy and develop explosive speed. A workout might include very fast repeats of 100, 200, and/or 300 meters. They are run at close to an all-out effort, with a good recovery after each repeat. For example, if you were doing 12 superfast 200s, you'd run very slowly for 200 meters after each one.

Do fast-paced intervals when your goal is to run a fast, short race—a 5-K or mile. Runners who have been doing regular interval training consistently each week can supplement that training with fast-paced intervals once a week.

Tempo Runs

Tempo runs help build "speed endurance" because they force you to run hard continuously, simulating the race experience somewhat. They're also known as threshold or lactate threshold training because they raise your lactate threshold (the point at which your body begins to work anaerobically). To do a tempo run, warm up, then pick up the tempo to a pace that feels hard but not fast—faster than a regular training run but slower than intervals. You should still be able to maintain a 3:2 breathing pattern, but you'll be on the edge of switching over to a faster 2:1 pattern. Maintain this pace for at least 10 minutes; 15 to 20 is preferable. Beyond 20 minutes, the training gains you'll make are negligible.

Because these workouts emphasize maintaining speed for an extended period of time, they are most useful when you are training for 10-Ks or longer races.

Hill Training

If you want to improve your running, head for the hills. They help you develop leg strength, power, stamina, speed, running efficiency, and mental toughness. Running hills is a teeth-gritting struggle with gravity, but it's worth it.

If you can, run on grass. Perhaps there's a college or high-school cross-country course nearby, or seek out hills in a nearby park or a public golf course where the golfers are few and friendly.

Hill training generally takes two forms: you can run a course with several challenging hills, or you can do hill repeats in which you run up and down one hill repeatedly—hard and fast on the way up, slow and easy on the way down.

The Long and Hilly Road

A good way to break into hill training, whether you have never really run hills before or haven't in a while, is to start with a hilly run. Begin with a route that takes you over gentle inclines. As you get stronger, search out courses that force you up longer and steeper climbs. Your goal should be to eventually run a course with several long hills—hills that take you at least 3 minutes to climb. Of course, the longer the better. Running long hills is a form of continuous resistance training for the legs. It builds strength and stamina and ultimately, a quicker pace. If you really want to spike up your speed, however, you'll do some hill repeats.

Do hill training anytime you want to work on leg strength, but back off of hills a month before an important race. You won't lose your strength gains; instead, you can turn your attention to sharpening your speed. You should plan to do hill running if you are training for a hilly race. It's also a good idea to run some hilly routes before attempting hill repeats, which are more strenuous.

Hill Repeats

If there's one running workout that will make you feel like you've become a bit masochistic in your training, it's hill repeats. To run hard up a hill once is no big deal, but to turn around and do it again and again and again and again . . . hope nobody's watching.

There are long hill repeats and short hill repeats. Do them both. Long hills (3 minutes or more to run) are like pace workouts. They will improve your $\dot{V}o_2$max and running economy and raise your anaerobic threshold. Your effort should be hard but controlled so that you can maintain your pace all the way to the top. If you have to slack off before you get to the top, you're running too fast. Run very slowly to the bottom of the hill and go again. Start with three repeats and work your way up to six.

When you are running repeats on short hills (about 200 meters in length), you *do* want to do them fast. Run them at just about an all-out effort, pushing at the very top as if you are trying to beat someone to the finish line. Short hill repeats improve your running economy and develop explosive speed in your legs (a speed that comes from a combination of quickness and strength). Aim for 5 or 6 in your first session and work up to 8 to 10 as you get stronger.

Try to find a location for repeats that offers both a short and a long hill so you can mix both in the same workout. Run a few short, fast ones first, then do a couple of long hills, and top off the session with a few more quick climbs. For your first session, try three short hills, one or two long, and three short. As you get stronger, work your way up to four short hills, three long, and four short. You could do this same workout on a long hill by running only partway up for the short portions of the session. As with any hard training run, be sure to warm up and cool down.

Since running hill repeats is similar to running intervals, you shouldn't do both workouts each week. Hill repeats are best done when you want to build strength and speed and you don't have any really special races coming up. In the month before a race in which you're hoping to run really well, however, drop them from your training and switch to intervals instead. Actually, hill repeats will get your legs ready to do high-quality speed training on the track.

Downhills

Running downhill fast offers certain unique benefits. It improves leg speed because your legs turn over quickly. (Think of your legs as spokes on a bike wheel. As the bike descends a hill, those spokes move much more rapidly in their circle; so do your legs when you run downhill.) More important, though, is that downhill running uses what's called an eccentric contraction of your muscles versus the usual concentric contraction. Research shows that regularly working your muscles eccentrically helps prevent the muscle soreness that comes with running hard. It's especially effective in preventing the soreness most runners experience after racing a course that has a lot of downhills or after running a marathon.

A *word of caution:* fast downhill running is not for everyone. It's especially hard on your legs because, with the eccentric contraction, your muscles are elongating and resisting at the same time. Only if you are a relatively injury-free runner should you consider fast downhill running in your training.

If you decide to give it a try, start on slight declines and gradually move to steeper slopes. When running downhills, you may be inclined to lean back—that's part of the natural tendency to "brake" so you don't go too fast—but resist this tendency. Relax, lean forward, shorten your stride a little and just allow your body to flow down the hill like a river. The more relaxed you are, the better.

Every now and then when you are doing a long hilly run, rather than running comfortably on the downhill portions, run them fast.

Rest

A day off from running . . . an easy 3-miler . . . doesn't seem like you're doing much at all on rest days that will help you become a better runner, but beneath the surface, your body is working hard to rebuild after those six quarter-mile hill repeats you did yesterday. A crew of hundreds of little construction molecules is scurrying around to shore up your bones, repair tiny muscle tears, restock your spent glycogen stores, and clear up any debris—waste products left lying around after the energy combustion needed to power your muscles.

It's on the rest days of training that your body actually gets stronger and faster. Rest is just as important to improvement as long runs, intervals, and hill repeats are. Those runners who don't believe this and who run hard day after day soon learn this lesson. They become fatigued and sluggish when running, and their race performances decline. If they keep up this pattern of relentlessly hard training, they'll become injured.

What qualifies as rest? A day off from running and all other exercise, cross-training, or a short, easy run. What's best? That depends on your level of training, but more important, on what fits your lifestyle and your physiology. Some runners find they are healthier and happier if they run every other day and do cross-training or take days off in between. Other runners prefer to run 6 or 7 days a week, resting with very easy runs between their hard training days.

New runners who have done little physical activity of any kind in their recent past would be best to take 2 or 3 days off each week. As you gradually increase your mileage, you can experiment with cross-training or a mix of hard and easy runs.

Rest after every hard workout you do, whether it's a long run, a speed session, a challenging hilly course, or hill repeats.

Putting the Pieces Together

Okay, so now you have long runs, pace workouts, tempo runs, hill repeats, and long hilly runs. Yikes! When do you do what? Fortunately, you'll find training schedules in the next two chapters that will tell you exactly how to prepare for a 5-K, 10-K, half-marathon, or marathon—but, hey, maybe you want to take charge of your own training and write your own schedule. Maybe you don't have any races in mind, but you'd like to do some training to improve your speed and strength. Here are some principles to follow and some suggestions to consider in combining all these different types of training into your running plans:

- Add one new element of training at a time, whether that's a long run, a speed session, or a hill workout. Once you feel comfortable with that new element, you can add another. Give yourself 3 to 4 weeks to become accustomed to each element.
- If you aren't planning to race for several months, consider adding these training elements in the following order: long runs, hills, and then speed. The long runs and hills build your endurance, strength, and pace and prepare you for pace workouts (intervals), which are the ultimate way to sharpen your speed and make you fast.
- Limit yourself to three hard runs a week: one long run, one speed session, and one hill run, for example. When you want to focus primarily on getting faster, you can drop the hill run and do two speed workouts.
- If you choose to do two speed workouts a week, mix them up: intervals and a tempo run or intervals and pickups or intervals and fast-paced intervals.
- The total distance you do in speed training each week should not exceed 10 percent of your total weekly mileage. If you run 20 miles a week, that's 2 miles.
- When you begin speed training—whether you've never done any or haven't done any in a few months—it's a good idea to do pickups or *fartlek* for a few weeks before running more formal intervals. Once you move on to intervals, begin with short distances and low total mileage (for example 200s and 400s for a total of 1½ miles of speed) and work up to longer distances (half-mile, three quarters of a mile, mile) and more total mileage.
- Tailor your interval workouts to the type of races you want to do. Run short, fast distances if you like 5-Ks; run longer distances for half-marathon and marathon training.
- Plan at least 1 rest day after every hard run. Don't do hard runs back to back.

- Fatigue, irritability, sluggishness during runs, and nagging aches and pains are signs of overtraining. Cut back on your quality workouts, reduce your mileage, and consider taking a few days off until your energy comes back; then gradually return to a higher level of training if that is your plan.

SAMPLE TRAINING WEEK

A week that includes all the training elements discussed in this chapter might look like this:

- Sunday: long run
- Monday: day off
- Tuesday: relaxed run
- Wednesday: speed session
- Thursday: relaxed run
- Friday: hills
- Saturday: day off

Training to improve isn't just a lot of hard work. Yes, running hills, long distances, and speed workouts is difficult, and you'll experience discomfort with each of them. But every time you finish a long run or climb to the top of a challenging hill or run fast, you enjoy the exhilaration of accomplishment. The rewards of training don't come with just one final excellent race; you receive them every week, with every challenging run you take.

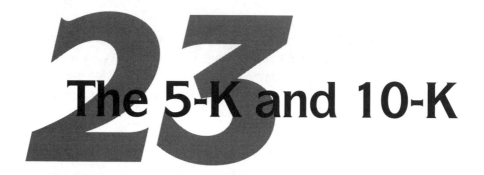

The 5-K and 10-K

THE 5-K IS THE MOST POPULAR RACE distance of all. It's short, quick, and you don't have to be able to run very far or very fast to participate in one. If you can run 3 miles, you can run a 5-K (3.1 miles). A 10-K is twice as far (6.2 miles) but doesn't require any more training than a 5-K does. You can run either distance simply for the fun of it on 12 to 15 miles a week, but if your goal is also to run fast, you'll need to do some specific training.

The challenge of racing a 5-K or 10-K is to run quickly for a relatively long time. In training, there are three quality runs you should do each week: a long run for endurance, a pace workout for speed, and strides, also for speed. As for weekly mileage, you can train on as little as 12 to 15 miles or as much as 45, but keep your long run to 16 miles or less. Any longer and the fatigue from that run will detract from the quality of your speed training. The amount of mileage you decide to run each week depends on how much time you have to train and how many miles you want to do. Following are three schedules to choose from.

COACH COATES

All the training schedules in this book were designed by Budd Coates, marathoner, coach, corporate fitness director for Rodale Press in Emmaus, Pennsylvania, and advisor to *Runner's World* magazine. There are many excellent coaches and many excellent training schedules available to runners. Why did I choose Budd to design the schedules for this book?

He has coached runners of all levels, from beginners training for their first 5-K to marathoners hoping to qualify for the Olympic trials. Budd himself is a nationally ranked marathoner with a best time of 2:13, and he has qualified for and run the Olympic marathon trials four times. That he has been able to maintain such a high level of performance for so many years is a tribute to his own well-planned training. Budd has a master's degree in exercise physiology, but he takes his education onto the street and practices everything he preaches.

Budd's training schedules are designed for "real people." He takes into account that most runners have busy lifestyles that demand a lot of time and energy, and he offers plans that will help you run your best given the time you have to train—they are high-quality programs that are also practical.

My biggest reason for asking Budd to design the training programs in this book, however, is that I know his plans work. By following Budd's schedules and advice, I lowered my 5-K time from 27 minutes to 21 and my 10-K time from 54 to 43 minutes, and I went from being a 4-hour marathoner to a 3½-hour marathoner and qualifying for and running the Boston Marathon twice. I've won one local 10-K, have finished second in another, and have placed often in my age group at races of all distances. In my 13 years of running and racing so far, I've had only one injury. I am not a natural athlete. My running accomplishments have come through my commitment to running my best and following Budd's good training programs. May you achieve success with them, too.

5-K and 10-K Training Schedules

The three schedules presented here will prepare you to run either a 5-K or a 10-K. The bronze schedule is for runners who don't have a lot of time to train, for those who haven't been running very many miles, or for runners who don't want to run very many miles each week. The silver schedule is a step up in mileage and intensity, and the gold plan takes you to an even higher level of training.

Does this mean the gold schedule is the best and that you'll run your fastest if you follow its workouts? Not necessarily. If your lifestyle allows for it, the more challenging training plan would produce the best race performances, but you cannot separate running from the rest of your life. You have only so much time and energy for career or school, family, friends, and other interests, including running. If you live a very demanding or stressful lifestyle, running high mileage and/or at high intensity might just push you beyond the anaerobic threshold of your life. Eventually, you'll become fatigued and overtrained and your performances won't meet your expectations. In such situations, you'll race better on a less-intense running schedule that doesn't overload your energy capacity. Only you can decide the right balance and the right running program.

The following plans designate specific amounts of mileage on specific days of the week. You can shift the schedules up or back a day, depending on what works best for you, but keep the workouts in the same order with the same rest days between.

Bronze

The Bronze schedule is an 8-week training plan based on 12 to 17 miles a week.

MILES

Week	Sun.	Mon.	Tues.	Wed.	Thurs.	Fri.	Sat.
1	3	2	0	3P	2	2	0
2	4	2	0	3P	2	2	0
3	5	2	0	4P	2	2	0
4	5	2	0	4P	2	3	0
5	6	2	0	4P	2	3	0
6	7	2	0	4P	2	3S	0
7	6	2	0	4P	2	3S	0
8	8	2	0	4P	2	3S	0
Race preparation	6	2	0	3P	2	0	2
Race/recovery **Race**		2	0	3P	2	3S	0

P = pace workout (3P = 3-mile pace workout); S = strides (3S = 3 miles with strides).

PACE WORKOUTS

See How to Run Pace Workouts below so that you'll be able to understand exactly how to do the following workouts.

- **Week 1:** 1 mile easy; 4 × 400 meters (recover for 200 meters); ½ mile easy
- **Week 2:** Same as week 1
- **Week 3:** 1 mile easy; 2 × 400 meters (recover for 200 meters); 1 × 800 meters (recover for 400 meters); 2 × 400 meters (recover for 200 meters); ½ mile easy
- **Week 4:** Same as week 3
- **Week 5:** 1 mile easy; 2 × 400 meters (recover for 200 meters); 2 × 800 meters (recover for 400 meters); ½ mile easy
- **Week 6:** 1 mile easy; 1 × 400 meters (recover for 200 meters); 1 × 800 meters (recover for 400 meters); 1 × 1,200 meters (recover for 400 meters); ½ mile easy
- **Week 7:** 1 mile easy; 1 × 400 meters (recover for 200 meters); 1 × 1 mile (recover for 400 meters); 1 × 400 meters (recover for 200 meters); ½ mile easy
- **Week 8:** 1 mile easy; 6 × 400 meters (recover for 200 meters); ½ mile easy

HOW TO RUN PACE WORKOUTS

Let's use week 3 from the Bronze schedule as an example: 1 mile easy; 2 × 400 meters (recover for 200 meters); 1 × 800 meters (recover for 400 meters); 2 × 400 meters (recover for 200 meters); ½ mile easy.

- **1 mile easy:** This is the warmup, which is run relaxed at a 3:2 breathing rhythm (see chapter 22 if you need to review rhythmic breathing).

- **2 x 400 meters (recover for 200 meters):** This is the fast stuff. Run 400 meters (about 400 yards or ¼ mile) at your anaerobic pace, which puts you into the 2:1 breathing rhythm. This is also equivalent to your 5-K race pace. Do two of these, and after each, recover by running half the distance (200 meters) very slowly.

- **1 x 800 meters (recover for 400 meters):** Run 800 meters (about 800 yards or ½ mile) at pace and recover by running half the distance very slowly.

- **2 x 400 meters (recover for 200 meters):** This is the same as above.

- **1/2 mile easy:** Cool down with a ½ mile of relaxed running.

- **Race preparation week:** 1 mile easy; 4 × 400 meters (recover for 200 meters); ½ mile easy
- **Race/recovery week:** 1 mile easy; 2 × 200 meters (recover for 200 meters); 2 × 400 meters (recover for 200 meters); 2 × 200 meters (recover for 200 meters); ½ mile easy

STRIDES

Warm up with 1 mile of easy running, then alternate 20 seconds of fast running (same speed as pace workouts) and 40 seconds of easy running eight times; finish running at an easy pace.

BEYOND BRONZE

Where do you go from here? You can simply continue training at this level, following the workouts for week 8 and switching to the race preparation and race/recovery weeks any time you decide to race. For pace workouts choose from those given for weeks 6, 7, and 8. If you want to increase your level of training, you can move to the Silver schedule in this chapter or the Bronze half-marathon schedule in the next chapter.

Silver

The Silver schedule is an 8-week program that builds from 17 to 32 weekly miles.

MILES

Week	Sun.	Mon.	Tues.	Wed.	Thurs.	Fri.	Sat.
1	6	2	0	4P	2	3S	0
2	8	2	0	4P	2	4S	0
3	6	3	0	5P	2	4S	0
4	10	3	0	5P	3	4S	0
5	8	3	0	6P	3	5S	0
6	12	3	0	6P	3	6S	0
7	8–10	3	0	6–8P	3	6S	0
8	12–14	3	0	6P	3	6S	0
Race preparation	6–8	3	0	6P	2	0	2
Race/recovery **Race**	3	0	6–7P	3	4–6S	0

P = pace workout (4P = 4-mile pace workout); S = strides (3S = 3 miles with strides).

PACE WORKOUTS

See How to Run Pace Workouts on page 295 so that you'll be able to understand exactly how to do the following workouts.

- **Week 1:** 1 mile easy; 2 × 400 meters (recover for 200 meters); 2 × 800 meters (recover for 400 meters); ½ mile easy
- **Week 2:** 1 mile easy; 1 × 400 meters (recover for 200 meters); 1 × 800 meters (recover for 400 meters); 1 × 1,200 meters (recover for 400 meters); ½ mile easy
- **Week 3:** 1 mile easy; 1 × 400 meters (recover for 200 meters); 1 × 800 meters (recover for 400 meters); 1 × 1,200 meters (recover for 400 meters); 1 × 800 meters (recover for 400 meters); 1 × 400 meters; 1 mile easy
- **Week 4:** 1 mile easy; 1 × 400 meters (recover for 200 meters); 1 × 1 mile (recover for 400 meters); 1 × 400 meters (recover for 200 meters); 1 × 1,200 meters (recover for 400 meters); 1 × 400 meters; 1 mile easy
- **Week 5:** 1½ miles easy; 1 × 400 meters (recover for 200 meters); 2 × 1 mile (recover for 400 meters); 1 × 400 meters; 1 mile easy
- **Week 6:** 1½ miles easy; 1 × 400 meters (recover for 200 meters); 1 × 1½ miles (recover for 800 meters); 1 × 800 meters (recover for 400 meters); 1 × 400 meters; 1 mile easy
- **Week 7:** 1½ to 2 miles easy; 1 × 400 meters (recover for 200 meters); 4 × 800 meters (recover for 400 meters); 1 × 400 meters; 1 to 2 miles easy
- **Week 8:** 1½ to 2 miles easy; 6 to 8 × 400 meters (recover for 200 meters); 1 to 2 miles easy
- **Race preparation week:** 1 to 2 miles easy; 6 × 300 meters (recover for 100 meters); 1 to 2 miles easy
- **Race/recovery week:** 1 to 2 miles easy; 2 × 400 meters (recover for 200 meters); 1 × 800 meters (recover for 400 meters); 2 × 400 meters (recover for 200 meters); 1 to 2 miles easy

STRIDES

Warm up with 1 mile of easy running, then alternate 20 seconds of fast running (same speed as for pace workouts) and 40 seconds of easy running eight times; finish running at an easy pace.

BEYOND SILVER

After recovering from your race, you can continue to train, alternating the routines for weeks 7 and 8. For pace workouts, select from any of the ones described. You can also move up to the Gold schedule in this chapter or to the Silver half-marathon program in the next chapter.

Gold

The Gold schedule is an 8-week program that starts at 28 miles in the first week and builds to a maximum of 46.

MILES

Week	Sun.	Mon.	Tues.	Wed.	Thurs.	Fri.	Sat.
1	8	3	2	6P	3	6S	0–3
2	10	3	2	6P	3	6S	0–3
3	8	3	4	6P	3	6S	0–3
4	12	3	4	6P	3	6S	0–3
5	10	3	4	6–8P	3–4	6S	0–3
6	12	3	4	6–8P	3–4	6–8S	0–3
7	10–12	3	4	6–8P	3–4	6–8S	0–3
8	14–16	3	4	6–8P	3–4	6–8S	0–3
Race preparation	8–12	3	4	6P	3	0	3S
Race/recovery **Race**		3	3–4	6P	3–4	6–8	0–3

P = pace workout (6P = 6-mile pace workout); S = strides (6S = 6 miles with strides).

PACE WORKOUTS

See How to Run Pace Workouts on page 295 so that you'll be able to understand exactly how to do the following workouts.

- **Week 1:** 1½ miles easy; 1 × 400 meters (recover for 200 meters); 1 × 800 meters (recover for 400 meters); 1 × 1,200 meters (recover for 400 meters); 1 × 800 meters (recover for 400 meters); 1 × 400 meters; 1½ miles easy
- **Week 2:** 1½ miles easy; 1 × 400 meters (recover for 200 meters); 1 × 800 meters (recover for 400 meters); 1 × 1 mile (recover for 400 meters); 1 × 800 meters (recover for 400 meters); 1 × 400 meters; 1½ miles easy
- **Week 3:** 1½ miles easy; 1 × 400 meters (recover for 200 meters); 1 × 1 mile (recover for 400 meters); 1 × 400 meters (recover for 200 meters); 1 × 1,200 meters (recover for 400 meters); 1 × 400 meters; 1½ miles easy
- **Week 4:** 1½ miles easy; 1 × 400 meters (recover for 200 meters); 2 × 1 mile (recover for 400 meters); 1 × 400 meters; 1½ miles easy
- **Week 5:** 2 miles easy; 1 × 400 meters (recover for 200 meters); 1 × 1 mile (recover for 400 meters); 1 × 800 meters (recover for 400

meters); 1 × 1 mile (recover for 400 meters); 1 × 400 meters; 2 miles easy

- **Week 6:** 2 miles easy; 1 × 400 meters (recover for 200 meters); 1 × 2 miles (recover for 1 mile); 1 × 800 meters (recover for 400 meters); 1 × 400 meters; 2 miles easy
- **Week 7:** 2 miles easy; 1 × 400 meters (recover for 200 meters); 6 × 800 meters (recover for 400 meters); 1 × 400 meters; 2 miles easy
- **Week 8:** 2 miles easy; 8 to 10 × 400 meters (recover for 200 meters); 2 miles easy
- **Race preparation week:** 2 miles easy; 6 to 8 × 300 meters (recover for 100 meters); 2 miles easy
- **Race/recovery week:** 2 miles easy; 2 × 400 meters (recover for 200 meters); 2 or 3 × 800 meters (recover for 400 meters); 2 × 400 meters (recover for 200 meters); 2 miles easy

STRIDES

Warm up with 2 miles of easy running, then alternate 20 seconds of fast running (same speed as for pace workouts) and 40 seconds of easy running eight times; finish running at an easy pace.

BEYOND GOLD

You can continue to train with this schedule by alternating the routines for weeks 7 and 8 and using the pace workouts described. You can also move up to half-marathon or marathon training as explained in the next chapter.

Notes and Variations

As you are following a training plan, if you notice signs that you are doing too much—fatigue, sluggishness, irritability—go back to an easier week of training. When you feel recovered and ready to do more, then you can progress to the next level.

When you miss a workout, *don't* try to make it up; just continue with whatever comes next on the schedule. If you should miss a whole week of training, however, do begin with that week's plan when you start running again. Whenever you stop running for several weeks because of injury or an overabundance of commitments other than running, you may need to start back with some walk–runs and gradually build up to your previous level of fitness.

The training schedules in this chapter will prepare you to race well at either the 5-K or 10-K distance. If you don't have a race coming up in 8 weeks, though, you can use these schedules as a basic blueprint for your running and make some alterations based on your overall goals and interests. For example, if you want to run on hills to get stronger, you could do a hilly run on Friday in place of strides. If you'd rather do hill repeats, substitute those for the pace workouts on Wednesdays. Are you tempted by tempo runs? Do them on Fridays in place of strides or even Wednesdays as a break from pace workouts. The Wednesday pace session is the highest-quality run you do each week, so if you want to improve, stick with it. If you need a break from the intensity of pace sessions, however, do *fartlek* or pickups instead. One other note: the best time to do strength training in the schedules given is on Tuesdays and Thursdays, and if you want to do a third session, Saturday.

It's a good idea to keep a training log and write down what you've run each day, along with notes about how you felt. Record every race you participate in and your time. After several months, review what you've written and look for patterns that will help you learn what training methods work best for you. With experience, too, you develop an intuitive sense of what kind of workouts you should do and when you should do them to help you achieve your goals.

TEN TOP U.S. RACES

The following races have a reputation among runners for being well organized, well attended, fast, and fun. All of these regularly appear on the *Runner's World* list of top 100 races published each February.

Bay to Breakers 12-K

Where: San Francisco, California

When: May

What: A zany "costume party" for 7.4 miles through the streets of San Francisco. About 70,000 runners participate in this event, which literally leads them from the bay to the ocean and then to a massive party in Golden Gate Park.

Contact:

> *Examiner* Bay to Breakers
> P.O. Box 429200
> San Francisco, CA 94124
> phone: (415) 512-5000, x2222

Bix 7-Mile

Where: Davenport, Iowa

When: July

What: A hot one with a monster hill, but runners love this event named for jazz musician Bix Beiderbecke.

Contact:

> Ed Froelich
> 2685 E. Kimberly Road
> Bettendorf, IA 52772
> phone: (319) 359-9197

Bolder Boulder 10-K

Where: Boulder, Colorado

When: May

What: Another popular race even though it's at high altitude (don't expect a personal record [PR] here) in one of the country's running meccas

Contact:

> Bolder Boulder
> P.O. Box 9125
> Boulder, CO 80301
> phone: (303) 444-7223

Carlsbad 5000

Where: Carlsbad, California

When: April

What: A flat, fast 5-K with lots of runners and spectators in a great setting

Contact:

> Elite Racing
> 10509 Vista Sorrento Parkway, suite 102
> San Diego, CA 92121
> phone: (619) 450-6510

Crescent City Classic 10-K

Where: New Orleans, Louisiana

When: March

What: A 6.2-mile party with great food and music afterward

Contact:

> Crescent City Classic
> P.O. Box 13587
> New Orleans, LA 70185
> phone: (504) 861-8686

Falmouth 7.1-Mile

Where: Falmouth, Massachusetts

When: August

What: One of the oldest races in the country; a Cape Cod course that offers some beautiful scenery

Contact:

> John Carroll
> P.O. Box 732
> Falmouth, MA 02541
> phone: (508) 540-7000

Lilac Bloomsday 12-K

Where: Spokane, Washington

When: May

What: A 7.4-mile race and one of the biggest in the country with more than 55,000 finishers

Contact:

> Lilac Bloomsday Association
> P.O. Box 1511
> Spokane, WA 99210
> phone: (509) 838-1579

Peachtree Road Race 10-K

Where: Atlanta, Georgia

When: July 4

What: Kick off the fourth with a blast at Peachtree. Finish in under an hour and you'll receive a special, much-coveted T-shirt.

Contact:

> Peachtree Road Race
> 3097 Shadowland Avenue
> Atlanta, GA 30305
> phone: (404) 231-9065

Runner's World Midnight Run 5-K

Where: New York, New York

When: December 31

What: One of the best ways to celebrate New Year's Eve—a fun run in Central Park

Contact:

> New York Road Runners Club
> 9 E. 89th Street
> New York, NY 10128
> phone: (212) 860-4455

Utica Boilermaker 15-K

Where: Utica, New York

When: July

What: Almost 10 miles. This race is loved by its enthusiastic participants, who claim it to be the best race in the country.

Contact:

Earle Reed

P.O. Box 4729

Utica, NY 13504

phone: (315) 797-1310

ROAD RUNNERS CLUB OF AMERICA

Traveling to another state and want to find a race to run? Check with the Road Runners Club of America (RRCA). They have listings of events and running clubs around the country. Contact them at 1150 S. Washington Street, suite 250, Alexandria, VA 22314, or check out their web site: **www.rrca.org.**

The Final Countdown

It's 7 days until the big race, time to hone your readiness. Refrain from doing any hill running or weight lifting; you need to rest so that you will be fresh and at full force on race day. Even your running training lightens up in the last week. This is called the taper, and it's essential to a good performance.

Don't think you can cram in any more speed training to make you race faster. You have built all the speed, strength, and endurance you're going to for this event. By running too much or too fast in this final week, you can only hurt your performance. There is, however, some mental training you can do.

Visualization

If you have seen the course you'll be running, visualization can be an especially effective mental technique to prepare you for the race. You only need 10 to 15 minutes. Find a quiet place where you won't be interrupted. Begin by taking five deep abdominal breaths to help you relax and focus. Close your eyes and imagine the race in your mind.

See all the details: you're standing at the starting line, excited yet calm, a little nervous but confident; the horn blows and you're running carefully among the throng of runners; eventually, everyone

PRACTICE TACTICS

A friend of mine, Megan Othersen Gorman, a runner and assistant coach of a women's running group, occasionally has the group practice the following race tactics during a training session.

- **Catch a runner:** A tactic that can help you maintain your pace or even pick it up when you are getting tired is to focus on catching the runner just ahead of you. Plan a workout with a friend in which one of you runs 25 to 30 feet in front of the other at a relaxed pace. After a few minutes, the runner in back picks up the pace to gradually catch the runner in front and then go ahead 25 to 30 feet. Then whoever's in the back must catch the runner in front, and so on.
- **Passing:** Sometimes you catch up to a runner and you suddenly find yourself in competition with that person. You want to pass, but you're a little nervous about the effort it requires. By practicing passing during training, you'll learn that it doesn't take much effort at all. Enlist a friend for a casual run; after 1 or 2 miles, run one just ahead of the other and take turns passing each other for a few miles.
- **A strong finish:** It's not easy to run strong at the end of a 5-K or 10-K; if you've been racing at your best effort, you're really tired. This is where your mental power can pull you through. During one of the last couple of speed workouts before your race, as you run each fast interval, imagine that you are running the final few hundred meters of a race. See yourself pushing toward the finish, picking up speed, and sprinting across the line. When you're approaching the real finish line, recall how you trained for this and go for it.

spreads out along the road and you have room to run and get into your pace. Your breathing is hard but not labored, your form is smooth and even. Picture yourself at each hill in the course, pushing smoothly up and over and gliding down the other side. With each mile, you get a little faster. You're running strongly and smoothly in good form. You're passing other runners. You come to the stone church, and you know there's only a quarter-mile left to go. Fatigue is coming on, but you're still running strong, and you push a little harder. Finally, you turn the corner onto Main Street and the last 200 yards. You accelerate smoothly until you are in a sprint to the finish, and you burst across the line in your best 5-K time ever!

Even if you don't know the course, simply imagine yourself racing fast and powerfully. Picture a runner whose form you admire and see yourself running with that same grace, stride, and efficient movement. Recall race strategies that have worked in the past, such as focusing on a runner in front of you, catching that person, and then running by.

Many of the country's best runners use visualization successfully, and most sports psychologists recommend it. It works because your body is easily fooled. Whether the image it's presented with is real or imagined, your body produces the same physiological response. By visualizing yourself racing well, both your mind and body will become conditioned for a good performance, and then you'll produce one when the real race arrives. Try to practice visualization once a day every day in the week preceding an important race.

Nutrition

When your upcoming race is a 5-K or 10-K, you don't need to be too concerned about what you eat the week before. Follow your usual high-carbohydrate, low-fat diet and drink plenty of fluids—the nonalcoholic, noncaffeinated kind—so you'll be well hydrated, especially if the weather's warm.

The day before your race, be careful to eat foods that digest easily and won't cause you intestinal problems the next day. The intensity of effort that goes into racing a 5-K or 10-K places more stress on your gastrointestinal tract than running a longer, slower race would. You need to be even more careful during your menstrual period, when changing hormones can cause looser bowel movements. Avoid very spicy meals and foods high in fiber.

Should you eat the morning of your race? For a 5-K, it's not necessary. Over such a short distance, your glycogen stores will not be depleted, but if you will feel better prepared by fueling up beforehand, then have a snack—toast, a bagel, or an English muffin—1 or 2 hours before you race.

Before a 10-K, a light breakfast can help you perform better. Cereal with milk, a bagel, and a banana—or any high-carbohydrate meal of about 400 calories that you know will digest easily—is appropriate. If real food doesn't sit too well with you, try sports bars, which are formulated for easy digestion, or a high-carbohydrate sports beverage. You can make your own liquid meal in a blender—a fruit smoothie, for example. Consume this light meal 2 to 4 hours before race time. Through trial and error, you'll learn what foods you can tolerate and how much time you need for digestion. If you can't tolerate any food the morning of your race, don't worry about it. Eat a good-size dinner the evening before and a high-carbohydrate snack before bedtime.

Sleep

Try to get your usual requirement of sleep during the final week, and then don't worry if you have insomnia the night before your race. As long as you've rested well on the previous days, your performance will not be affected.

Race Day Tips and Strategies

First and most important, know that you have trained well for this race. You can go to the starting line confident that you are prepared to run your very best. Following are several tips to help further your racing success.

Don't Try Anything New

Don't try any new foods, beverages, shoes, or clothing. A fresh pair of running shoes—even a different style of sock than you're used to wearing—might just cause blisters bad enough to ruin your race.

Warm Up Just Before the Start

Run slowly for 10 to 20 minutes before the race to loosen your muscles and rev up your metabolism. If you want to stretch, do so

DRESS FOR SUCCESS

What should you wear for your race? Whatever you find comfortable for your speed workouts will be best for racing. Usually a singlet and shorts or a T-shirt and shorts will be fine, even when the temperature is in the midforties. You'll warm up quickly once the race is underway. On a cool day, wear long pants or tights over your shorts and a long-sleeved shirt or jacket over your T-shirt to keep warm before the race and then climb into them again afterward.

When the degrees dip into the low forties or thirties, wear a long-sleeved shirt and a pair of gloves. Change shorts to tights as the mercury in the thermometer approaches freezing. Fabrics should be breathable so that the sweat you generate will quickly evaporate.

It's better to be a bit underdressed than overdressed because you will get warm once you start running. If you tend to get cold easily, however, consider wearing two tops—a singlet or T-shirt and a long-sleeved breathable shirt that you can take off and tie around your waist if you become too warm.

after you've run for a mile or so when your muscles are more flexible. Experts recommend that you keep moving even when you are lined up waiting for the start. You can do this by running in place.

Use the Porta Potti Early

Long lines always form outside the portable toilets. You don't want to get caught inside when the gun goes off, so use the Porta Potti early.

Don't Go Out Too Fast

The single most important piece of advice to follow when racing is don't start too fast. Many runners think that they should run as hard as they can and try to hold on to that pace. It doesn't work very well. What happens is that you just become fatigued early in the race and end up slowing down and finishing poorly. Trust me—I know; I've done it.

Surprising to most runners is the fact that you can start out a little slower than your goal pace and get faster along the way. It's true; I've done this also. It makes for a great race experience. Think about it: you start at a hard but controlled pace while all the inexperienced runners around you are flying wildly down the road as if they're in a sprint. By the second half of the race, though, they're slowing down, their form's a little wobbly, and they're breathing hard. Meanwhile, you're feeling good and running powerfully, you've picked up your pace, and you smoothly pass runner after runner as you cruise on down to the finish line.

That's great, but what's the right pace to start at? Using rhythmic breathing as your gauge (see pages 280 through 282 in chapter 22 for details), you should be running at an effort that puts you just into the 2:1 breathing pattern for a 5-K. It should feel hard but not all-out. Remember, you have to keep it up for 3 miles.

For the 10-K, your effort should be a little more relaxed so that you are still breathing in a 3:2 rhythm—although close to having to cross over into a faster 2:1 rate. You will probably move into the 2:1 rhythm by about mile 3. If you've been timing your pace workouts during training, you can also use the table "Pace per Mile" on page 416 of the appendix to determine what your per-mile race pace should be. The more experience you gain at racing, the more attuned you will become to your body and the easier it will be to instinctively know if you are running at the right effort.

How important is it to take water during the race? Is a sports drink like Gatorade even better than water?

The 5-K is short enough that if you are well hydrated beforehand, you don't have to take water during the race unless it's a hot day, but do drink during a 10-K. Water can take anywhere from 10 to 20 minutes to pass through your digestive tract and then out through your body, so drink early in the race. Sports beverages can be helpful in races that last 90 minutes or more when you'll be burning lots of carbohydrates, but you won't need them for either a 5-K or 10-K.

Feed Off the Energy of Other Runners

You are racing among hundreds of other runners, and you can all help each other. Try to run near or with a group of runners who seem to be of the same ability as you. It'll keep your energy up and make the effort feel easier.

Maintain Effort on Hills

Don't do a heart-pounding, panting charge up the hills. Run with the same effort you used on the flats. Shorten your stride but don't change your stride rate. Yes, you'll be running more slowly, but you'll reach the top with energy to run faster on the downhill and through the rest of the race. If you expend all your effort on the hills, your race will be over way before you get to the finish line.

Relax

In the later miles of a race as you start to fatigue and the effort feels harder, it is not uncommon for your muscles to tighten and your form to deteriorate. When you start to notice discomfort, make a conscious effort to focus on your form, correct your posture if it's slumped, bring your arm swing into proper position if it has become too high or if your arms are crossing too far over your body, and concentrate on relaxing.

Relax? While you're running as hard as you can? It sounds like a contradiction, but it is possible, and it will help you perform better. Tension takes energy and it holds your body back from running smoothly. By relaxing your muscles, you can release that energy to the task of running.

RELAXATION RESPONSE

Jerry Lynch, Ph.D., sports psychologist and author of *Thinking Body, Dancing Mind* (New York: Bantam, 1992), offers a way to help calm your nerves before a race or to relax during a race. He calls it anchoring. Get yourself into a relaxed state. While you are in that state, repeat the word *relax* over and over again in your mind as you are experiencing this inner calm and peacefulness. Those feelings become tied to the word *relax,* so that when you think that word before or during a race, it will immediately trigger those same feelings and all the associated physiological responses of relaxation.

Lynch says you can also anchor the relaxation response to a physical cue. For example, when in a peaceful state, form a circle with your thumb and index finger. Tell yourself that whenever you make this circle, you will become relaxed just as you are now.

Start with your face: relax the furrowed brow. Move on to your neck and shoulders . . . think, *Relax* . . . allow your shoulders to drop down. Make sure your arms are swinging smoothly and close to your body; your hands should be loose, not clenched. Breathe fully from your abdomen and repeat the word *relax* again and again in your mind.

Divide the Course and Conquer

If you're having a difficult race and you feel like you want to drop out, pick a point on the course and say to yourself, *Okay, I'll run just to that point.* When you get there, pick another point, and so on. You may find eventually that you'll have a resurgence of energy that will carry you more easily through the rest of the race. Sometimes if you just push through a bad patch, you'll get to a point of renewed energy.

Reel Runners In on Your Way to the Finish

The last half-mile of any race is difficult. You're fighting muscle fatigue and working hard to pick up the pace or even maintain your speed to the finish. By focusing on trying to catch the runner ahead of you, you'll be more motivated to keep running hard. Also, by looking up rather than down at your feet, you'll run with a better stride. Even more important, though, is that if you catch and pass that person, you're one up in the race results. This can mean the difference in whether you win an age-group award if that runner is a woman.

Why do I sometimes feel nauseated at the end of a hard workout or competition?

"We don't really know why," says Ted L. Edwards, Jr., M.D., a gastroenterologist and sports medicine specialist who has worked with runners and cyclists in Austin, Texas, for 25 years. "But when you push yourself beyond the limit, it produces a vagal response—you feel exhausted and nauseated."

Edwards has been prescribing bromelain to the athletes he works with. It's a natural anti-inflammatory found in the stems of pineapple. You can purchase it in health-food stores as Bromelain 2000. "The runners take two two hundred fifty milligram capsules before and after a race, and it seems to be working," says Edwards.

Edwards also advises avoiding sports beverages and drinking only water in the 2 hours prior to a hard workout or competition. Finally, don't take ibuprofen or aspirin before an intense effort: they may contribute to heat exhaustion and nausea in some people, says Edwards.

After the Race

When you cross through the finish, drink some water or a sports beverage right away to start replacing fluids and keep moving to prevent your muscles from tightening up. Ideally, you should do a cooldown—a slow run of 1 or 2 miles—just as you would after a speed session. Then get something to eat. Sports nutritionist Nancy Clark, M.S., R.D., recommends that after a race, you consume 0.5 gram of carbohydrate per pound of body weight every 2 hours for 6 to 8 hours. For a 130-pound woman, that's 65 grams, or 260 calories.

The best foods to choose from are those with a moderate to high glycemic index, which digest quickly and speed through your bloodstream to your muscles for fast recovery. Bagels, cereals, bananas, and oranges—all the foods you typically find at a postrace celebration—are good choices. (See Glycemic Index on page 82 in chapter 8 for others.) A little protein—some milk or yogurt—along with those carbohydrates speeds recovery even more.

So eat, drink, share race stories with your friends, and congratulate yourself on your accomplishment. Oh, and stick around for the awards ceremony; you may just have placed first, second, or third in your age group. Besides, it's important to share in the success of those who have run along with you (even if ahead of you) for those 3 or 6 miles.

24
The Marathon and Half-Marathon

YOU WON'T BE ABLE TO RESIST DOING ONE. It's surrounded by intrigue, challenge, and risk and promises rewards of extraordinary accomplishment to all who complete its course. It's the marathon—26.2 miles—the ultimate distance event for runners.

The marathon has become more popular than ever, a testimony to our curiosity about the outer reaches of our strength and endurance— and women are running marathons like never before. "In the 80s, approximately 10 percent of the finishers were female," reports USA Track & Field in their newsletter *On The Road.* "By 1996, 28 percent of marathon finishers were women."

And the marathon just might be the race for us. Women have high thresholds of discomfort, as is evidenced every time a baby is born, and our endurance extends a long way. Look at Ann Trason, who has won outright several ultramarathons and has come very close to victory overall at the Western States 100-Mile Endurance Run, one of the most prestigious ultra trail runs around. Many studies have suggested that women burn more fat than men during exercise, which would be an advantage for long-distance events; however, experts have not yet concluded that we have greater endurance than men do.

Though the marathon tempts many new runners, it's best to get your feet warm with a year of running and racing before charging on into marathon training. You might want to consider doing a half-marathon on your way to the full distance.

Half-Marathon Training Schedules

The following training schedules will prepare you to race a half-marathon—13.1 miles. You'll see that the only significant differences between training for a 5-K or 10-K (discussed in the last chapter) and the half-marathon are the length of the long run and the amount of weekly mileage. You'll do the same speed workouts; what you need to develop now is endurance.

Bronze, Silver, and Gold designate plans of low, medium, and high mileage and intensity, respectively. Each is a continuation of the 5-K/10-K schedules in the previous chapter. Choose the plan that dovetails with your current level of training and fits in the available time you have for running. For example, if you've been running 15 to 20 miles a week and don't have time for much more, you should choose the Bronze schedule rather than the Silver or Gold.

Bronze

The Bronze half-marathon schedule is a continuation of the Bronze 5-K/10-K training plan in the previous chapter. Week 1 below is the same as week 8 from the 10-K plan. The weekly mileage for this program builds to a maximum of 25 miles.

MILES

Week	Sun.	Mon.	Tues.	Wed.	Thurs.	Fri.	Sat.
1	8	2	0	4P	2	3	0
2	10	2	0	4P	3	4S	0
3	8	3	0	5P	4	4S	0
4	12	2	0	5P	3	0	2
5	10-K race*	2	0	6P	3	0	3
6	8	2	0	4P	3	0	2
7	Half-marathon	0	0	2	0	3	0
8	4–6	0	2	4P	2	3	0

P = pace workout (4P = 4-mile pace workout); S = strides (4S = 4-mile run with strides).

*On this day, race either a 10-K or 5-miler or run 15 miles.

PACE WORKOUTS

Rotate the following pace workouts on Wednesdays. The length of the warmup and cool-down will depend on the total mileage required for that day's workout. (If you need to review how to do these workouts, see How to Run Pace Workouts on page 295.)

- **The roller coaster:** Warm up; 1 × 400 meters (recover for 200 meters); 1 × 1 mile (recover for 400 meters); 1 × 400 (recover for 200 meters); 1 × 1,200 meters (recover for 400 meters); 1 × 400 meters; cool down
- **Miles:** Warm up; 1 × 400 meters (recover for 200 meters); 2 × 1 mile (recover for 400 meters); 1 × 400 meters; cool down
- **The peak:** Warm up; 1 × 400 meters (recover for 200 meters); 1 × 1½ miles (recover for 800 meters); 1 × 800 meters (recover for 400 meters); 1 × 400 meters; cool down
- **Halves:** Warm up; 1 × 400 meters (recover for 200 meters); 4 × 800 meters (recover for 400 meters); 1 × 400 meters; cool down
- **Race preparation week:** Warm up; 6 × 300 meters (recover for 100 meters); cool down
- **Race/recovery week:** Warm up; 2 × 400 meters (recover for 200 meters); 1 × 800 meters (recover for 400 meters); 2 × 400 meters (recover for 200 meters); cool down

STRIDES

Warm up with 1 mile of easy running, then alternate 20 seconds of fast running (same speed as for pace workouts) and 40 seconds of easy running eight times; finish running at an easy pace.

Silver

The Silver half-marathon schedule is a continuation of the Silver 5-K/10-K training plan in the previous chapter. Week 1 below is the same as week 7 from the 10-K plan. The mileage required in this program ranges from 28 to 36.

MILES

Week	Sun.	Mon.	Tues.	Wed.	Thurs.	Fri.	Sat.
1	10	3	0	6P	3	6S	0
2	12–14	3	0	6P	3	6S	0
3	10	3	0	8P	3	6S	0
4	14–16	3	0	8P	3	6S	0
5	10-K race*	3	0	6P	4	6–8S	0
6	8–10	3	0	4P	3	0	3
7	Half-marathon	0	0	2–4	0	3	0
8	6–8	3	0	4P	3	4	0

P = pace workout (6P = 6-mile pace workout); S = strides (6S = 6-mile run with strides).

*On this day, race either a 10-K or a 5-miler or run 16–18 miles.

PACE WORKOUTS

Rotate the following pace workouts on Wednesdays. The length of the warmup and cool-down will depend on the total mileage required for that day's workout. (If you need to review how to do these workouts, see How to Run Pace Workouts on page 295.)

- **The roller coaster:** Warm up; 1 × 400 meters (recover for 200 meters); 1 × 1 mile (recover for 400 meters); 1 × 400 (recover for 200 meters); 1 × 1,200 meters (recover for 400 meters); 1 × 400; cool down
- **Miles:** Warm up; 1 × 400 meters (recover for 200 meters); 2 × 1 mile (recover for 400 meters); 1 × 400 meters; cool down
- **The peak:** Warm up; 1 × 400 meters (recover for 200 meters); 1 × 1½ miles (recover for 800 meters); 1 × 800 meters (recover for 400 meters); 1 × 400 meters; cool down
- **Halves:** Warm up; 1 × 400 meters (recover for 200 meters); 4 × 800 meters (recover for 400 meters); 1 × 400 meters; cool down
- **Race preparation week:** Warm up; 6 × 300 meters (recover for 100 meters); cool down
- **Race/recovery week:** Warm up; 2 × 400 meters (recover for 200 meters); 1 × 800 meters (recover for 400 meters); 2 × 400 meters (recover for 200 meters); cool down

STRIDES

Warm up with 1 mile of easy running, then alternate 20 seconds of fast running (same speed as for pace workouts) and 40 seconds of easy running eight times; finish running at an easy pace.

Gold

The Gold half-marathon schedule is a continuation of the Gold 5-K/10-K training plan in the previous chapter. Week 1 below is the same as week 7 from the 10-K plan. The mileage required for this program ranges from 41 to 47.

MILES

Week	Sun.	Mon.	Tues.	Wed.	Thurs.	Fri.	Sat.
1	10–12	3	6	8P	3	6S	0–3
2	14–16	3	6	8P	4	8S	0–3
3	10	3	6	8–10P	4	6S	0–3
4	16–18	3	4–6	8P	3	6S	0–3
5	10-K race*	3	6	8P	4	8S	0–3
6	8–10	3	4	6P	3	0	3S
7	Half-marathon	0	0–3	2–4	0	4	0
8	6–10	3	4	6P	3	4	0

P = pace workout (8P = 8-mile pace workout); S = strides (6S = 6-mile run with strides).

*On this day, race either a 10-K or a 5-miler or run 18–20 miles.

PACE WORKOUTS

Rotate the following pace workouts on Wednesdays. The length of the warmup and cool-down will depend on the total mileage required for that day's workout. (If you need to review how to do these workouts, see How to Run Pace Workouts on page 295.)

- **The ladder:** Warm up; 1 × 400 meters (recover for 200 meters); 1 × 800 meters (recover for 400 meters); 1 × 1 mile (recover for 400 meters); 1 × 800 meters (recover for 400 meters); 1 × 400 meters; cool down
- **The rollercoaster:** Warm up; 1 × 400 meters (recover for 200 meters); 1 × 1 mile (recover for 400 meters); 1 × 400 meters (recover for 200 meters); 1 × 1,200 meters (recover for 400 meters); 1 × 400 meters; cool down
- **Miles:** Warm up; 1 × 400 meters (recover for 200 meters); 2 × 1 mile (recover for 400 meters); 1 × 400 meters; cool down
- **The M workout:** Warm up; 1 × 400 meters (recover for 200

meters); 1 × 1 mile (recover for 400 meters); 1 × 800 meters
(recover for 400 meters); 1 × 1 mile (recover for 400 meters); 1 ×
400 meters; cool down
- **The 2-miler:** Warm up; 1 × 400 meters (recover for 200 meters);
1 × 2 miles (recover for 1 mile); 1 × 800 meters (recover for 400
meters); 1 × 400 meters; cool down
- **Halves:** Warm up; 1 × 400 meters (recover for 200 meters); 6 ×
800 meters (recover for 400 meters); 1 × 400 meters; cool down
- **Race preparation week:** 2 miles easy; 6 to 8 × 300 meters
(recover for 100 meters); 2 miles easy
- **Race/recovery week:** 2 miles easy; 2 × 400 meters (recover for
200 meters); 2 or 3 × 800 meters (recover for 400 meters); 2 ×
400 meters (recover for 200 meters); 2 miles easy

STRIDES
Warm up with 1 mile of easy running, then alternate 20 seconds
of fast running (same speed as for pace workouts) and 40 seconds of
easy running eight times; finish running at an easy pace.

Marathon Training Schedules

Training for a marathon is certainly challenging, but don't let
thoughts of it overwhelm you. If your goal is to complete the distance
whatever the time it takes (and this is an excellent goal for your first
26.2-mile journey), the training is very doable; the Bronze schedule
starts out with a 19-mile week and requires no more than 31 miles
for the hardest week of training.

The most important workout, of course, is the long run. If you have
the psychological energy for only one quality effort a week, this is the
one to do. Long runs build endurance, which is essential to completion
of a marathon. They also teach your body to burn fat and conserve
glycogen, another important asset when running long distances. Anytime you are running for 90 minutes or more, your metabolism shifts
to burn more fat so that you don't use up all your glycogen stores,
which are good to have on hand in an emergency when you need
energy fast and which are necessary to keep your brain functioning.
With several training runs of 10 miles or more, you'll practice fat burning again and again and your body will become more efficient at it.

The second quality run you'll do each week is a pace workout.
Though you don't have to do speed training to complete a marathon,

you'll run a stronger and better-paced marathon if you do. Speed work prepares you to run your best, given the training plan you follow, and you'll be much more pleased with your marathon if you give it your best effort.

Again, the schedules are designated Bronze, Silver, and Gold on the basis of the level of weekly mileage and the intensity of the pace workouts. Each will prepare you well for the marathon. Which one you choose is a matter of the amount of time you have to train and what you are comfortable doing rather than your level of ability. An experienced female runner who's chief executive officer of a major corporation might have the ability to train on the Gold plan but the time for only the Bronze.

Bronze

If you can run 15 miles a week, including a long run of 6 miles, you're ready to start the Bronze marathon program, which begins with a 19-mile week and reaches a maximum of 31 miles. Do the pace workouts and strides given on page 313 for the Bronze half-marathon schedule.

MILES

Week	Sun.	Mon.	Tues.	Wed.	Thurs.	Fri.	Sat.
1	8	2	0	4P	2	3S	0
2	10	2	0	4P	2	4S	0
3	8	3	0	5P	2	4S	0
4	12	2	0	5P	3	5S	0
5	8	3	0	6P	3	5S	0
6	15	3	0	6P	4	5S	0
7	12	3	0	6P	4	6S	0
8	18	2	0	6P	4	6S	0
9	12	3	0	6P	4	4S	0
10	20	2	0	4–6P	3	0	2
11	10-K race*	3	0	6P	4	3S	0
12	8–10	2	0	4P	3	0	2
13	Marathon	0	0	2–3	0	2–3	0

P = pace workout (6P = 6-mile pace workout); S = strides (6S = 6-mile run with strides).

*On this day, race a 10-K or 5-miler or run 15 miles.

Silver

The Silver marathon schedule begins with a 28-mile week and progresses to 35 to 40 miles a week. Do pace workouts and strides given on pages 314 to 315 for the Silver half-marathon schedule.

MILES

Week	Sun.	Mon.	Tues.	Wed.	Thurs.	Fri.	Sat.
1	10	3	0	6P	3	6S	0
2	14	3	0	6P	3	6S	0
3	10	3	0	8P	3	6S	0
4	16	3	0	8P	4	6–8S	0
5	12	3	0	8P	4	6–8S	0
6	18	3	0	8P	4	8S	0
7	12	3	0	8P	4	6S	0
8	20	3	0	8P	4	8S	0
9	15	3	0	8P	4	6S	0
10	20–22	3	0	6–8P	3	0	3
11	10-K race*	3	0	8P	4	6S	0
12	10	3	0	6P	3	0	3
13	Marathon	0	0	2–3	0	3	0

P = pace workout (6P = 6-mile pace workout); S = strides (6S = 6-mile run with strides).

*On this day, race a 10-K or 5-miler or run 15 miles.

Gold

For runners who want a challenge and have the time to put in a lot of training for the marathon, the Gold marathon schedule starts you out at 38 miles, but most weeks will have you running around 50 miles. There are three high-quality workouts: the Sunday long run, a long pace workout midweek, and a fairly long run with strides. Do the pace workouts and strides given on pages 315 to 316 for the Gold half-marathon schedule. You'll definitely be ready for a marathon (PR) when you've completed this program.

MILES

Week	Sun.	Mon.	Tues.	Wed.	Thurs.	Fri.	Sat.
1	12	3	6	8P	3	6S	0
2	16	3	6	8P	3	6S	0
3	12	3	6	8–10P	3	6S	0
4	18	3	6	8P	4	8S	0
5	15	3–5	6	10P	4	8S	0
6	20	3	6	10P	4	8S	0
7	12–15	3–5	6	10P	4	8S	0
8	20–22	3	6	10P	4	8S	0
9	12–15	3–5	6	10P	4	8S	0
10	22	3	6	6–8P	3–4	0	3
11	10-K race*	3	6	6–8P	4	6S	0
12	10–12	3	4	6P	3	0	3
13	Marathon	0	0	3	0	3	0

P = pace workout (8P = 8-mile pace workout); S = strides (6S = 6-mile run with strides).

*On this day, race a 10-K or 5-miler or run 15 miles.

BOSTON MARATHON

Having celebrated its one hundredth year on April 15, 1996, the Boston Marathon is the oldest and most prestigious marathon in the world, in part because of its rich history but also because runners must qualify to participate. To run the Boston becomes the ultimate goal for many marathoners; it is a symbol of their achievement at this challenging distance.

To qualify, you must run a marathon within a certain time based on your age in the year prior to the Boston Marathon that you hope to enter. Here are the qualifying standards for women:

Age Group (years)	Marathon Time (hours: minutes)
18–34	3:40
35–39	3:45
40–44	3:50
45–49	3:55
50–54	4:00
55–59	4:05
60–64	4:10
65–69	4:15
70 and over	4:20

For more information about participating in the Boston Marathon, write the Boston Marathon, 131 Clarendon Street, 8th floor, Boston, MA 02116 or call (617) 236-1652.

A DOZEN MARATHONS

Pick your marathon before you start training so that you can tailor your running program in the ways that help you run your best on that particular course. Here are 10 to consider. Those marked with an asterisk are excellent choices for first-time marathoners.

Avenue of the Giants Marathon

Where: Weoff, California

When: May

Comments: A small marathon on a flat out-and-back course that takes you through redwood forest

Contact:

> Gay Gilchrist
> Six Rivers Running Club
> 281 Hidden Valley Road
> Bayside, CA 95524
> phone: (707) 443-1226

Big Sur Marathon

Where: Carmel, California

When: April

Comments: Very hilly but spectacular; be sure to do some hill training. The course travels up Route 1 along the coast. This is a good one to do just for fun.

Contact: Big Sur Marathon, Box 222620, Carmel, CA 93922; (408) 625-6226.

California International Marathon*

Where: Sacramento, California

When: December

Comments: The course has some gentle hills but still has earned a reputation for being fast.

Contact:

California International Marathon
P.O. Box 161149
Sacramento, CA 95816
phone: (916) 983-4622

Chicago Marathon*

Where: Chicago, Illinois

When: October

Comments: Flat and fast (except on windy days), the course takes you through several of Chicago's neighborhoods. Thousands of runners participate each year.

Contact:

Chicago Marathon
P.O. Box 10597
Chicago, IL 60610
phone: (312) 243-0003 or (888) 243-3344

Columbus Marathon*

Where: Columbus, Ohio

When: November

Comments: A big event, well-organized, flat and fast; a good one to consider if you're aiming for a personal record (PR)

Contact:

Columbus Marathon
P.O. Box 26806
Columbus, OH 43226
phone: (614) 433-0395

Grandma's Marathon*

Where: Duluth, Minnesota

When: June

Comments: A popular, well-organized marathon; the course is flat and fast and temperatures are usually just right for running

Contact:

> Grandma's Marathon
> P.O. Box 16234
> Duluth, MN 55816
> phone: (218) 727-0947

Honolulu Marathon*

Where: Honolulu, Hawaii

When: December

Comments: Lots of fun, scenic, many first-time marathoners; plan a vacation around this one

Contact:

> Honolulu Marathon Association
> 3435 Wailae Avenue, #208
> Honolulu, HI 96816
> phone: (808) 734-7200

Marine Corps Marathon*

Where: Washington, D.C.

When: October

Comments: A stunning tour of the nation's capital, this is one of the largest marathons in the country. It's well-organized, relatively flat, and fast.

Contact:

> Marine Corps Marathon
> P.O. Box 188
> Quantico, VA 22134
> phone: (703) 784-2225 or (800) 786-8762

New York City Marathon

Where: New York, New York

When: November

Comments: One of the most exciting marathons in the world. Over 25,000 runners from all over the world participate, and thousands of spectators line the course to cheer you on. On marathon day, the Big Apple shines. Get your entry in early; this race is so popular, entry is by lottery.

Contact:

> New York Marathon Entries
> P.O. Box 1388, G.P.O.
> New York, NY 10116
> phone: (212) 423-2249

Portland Marathon*

Where: Portland, Oregon

When: September

Comments: In addition to the marathon, several other races take place, including a kids' run. The marathon is relatively flat and fast.

Contact:

> Les Smith
> P.O. Box 4040
> Beaverton, OR 97076
> phone: (503) 226-1111

Twin Cities Marathon*

Where: St. Paul, Minnesota

When: October

Comments: Billed as the most beautiful urban marathon, and it is. The course winds through several parks with trees ablaze in fall colors. This is a fast marathon.

Contact:

> Twin Cities Marathon
> 708 N. First Street, suite CR-33
> Minneapolis, MN 55401
> phone: (612) 673-0778

Walt Disney World Marathon

Where: Orlando, Florida

When: January

Comments: A fairly flat course that heads into the park for a few miles; a good choice if you have kids

Contact:

> Walt Disney World Marathon
> P.O. Box 10000
> Lake Buena Vista, FL 32830
> phone: (407) 939-7810

Training Notes and Variations

Depending on the marathon you are training for, you may want to make a few adjustments to the schedules in this chapter. The first change you might want to make is to shift the schedule up or back a day during the week. For example, you may prefer to do your long run on Saturday instead of Sunday. Shift all the other workouts accordingly so that they are in the same order.

Long runs and pace workouts are rather sacred. They are most important for a good race performance, so be as consistent as you can about doing them each week. That being said, if you find a group to run speed sessions with, join it even if members aren't planning to do exactly the workout you have in mind, although it should be similar—you don't want be running a lot of 200-meter repeats if your goal is the half-marathon or marathon). It's much easier to run fast-paced workouts with other runners than to do them on your own, and you'll gain greater benefit by doing them in a group.

Hills

If the marathon you've chosen is a hilly one, you should do some hill runs. They require a lot of effort and therefore should take the place of one of the high-effort workouts of your week. Don't add them to an already challenging training schedule. If you want to do hill repeats, do them in place of the Wednesday pace workouts. A long hilly run is best scheduled on Friday instead of the usual strides.

Training on hills builds strength and power, but because you can't run as fast uphill as you can on flat roads, it's not as effective at stimulating speed as pace workouts are. Therefore, if you decide to do hill repeats in place of pace sessions, limit them to 3 or 4 weeks in the first half of your training program and then use the pace workouts to sharpen your speed. You'll also want to back off of long hilly runs in the last 2 weeks before the marathon.

Tempo Runs

If you like tempo runs and find they benefit your running, do them in place of strides on Fridays.

Strength Training

Plan your resistance workouts for days that call for relaxed running—Tuesday and Thursday, or Tuesday, Thursday, and Saturday if you prefer three sessions a week. A month before race day, stop weight training altogether and allow your muscles to focus specifically on running. You won't lose the strength you've gained.

Do I need to follow a special diet during marathon training?

Assuming that your usual diet follows the nutritional recommendations given in chapter 8, you don't need to make any changes in what you eat—just in how much you eat. You'll be burning many more calories during marathon training, so be sure to replace them. That'll be a piece of cake, since your appetite will naturally increase along with your mileage.

Speaking of cake, don't fall into thinking that because you are burning so many calories, you can eat anything you want, including cookies, chips, and other high-calorie, low-nutrient goodies. Consume snacks and desserts in moderation.

The Final Countdown

In the last 7 days before your marathon, you'll run the lowest weekly mileage of your total 3-month training program, and it's going to feel weird. By this point, you have become so accustomed to running lots of miles that this easy week may seem a bit of a shock to your mental and physical systems, but don't be tempted to run 1 mile farther than what's on your schedule.

This is one of those "less is more" situations. Your running preparation for the marathon is complete. You have gained all the speed, strength, and endurance you're going to. Any attempt to fit in one more intense speed workout, long run, tempo run—whatever—will prevent your body from getting enough rest and can only harm your performance on race day. The running you do should be very relaxed. It serves simply to keep your muscles loose and remind them of the physiological processes of running.

Despite this low-key training—called the taper because you are tapering the mileage and intensity of your training—plenty of internal preparation is going on. Just as a rest day gives your body a chance to recover and rebuild before your next tough workout, this rest week provides the time your body needs to fully replenish glycogen stores and completely regenerate after months of intense training. By race day, you should feel fresh and ready for your 26.2-mile challenge.

Carbo-Loading

Runners have tried all kinds of dietary manipulation to load up their muscles with carbohydrates for optimum marathon performance, including a carbohydrate depletion and loading plan that required eating a high-protein, low-carbohydrate diet for a few days to "starve" the muscles of carbos and then consuming very high carbohydrate foods, which your muscles would hungrily suck up for maximum glycogen storage. That was the theory, anyway. What we have finally learned is that following your normal training diet but increasing the amount of carbohydrates you eat is the best strategy.

We've also learned that women and men are not equal when it comes to carbo-loading. Research reported in the *Journal of Applied Physiology* (Tarnopolsky, M. A., et al.: "Carbohydrate Loading and Metabolism During Exercise in Men and Women," 1995; 78: 1360–1368), showed that women do not store more muscle glycogen with typical dietary carbo-loading. The study compared a group of men and women fed a diet of 75 percent carbohydrates and a diet of 55 percent to 60 percent carbohydrates prior to an endurance event. Though the men did store more glycogen through carbo-loading and performed better, the women did not have higher muscle glycogen or better performances.

Researchers don't know why this is so, and until they do, we won't have a definite solution. One of the theories, however, is that female runners may not be getting enough calories in the first place, which would mean we don't have a whole lot of extra calories to store away as muscle glycogen. Therefore, make sure you're regularly eating adequately. Tarnopolsky and colleagues also recommended that female runners be conscientious about eating a high-carbohydrate snack (200 to 300 calories) within 20 minutes after a hard run or race when muscles *will* soak up carbos. During the week before your marathon, consume *extra* carbohydrates, in addition to your usual diet, for about 300 extra calories a day—equivalent to a piece of fruit and a bagel.

The night before a marathon, many runners traditionally sit down to a big plate of pasta and bread, but any combination of foods high in carbohydrates and low in fat will be fine. A meal that includes low-fat meat, such as poultry or fish, and vegetables, along with a typical starchy side dish of rice, potatoes, or pasta, is just as appropriate as a bowl of spaghetti. Simply avoid buttery, cheesy, or creamy sauces or toppings.

What's most important is that you've eaten these foods before in training and you know they will not cause you intestinal problems when you are running. This is also why you should avoid foods that are very high in fiber.

Fluids

Carbohydrates hold onto water, so as you are stocking your muscles with glycogen, you will also be retaining water, which is good because you need to be well hydrated before the marathon. Be conscientious about drinking plenty of noncaffeinated, nonalcoholic beverages throughout the week before the marathon.

How do you know if you are drinking enough? The easiest way is to check the color of your urine: if it is very pale or clear, you are well hydrated. One caveat: taking vitamin supplements will turn urine bright yellow. You can also follow the guideline of drinking a quart for every 1,000 calories you expend each day. Assuming you burn the calories you consume, you can figure the amount of water on the basis of how many calories you take in each day.

By the end of this final week of marathon preparation, you are likely to feel a bit bloated and to have gained a couple pounds. This is a good sign; it means you are appropriately stocked with fluids and carbohydrates for your long journey.

Finishing Touches

Here are a few more tips for your final week of preparation:

- Take 10 to 15 minutes every day to visualize your upcoming race. (For information on visualization, see pages 303 through 305 in chapter 23).
- Don't become concerned if you happen not to feel particularly spunky when you do run. Many runners experience some sluggishness in the final week and then run the best marathon of their lives.
- Keep all activity levels low. This isn't a good time to help a friend move or plan an excursion that requires lots of walking. See what life is like as a couch potato for a change.
- Get your usual amount of sleep during the week, and then don't worry if you toss and turn the night before the marathon—you'll still be well rested.
- The evening before race day, gather together the clothing you'll be wearing and your race number so that the next morning, you simply have to get up and get dressed.

Race-Day Tips and Strategies

You can't help but be a little nervous on race day; after all, the marathon is an imposing distance. Trust that you are well prepared. You've done the training. You've rested well during the past 7 days. Now it's up to you to run a smart race. The rest is in the hands of fate.

Begin with a Warm Shower and a Meal

A race-morning shower leaves you feeling fresh and renewed after a good (or even not-so-good) night's sleep. Eat a light breakfast 2 to 3 hours before the start of the marathon—300 to 400 calories' worth: a bowl of cereal, oatmeal, a plain bagel, or dry toast, along with some juice, are good choices.

Sports bars, high-carbohydrate beverages, or even energy gels, such as GU, are other ways to top off your carbohydrates before the marathon. Stick to foods or food products that you have tried before your long training runs and that you know will digest easily and not cause an upset stomach or intestinal problems.

One of the most important reasons to consume carbohydrates before the marathon is that though your muscle glycogen stores should still be full from the previous night's dinner, the glycogen levels in your liver will have become lower, and it's this form of carbohydrate that fuels your brain. During a long event like the marathon, if you run low on liver glycogen, you'll become a bit fuzzy in the head.

If you cannot tolerate any food the morning of your run, try liquids—juices or sports beverages. If those don't sit well in your stomach, make sure to have a high-carbohydrate snack (300 to 400 calories' worth) before you go to bed the night before.

If you're used to a cup of coffee before you run, go ahead and have one. Though caffeinated beverages are diuretics, one cup won't do any harm, especially since you'll be drinking other fluids as well before the start of the race.

Dress for Success

You should be comfortable running in shorts and a singlet or T-shirt. If the temperature dips below 50° Fahrenheit and you expect to be running slowly and for 4 hours or more, you may prefer a long-sleeved T-shirt. Below 40° to 45°, think about wearing running tights, depending on your cold tolerance.

RAIN GARB

What if it's raining on race day? Take a big plastic garbage bag and make holes for your head and arms. When the rain stops or you've become warm enough running that you don't need coverage, simply slip the bag over your head and toss it off the side of the race course, preferably at a water stop, where a volunteer can pick it up and dispose of it.

Because the marathon is such a long event, the temperature often gets warmer as the day progresses. Consider wearing a long-sleeved shirt over your T-shirt or singlet that you can take off and tie around your waist when you get too warm. Of course, wear clothing made from breathable fabrics, so you'll stay dry and comfortable.

On a cool day, wear enough layers over your racing outfit to keep you warm before the marathon starts. Most events will transport your extra clothing to the finish line, or you can toss them to a friend or partner before the start. Wear gloves; you can take them off and tuck them under the waistband of your shorts if your hands become too warm.

Don't Try Anything New

Though it may be tempting to go buy new running shoes and clothes, especially for your marathon debut, don't do it. A new sports bra can cause chafing. New shoes can cause blisters, and even socks that aren't the style and fabric you're used to can rub your feet raw. Instead, treat yourself to some new running gear after the race as a reward for completing the marathon.

Start Slowly

Even if your goal is to run a PR, hold back at the beginning. In fact, run a little slower than your goal pace. (You can use the "Pace per Mile" table on page 416 of the appendix to determine your appropriate marathon pace.) It's easy to go out too fast in the marathon. You're well rested, your legs are fresh, and you're eager to run after sitting around the past 7 days filling up on fluids and pasta. Also, the marathon race pace is slow compared with the pace you run for a 5-K or 10-K, and it will feel easy those first few miles—too easy. You'll want to run faster, but hold back.

Let's say your goal pace is to run about 9 minutes a mile. You may discover much to your delight that an 8½-minute pace feels easy—until mile 16, and then your legs start to feel tired, and you run slower. An 8½-minute pace becomes 9, 9:30, 10:00, 11:00 . . . You find yourself crawling through the last few miles and finishing the marathon in a time slower than you were capable of had you run a 9-minute pace the whole way. (I know this to be true. It happened to me.)

I also know that by starting off at a pace that's slower than your goal pace and running the first half of the marathon comfortably, you can run the second half faster and finish in a better time than you had hoped for. (This also has happened to me.) It's called "negative splits," and it simply means that you ran the second half of a race faster than the first. Most runners don't believe in such a thing. They think it's not possible to run a faster second half because you'll be tired from having run 13 miles. If you are running just a little slower than you are capable of in the early miles, though, you are conserving energy that you can then use to pick up the pace later. Think of it like this: the first half is an extended warmup and the second half is the race.

Your effort at the beginning of the marathon should feel very comfortable. You shouldn't be breathing hard at all. In the second half, if you want to pick up the pace and you can do so while still running at a comfortable effort—this shouldn't feel like a 5-K or 10-K race—then go for it.

Drink Fluids Regularly

Take liquids at every water stop, even if you're not thirsty. You will lose a lot of water running 26 miles even on a cool day, and even a slight deficit in your body's hydration level can adversely affect your performance, say the experts. How much water you'll need depends on your weight and how much you sweat. (To figure out your specific requirements, see "Hydration" and "Rehydration" on pages 77 to 78 in chapter 8.) The general guideline for taking fluids during a race is to drink about 8 ounces every 15 minutes.

Many marathons offer sports beverages, such as Gatorade or Exceed, along with water. These sports drinks can offer two advantages to marathoners: the small concentration of sugar and salt helps your body to absorb the fluid faster than plain water, and that sugar can help fuel your muscles. Do not take a sports beverage during a marathon if you haven't tried it during a training run, however. Though these drinks

MANAGING A WATER STOP

Getting water at an aid station and then drinking it while running is one of the arts of racing. Here are some hints:

- The water stop will be crowded when you first approach it, so keep running in the middle of the road and then take a cup toward the end of the station, where there are fewer runners and it will be easier to move in to the table and back out onto the course.
- Squeeze the cup at the top to form sort of a spout so it will be easier to pour water into your mouth while you are running.
- Drink as much as you can, carrying the cup with you for a few yards and taking several sips.
- If it becomes too troublesome to drink on the run, stop and walk. It only takes a few seconds to swallow a cup of water and it won't affect your finishing time. By not taking fluids, however, you can be certain you'll run slower than you had hoped.

are formulated for easy digestion, they do cause stomach problems for some runners. This isn't something you want to learn at mile 18 of your marathon. If you discover in training that you can't tolerate a sports drink, don't feel you'll be at a disadvantage during the marathon. Water will keep you well hydrated, and if you have eaten plenty of carbohydrates prior to the marathon, you won't run out of fuel.

Use Your Mental Power

Even if you've done everything right, prepared properly the week before, run the appropriate pace, and taken fluids at all the water stops, you will come to a point in the marathon where discomfort sets in. Let's be honest: eventually, every part of your body starts to hurt. This isn't a sign necessarily that you are about to "hit the wall"; it means that you've been exerting a good physical effort for a long time. Your body wants to stop, but you must keep going.

Let your mind come to the rescue. First, accept the pain and fatigue. Don't give in to it; just acknowledge that this is part of what running a marathon is all about. Once you've accepted the discomfort as normal, you stop worrying about it as something that's going to prevent you from getting to the finish line.

Remind yourself that you have prepared well for this day. Three months of training have toughened you for this challenge. You have

EXTRA ENERGY

First, it was candy. Marathoners would sometimes stuff a few hard candies in their shorts pocket to give them an energy boost for the last few miles of the race. Then came sports bars to chew on when you felt you needed a boost. Now we have energy gels: GU, ReLode, Squeezy and Pocket Rocket are a few brands. These high-carbohydrate products have the consistency of pudding or cake frosting and come in small packets that you can carry in a pocket and that rip open easily for a quick supply of energy. Individual packets deliver 70 to 100 calories, or 17 to 25 grams of carbohydrates. You should take them with 8 ounces of water to aid digestion and absorption.

Do you need to take one of these products with you? No, but some runners find that carbohydrates taken in the second half of the marathon help them maintain their pace. It's another matter of personal preference—and tolerance. You may not be able to stomach sour balls, sports bars, or energy gels while you are running. Test them out in training before trying them during a race.

the power and ability to run the whole distance. Say to yourself over and over again that you are strong.

Take a few minutes to check your running form as described on page 35 in chapter 5. Make any necessary corrections in posture or arm swing. Relax muscles that are tense. (See pages 308 to 309 in chapter 23 for a discussion of how to relax during a race.) Picture yourself running smoothly, fluidly over the road. Banish all negative thoughts by replacing them with positive ones, such as changing *I'm not sure I can make it* to *I know I can; I know I can.*

If despite your efforts you think you can't go any farther, pick a point ahead of you and say to yourself that you will just get to that point; it will arrive sooner than you think. Then pick another landmark and keep moving until you reach that one. Continue on in this way, and before you know it, you'll be looking at the finish-line banner.

I've seen marathoners have to stop because of a muscle cramp. What should I do if this happens to me?

"What's happening is that your muscles have gone into a spasm," says Budd Coates, marathoner and coach. "Stop and massage your leg to try to get it to relax, and then try to stretch it."

THE WALL

It's the dread of every marathoner: hitting "the wall." What happens is that you run out of glycogen to fuel your muscles and brain. You become overwhelmed with mental and physical fatigue and your pace slows dramatically until you are struggling just to keep running at all.

Most often, this occurs at around the 20-mile point. The reason? Your body can store only enough glycogen to fuel about 20 miles of running. Fortunately, we can also burn fat for energy. Your muscles prefer glycogen because it is an easier and faster source of energy; however, after you've been running for a long time, your muscles will cut back on carbohydrate consumption and burn more fat. Still, you need some glycogen to help you maintain your pace and to feed your brain.

If you haven't loaded up on enough carbohydrates before the marathon, you could very well become glycogen depleted and—*smack*. Proper and consistent training is also essential to avoiding "the wall." Well-trained muscles can store more carbohydrates than poorly trained muscles can: plus, those weekly long runs will teach your body to become more efficient at burning fat and sparing precious glycogen.

Steps to Recovery

Don't be surprised if, after you cross the finish line of the marathon, you want to keep moving because it hurts more to stand still. This will be to your benefit because walking keeps your muscles from tightening up and helps prevent muscle soreness later on. To further prevent muscle soreness and speed your recovery from the marathon, follow these steps:

1. **Get something to drink.** Even if you took water at every aid station, you'll need to replenish fluids lost through sweat. Either water or a sports drink will do, although the latter will be absorbed more quickly and will begin sooner to replenish your spent carbohydrates.
2. **Get something to eat.** Foods or drinks with a high glycemic index are best because their carbohydrates are quickly absorbed into your bloodstream and delivered to depleted muscles. Baked potatoes have a very high glycemic index; however, you don't usually find them among postmarathon fare. Bagels, watermelon, breads, muffins, orange juice, and ripe bananas are good choices (see The Glycemic Index on page 82 for other suggestions). Try to consume about 300 calories' worth of carbohydrates. If you can't tolerate solid foods, drink juices or sports beverages.

3. **Take a cold shower.** No kidding. Cold water decreases blood flow to the muscles, which reduces inflammation and pain. The legs of thoroughbred horses are iced down after a race for the same reason. If you absolutely refuse to chill your well-run legs, at least refrain from taking a *hot* shower, which has the opposite effect—increasing blood flow, inflammation, and muscle soreness.

4. **Continue walking, eating, and drinking throughout the rest of the day.** The snacks and beverages you consumed at the finish of the marathon only begin to refill your dwindled stores of muscle glycogen and to rehydrate your parched body.

5. **Congratulate yourself.** Whether or not you ran your best marathon, you completed the distance. It is a daunting feat and an extraordinary achievement at any pace. You should be proud.

Will a massage help me recover quickly and prevent muscle soreness?

Yes, a massage will speed recovery and ease the pain; however, studies suggest that you are better off waiting 1 or 2 days after the marathon rather than hopping on the massage table immediately after the race. Recovery seems fastest for those who keep walking after the run, so hobble along for 10–15 minutes before you put your feet up.

The Days After

How sore you'll be in the days after the marathon depends on the difficulty of the course, the kind of training you did, whether you took the proper recovery steps outlined above, and how your body responds to the effort of running a marathon. If you ran a hilly marathon but didn't train on hills, count on hobbling around for a few days. Some courses—the New York City Marathon is one—are run on roads built from asphalt over concrete, making them extra hard on your legs.

You'll find that going down steps will be the most painful of all activities. Turn around and descend them backward and it'll feel much easier. Continue to eat as your appetite dictates and drink plenty of fluids. You may find that you're hungrier the day after the marathon than you were at dinner the evening of the race. This means your body is still replacing spent carbohydrates.

Light activity—easy cycling or walking—in the first couple post-marathon days can be healing. It will keep your muscles loose and circulate blood more quickly through your muscles to remove the waste products of endurance exercise. Later that week, you can run an easy 2 to 3 miles if you want and then gradually add mileage. If you'd rather, take a couple weeks' break from running. Listen to your mind and body. When you're ready to start running again, you'll know.

Champions

BY MEGAN OTHERSEN GORMAN

I USED TO BE A WORLD CHAMPION.

In the fall of 1994, my friends Jane and Kate and I competed as a team in the finals of the 3.5-mile Chemical Bank Corporate Challenge. Kate and I were in our early thirties, Jane her midforties. We called ourselves the "old bats"—even though Jane, our elder stateswoman, wore bun-hugger shorts, and all three of us could still string together sixes (6-minute miles) like pearls around our necks.

But none of our stars was exactly rising. Jane had run in the 1984 Olympic marathon trials, the first for women, and I'd done the same in 1988—the year Kate conquered the Ironman Triathlon, which she'd finished in an in-your-face thirty-fourth. We were talented, yes, but we were years beyond our peaks. We huddled at the start in Midtown Manhattan not because we considered ourselves contenders, but because the race was a freebie—a company-funded trip.

The gun sounded.

Adrenaline surged.

Twenty minutes later, it was over—for everyone else. The sum of our three times was lower than that of all the other women's teams, so Chemical Bank declared the old bats world champions.

A lot has changed in the 4 years since that day. I run trails now to spare my tibias the smack of impact on asphalt. Careful of rocks, roots, and a floppy, rag-dolly right ankle, I move with less flash and finesse. My stride is heavier, as am I, more workmanlike—and I don't do speed work or long runs.

I don't even run every day. I am not fast.

But when I push past my husband, elbows slicing air, on the wicked hills in Philly's Wissahickon Park . . . When I slip, seemingly by accident, into a rhythm my heart and mind remember—call it a 6:30-pace déjà vu—on a once-in-a-blue-moon magnificent day . . . When I'm out there—huffing, spitting, slogging, sweating—despite deadlines, leg-length to-do lists, laundry, life . . . I'm a champion—still.

It may sound conveniently self-serving or even irritatingly politically correct, but I've come to realize that success in running isn't most accurately measured by titles or trophies or even times, but by sweat. By balls. By what I call *teeth*. Sometimes, maybe even more often than not, it's when you're on that far, pock-marked side of your peak that you show the most teeth. When I pass the occasional jogger picking her way along the trail these days, I nod, smile, show some respect. I am her. She is me. You never know a world champion—past, present, or future—when you see one.

Megan Othersen Gorman is a writer living in Plymouth Meeting, Pennsylvania.

PART VIII

Injury Prevention and Treatment

25 Preventing Injury

HAVE YOU EVER BEEN TALKING AMONG A group of people about your running when someone piped, "You're going to ruin your joints with all that running"? Rest assured that running does not cause arthritis or wear your joints thin, and it will not leave you hobbling through your older years. On the contrary, running keeps you spry. Yes, some runners get arthritis, but those who do were going to end up with this disease whether they ran or not. In fact, running may postpone the onset of their arthritis.

Running gets a bad rap when it comes to injury. Injuries to runners do happen, but most are relatively minor—strains and inflammations. You're not likely to break a leg, sever a tendon, or suffer a concussion, and though knee problems are a fairly common complaint among female runners, they usually are not as severe as those incurred playing soccer, basketball, or volleyball.

The body was meant to move, and our history as runners is as old as the human race, springing from our days as hunters and gatherers. Running is a natural activity. Though the force of impact as we strike the ground is great (three times our body weight), the motion of running is fluid, which lessens that impact, and our bodies have ways to absorb and disperse the impact.

Still, injury happens, in part because running is such a repetitive activity. Although repeating the same movements over and over makes you stronger, faster, and more resistant to injury, if you overdo it you'll wear your body down and become prone to strains, sprains, and stress fractures. Most injuries aren't caused by running itself but by running too much relative to what your body is ready to handle. This doesn't mean you can't run long or hard; it's just that you need to increase mileage and intensity gradually.

Are Women More Susceptible to Certain Injuries?

Several reports indicate that knee injuries in particular are more common among women than among men. The reasons given have to do with leg alignment, muscle strength, and joint laxity or looseness. In general, women have wider pelvises than men do, which makes for a corresponding larger quadriceps angle (Q-angle), meaning the hips come down to the knees at a sharper angle. This puts more stress on the knees, making them more vulnerable to injury. Sports physicians often refer to a condition common in women called "the terrible triad," in which a wider pelvis causes legs to be more knock-kneed; the tibia (shinbone) tends to rotate toward the inside; and feet tend to be flat. The result is overpronation and increased stress to the knees during running. Despite all this, there are very few studies that show that a larger Q-angle in fact causes knee problems.

Experts speculate that perhaps differences in hamstring versus quadriceps strength between women and men account for a higher incidence of knee injuries in female athletes. In men, the hamstrings (muscles in the back of the thigh) are stronger and more dominant than the quadriceps (muscles in the front of the thigh). In women, the reverse is true. Again, how this affects knee stability and risk of injury needs to be studied further before any definite conclusion can be reached.

Another factor that might contribute to injuries in women is looseness of the joints, particularly around the time of ovulation, when estrogen is high, and during pregnancy, when production of the hormone relaxin causes the ligaments surrounding joints to relax. Here, too, however, evidence hasn't been gathered to show that this looseness leads to injury.

Scoliosis is more common in women than men and results in a tilted pelvis, such that one leg appears slightly shorter than the other. Such a discrepancy may not be obvious; see Short Leg, Long Leg (page 358) in the next chapter for a test you can do at home to check if your pelvis is level. If you have scoliosis, you can still run, but depending on the extent of the resulting leg length discrepancy, you may need a heel lift.

Sports physicians also report that stress fractures, shinsplints, and foot problems are more common among women than men. Regardless of the potential problem or its specific cause, there are certain measures you can take that will help prevent injuries of all types.

Injury Prevention

You can't change your Q-angle or the laxity of your joints, but by following the basic principles of injury prevention, you can minimize whatever adverse effects these factors might have on your running.

Wear Quality Running Shoes

I've heard runners complain about shinsplints only to look down at their feet and see that they're wearing cross-training shoes. You can do everything else right and ruin your running with the wrong or a worn-out pair of shoes. No matter how few miles you run each week, do not run in tennis shoes, aerobic shoes, or cross-trainers. Athletic shoes are designed to complement the type of activity you will be doing. Tennis requires a lot of lateral movement. Running involves strictly forward motion. Not only is it important that you wear running shoes, but they should be of a design appropriate to your running style. For example, overpronators require a different

WHEN THE SHOE DOESN'T FIT . . .

. . . don't wear it. Running shoes that fit improperly can cause bunions, Morton's neuroma (a pinched nerve between the bones of the foot), hammertoe, and black toenails (blood under the nail from the toe's banging into the top of the shoe during running). For details on finding the right fit, see chapter 14.

type of shoe than underpronators do. (See chapter 14 to learn more about pronation and shoe selection.) Shop at a specialty running store where the salespeople have the knowledge to help you find the best shoe and the right fit.

And replace your shoes regularly. When the midsoles—the supportive layer of the shoe between the bottom of your foot and the outsole—break down, your foot motion during running will be affected, which in turn can place stress on the tendons and ligaments of your legs and lead to injury. Unfortunately, you can't really see the midsole of the shoe to know whether it is worn out. Therefore, experts recommend simply that you replace running shoes after you've worn them for 500 miles.

Increase Mileage Gradually

The guideline to follow when increasing mileage is to add no more than 10 percent to 15 percent each week. If you currently run 20 miles a week, you could step it up to 22 or 23. The point is to allow your body to gradually strengthen itself for higher mileage rather than to overload your muscles by running a lot farther than what you're accustomed to handling.

Also, rather than continuously increasing your mileage each week, raise it for a just 1 or 2 weeks and then do a shorter week. Follow the short week with another increase. For example, if you were to increase from 20 miles to 23, stay at that distance for a couple of weeks and then drop back to 20 miles for a week. Then you could jump to 25 miles and follow that with a 22-mile week. It's the same principle behind hard–easy training applied to weekly mileage: you push your body, then you rest, push, then rest.

Gradual increases in mileage apply to your speed sessions, too. For your very first pace workout, limit yourself to 1½ miles of fast running and build from there. You can look at the training schedules in chapter 23 for examples of how to increase weekly mileage and speed distance appropriately.

Add New Training Elements Gradually

Don't get so excited about training that you go from running 5 miles 4 days a week to adding a long run of 10 miles and a hard hilly run and a speed workout to your week's schedule. Introduce one new element at a time. Begin by extending one of your runs into a long run to build endurance. When you feel comfortable with that change in your running—meaning that it doesn't leave you sore or tired the way it did the first few times you ran it—add a hill run once a week or a pace workout. Once you've adapted to that new run, you can consider adding a third challenging run. Stop at three quality workouts a week and keep all of your running in between nice and easy. If you run hard every day, you'll fall victim to an overuse injury.

Don't Overdo Those Challenging Runs

If you haven't run on hills in a while, pick a course with short, gentle slopes to start and gradually work your way up. The same goes for long runs: as you increase the distance of these runs, do so by 2 or 3 miles at a time. When it comes to pace workouts, begin by running fast 200 meters or 400 meters rather than miles.

Rest

The day after every challenging run, go easy, cross-train, or take the day off. Giving your body time to recuperate from the intense effort of a long run, hilly run, or speed training is essential to preventing injury. After running hard, your muscles will need to do some minor repair work and refuel before they'll be ready to produce another strong effort.

Even if you don't do hills or speed or especially long runs, alternate harder and easier days of running, whether by pace or distance. Alternating gives your muscles the rest they need to stay strong and healthy. Running hard every day would be like not taking any time off from your job, working 7 days a week, morning, noon, and night. Before long, you'd burn out.

How do I know if I'm overtraining?

You'll feel tired and irritable. Your runs will be sluggish and slow, and you'll have a hard time getting motivated to do them. Race performances will fall short of expectations. Though running generally strengthens your immune system, too much running can wear it down, which is why it is not uncommon for a runner to catch a cold after completing a marathon.

Warm Up with Every Run

Even if you are headed out on a relaxed 5-miler, ease into it. Run slowly the first mile or so to increase the rate of blood flow and quicken your metabolism, which literally warms and loosens your muscles for the activity ahead. Then gradually settle into a comfortable pace.

Cooling down at the end of a run or race with slow running or walking helps prevent your muscles from tightening up in response to hard effort, prevents blood from pooling in your legs, and aids recovery.

Stretch After Running

Though there's no scientific evidence to prove that stretching prevents injury, most experts intuitively believe it to be a good practice after running to maintain overall flexibility. Muscles that become too tight are more easily torn with any quick or forceful movements. Don't stretch before running, however, because muscles are tightest then. You can stop and stretch after 1 or 2 miles when you're more flexible; otherwise, wait until the end of the run. If you don't have the time to stretch immediately after running, wait until later in the day or at night while you're watching the evening news, but do try to make stretching part of your daily routine. (For a complete program, see chapter 17.)

Choose Good Running Surfaces

What's a good running surface? It's one that's even and neither too soft nor too hard. When you run on uneven ground—grass surfaces or trails, for example—your feet don't land evenly as they would on flat terrain, and this causes more twisting and turning of the joints and muscles of the lower legs. Uneven surfaces can be particularly hazardous for those prone to ankle sprains.

This doesn't mean you shouldn't run on trails and grassy terrain. The extra work your muscles must go through to run on these surfaces builds strength in your feet, ankles, and legs and ultimately will make you *less* prone to injury. In addition, the softness of these surfaces reduces the force of impact as you run. Choose terrain that's not too lumpy, rocky, or root strewn, however. Take to the challenging trails when you've become stronger and more experienced at off-road running.

On the roads, you need to be careful of cambered surfaces. This is when the road is built such that the center of the road is higher than the sides, forming a bit of a slope. While you are running facing traffic, your right foot lands and then rolls inward farther than it normally would, causing overpronation. When your left foot lands, it will roll more to its outside, a sort of underpronation. Over time, running in this way causes uneven stresses to your muscles and joints and may result in injury.

If you must run on cambered roads, this is one time that you can break the rule about always running facing traffic. For example, on an out-and-back route, run against traffic on the way out and with it on the way back so that each leg shares evenly the stress of running across a slope—but be very careful of traffic when running with it.

Also, try not to do too much running on very soft (sand) or very hard (concrete) surfaces. Running on the beach can be beneficial when done occasionally; it's more difficult than running on a firm surface and can help build leg strength. Your heels sink in sand, however, which pulls on your Achilles tendons (the tendon just above the heels at the bottom of the calves), and too much of this can cause Achilles tendinitis. As for running on concrete sidewalks, do so only when you need to avoid traffic.

Incorporate Strength Training into Your Weekly Routine

Exercises for the hamstrings and quadriceps can correct muscle imbalances that could lead to injury. Also, by strengthening the quadriceps and the tendons and ligaments around the knees, you will help make your knees more stable and resistant to injury. Abdominal exercises strengthen your lower back and can help prevent back pain. Weight training in general builds bone, making you less susceptible to stress fractures. It strengthens your upper body so that you can maintain good form during running. The better your form and posture, the more evenly the stresses of running are distributed throughout your body and the less likely you are to develop strains from a particular muscle's having to work to excess. (See chapter 18 for a complete strength-training program.)

Pay Attention to Pain

By learning to recognize pains that are a sign of *potential* injury, you can resolve them before they develop into problems. Not all pain signals injury. Muscle soreness will occur any time you try something new—hills, a long run, or speed training—or when you increase the length or intensity of running. Most runners are sore after racing. This is a normal and natural response to the extra effort that your muscles exert. The pain will gradually fade in a day or two.

Take note of where the pain is. Soreness, stiffness, and aches that you feel within your muscle usually mean simply that you've been running harder than usual; they are not a sign of injury. Pain felt near your joints where tendons attach muscle to bone may be a sign of inflammation or tendinitis. Pain in the joints—knee, hip, or ankle—also may be a precursor to injury. Sharp pains usually indicate a more severe situation than dull aches and soreness.

Finally, pay attention to the persistence of pain. Stiffness or soreness at the beginning of a run that disappears as you warm up is nothing to be concerned about. Pain that stays with you or gets worse as you run and causes you to alter your gait is a strong indicator of a problem. The more experience you gain as a runner, the better you will become at distinguishing whatever aches and pains might develop.

I've heard the phrase "delayed-onset muscle soreness." What does it refer to?

The muscle soreness and fatigue of a hard run or race takes a little while to set in. You won't feel much pain right after you run, but be prepared for some stiffness and soreness in the next day or two.

Anytime you become concerned about pain or soreness, take 1 or 2 days off from running and follow the treatment procedures described later in this chapter and in the next chapter on specific injuries. If the pain doesn't go away, consult a sports physician or trainer knowledgeable about running.

Injury Treatment

The prevention and treatment of specific injuries is covered in detail in the next chapter, but certain procedures apply to all injuries. Remember one word—*RICE*—and you have the key to the first and most important steps for treating any injury or developing injury. *RICE* stands for rest, ice, compression, and elevation.

Rest

Resting doesn't mean you have to stop all physical activity and turn into a couch potato until you're healed. You can keep active by cross-training—swimming, cycling, stair climbing—whatever does not cause you pain and will not aggravate your running injury. Cross-training will help keep you cardiovascularly fit for your return to running, and psychologically, it will ease some of the disappointment of not being able to run. (For more on cross-training, see chapter 19.)

Ice and Compression

Put your injury on ice as soon as you can. Ice reduces inflammation and pain by decreasing blood flow and swelling to the injured area. Heat increases circulation, aggravates inflammation, and can worsen your pain.

When using ice, do not put it directly on your skin. Cover the area with two layers of plastic wrap. Use a bag of crushed ice, a gel pack (which you can get at sporting goods stores or through mail-order companies), or even a bag of frozen vegetables (corn or peas are best because the package will mold better around the injured area). Place the ice on top of the injured spot and wrap it with an Ace bandage to compress the area, which helps keep swelling down. Warren Scott, M.D., chief of sports medicine at Kaiser Permanente Medical Center in Santa Clara, California, recommends that you keep ice on the injured area for 20 minutes at a time. After the first 20 minutes, take it off for 10 minutes, and then apply it again for 20 minutes; remove the ice for 10 minutes and then reapply for one last 20-minute chill. "If you can do this three times a day for three days in a row, you'll get a tremendous anti-inflammatory effect," says Scott.

Elevation

If you can, keep the injured area elevated. This allows excess fluids to drain and helps reduce swelling.

Anti-Inflammatories

Ice is the first and best way to treat inflammation, but you can also take anti-inflammatory medications to reduce pain and swelling. Doctors usually recommend ibuprofen or naproxen sodium first, but aspirin works, too. Acetaminophen (Tylenol) is not an anti-inflammatory. It does relieve pain that is not caused by inflammation, such as that produced by osteoarthritis, and is a better choice in those situations because it is gentler on your stomach.

What about sports creams? Will they reduce inflammation and relieve pain?

No. In fact, sports creams are irritants—meaning not that they will make your injury worse but that they create a tingling or burning sensation in your skin, which simply diverts your brain's attention from the pain of the injury. If they make you feel better, go ahead and use them, but sports balms produce no healing effect.

Some runners take anti-inflammatories before running or racing to prevent pain, but it's best not to. Pain can protect you from injury by warning you that perhaps you're running too far or too hard. Plus, anti-inflammatories may cause nausea in some runners.

Return to Running

When can you start running again after you've been injured? Clearly, that depends on the severity of your injury. One or 2 days of no running may be all you need if you are trying to prevent a nagging pain from becoming an in-your-face problem. If you have an injury, take a week off and then try a test walk–run of up to 3 miles, stopping as soon as you feel pain. If running hurts, take more time off. If you feel no pain, you can gradually return to your normal routine.

Always build up mileage slowly after a layoff, even if you've been cross-training. The safest way is with a walk–run combination. As you get stronger, increase the running and decrease the walking. (You can find a walk–run program on page 47 in chapter 5.) Just because you don't feel pain doesn't mean you are completely healed. Go ahead and run, but do so comfortably and increase mileage slowly to allow for a full recuperation.

Don't worry about losing your running fitness—that takes 3 weeks of inactivity, and most minor injuries are resolved by then. If you happen to have a stress fracture or some other injury that knocks you off your feet for a while, there are cross-training activities that can keep you almost as fit as if you had been running the whole time. Once you get back on the roads, trails, or treadmill, your running fitness will return quickly.

26 Common Injuries

YOU'RE TRAINING FOR A MARATHON,
you've been careful to increase your mileage
gradually, you take a day of complete rest each
week, and you stretch after every run. Then a
friend convinces you to join her on a long, hilly
run even though you just ran hills yesterday.
The two of you get caught up racing the
downhills. The next morning, you get out of bed
and your knee hurts.

Women are by no means fragile, but push the
body too far, too often and something's going to
give. The quicker you attend to an injury,

349

the faster you'll get over it. As soon as you notice pain that does not seem like the usual muscle soreness after a hard effort, pay attention. If it doesn't go away in a few days or if it is aggravated by running, you may have the beginnings of an injury. If you experience pain during running, stop and try to figure out what the problem may be.

Clearly, the first step in treating any injury is proper diagnosis. The symptoms of 10 common running injuries are described in this chapter. If you can determine on the basis of these descriptions what's causing your pain, follow the guidelines listed for treatment compiled from the advice of various sports physicians and podiatrists. If none of them seem to fit your situation or you simply aren't sure, consult a sports physician knowledgeable about running.

Most running injuries involve an inflammation of a tendon or liga-

DR. RIGHT

Whom should you consult about a running injury—a podiatrist, an orthopedist, or a sports medicine specialist? Depending on the particular expertise of the physicians you are considering, all three of these specialists can treat most common running injuries, but there are a few distinctions. Clearly, a sports med doc will be knowledgeable about athletic problems, whereas orthopedists and podiatrists who do not limit their practices to athletes will vary in their expertise. Look for one who treats a lot of runners. The best way to find the best physician is by referrals. Ask your running friends who they like.

- **Orthopedists:** Experts of the musculoskeletal system, these medical doctors know a lot about bones, joints, muscles, tendons, and ligaments. They can treat injuries of the foot, ankle, lower legs, knees, hips, and back. Some orthopedists specialize in particular areas, such as the knee, hip, or spine, but most treat the whole body. See an orthopedist for acute and severe injuries, including knee pain, stress fractures, muscle tears, and iliotibial band (ITB) syndrome. They also treat Achilles tendinitis and plantar fasciitis.
- **Podiatrists:** These doctors specialize in the foot. Call on them to treat bunions, hammertoes, Morton's neuroma, stress fractures of the foot, and plantar fasciitis, as well as Achilles tendinitis. A podiatrist knowledgeable in biomechanics can also diagnose problems of the leg and hip, since many such problems begin with improper foot motion.
- **Sports medicine physicians:** These medical doctors are specialists in sports medicine. They are experts in diagnosing and treating all kinds of sports-related injuries among all types of athletes. You can consult them to treat anything from black toenails to back pain.

ment, which is best treated with RICE—rest, ice, compression, elevation (see chapter 25 for a review of the basics of injury treatment). Some of the treatments below call for stretching or strengthening exercises; for specifics, refer to the chapters on strength training (chapter 18) and stretching (chapter 17). If despite your efforts at treating the injury it doesn't heal in 2 to 4 weeks, or if pain worsens, see a podiatrist, orthopedic surgeon, or sports medicine physician who knows running.

Achilles Tendinitis

The Achilles tendon attaches the calf muscles to the heel bone. When it becomes overstressed, some of the fibers making up the tendon become damaged, and inflammation occurs. If Achilles tendinitis is allowed to progress, scar tissue will form over the inflamed area, making it less flexible. In severe cases, the tendon can tear or rupture.

Symptoms

You'll recognize Achilles tendinitis by dull or sharp pain anywhere along the tendon that is usually worse in the morning when you are most stiff and eases up as movement warms and loosens the calf. When you are running, your Achilles will hurt the most at the start and feel better as you continue. The area of injury will be painful to touch and it may be red and warm.

Treatment

Treat Achilles tendinitis as follows:

- Use RICE.
- Take anti-inflammatory medications as directed on the containers' labels.
- Stretch your calf muscle several times a day. Also stretch the Achilles tendon; however, because this may cause irritation, ice the tendon immediately afterward.
- Wear street shoes with a heel to relieve tension on your Achilles. The height of the heel depends on what feels most comfortable. You may find that your running shoes are best.

Running

In the early stages of Achilles tendinitis, pain may not occur during running; you may notice it only in the morning when you get out of bed. If this is the case, you can continue to run. If the injury has progressed to the point of causing pain during running, however, stop and cross-train instead. Begin running when you can do so with no pain.

Appropriate Cross-Training

You can do cycling, swimming, or aquarunning or use an elliptical trainer—whatever does not cause pain.

Possible Causes

Achilles tendinitis can be caused by any of the following:

- Sudden, dramatic increases in mileage or intensity of running
- Running too often or too many miles on very soft surfaces such as sand
- Tight calf muscles, which put extra strain on the Achilles during running
- Overpronation
- Frequent wearing of high-heeled shoes, which allows the calf muscles to shorten so that when you put on running shoes and go for a run, your calf and Achilles are forced to stretch quickly

Prevention

To prevent Achilles tendinitis, do the following:

- Regularly stretch your calves and Achilles tendons.
- Wear street shoes with low heels.
- If you are an overpronator, make sure you wear running shoes that control pronation (see chapter 14).
- Limit the amount of running you do on soft surfaces, especially if you are not accustomed to it.
- Follow appropriate guidelines for increasing the mileage and intensity of your running.

Ankle Sprains

Ankle sprains occur when the ligaments of the ankle tear because of twisting.

Symptoms

If you sprain your ankle, it will be painful and will swell. It may turn black and blue, depending on the severity of the sprain.

Treatment

Treat sprained ankles as follows:

- Use RICE.
- Get some chewing tobacco—an amount that fits in the palm of your hand—and wrap it in a white T-shirt or some cheesecloth to make a compress. Moisten the compress and put it over the swelling, wrapping the ankle with an Ace bandage. Then put your foot in a plastic bag, as tobacco stains. Within 6 to 12 hours, the swelling will be gone. *Notes:* Don't do this if you have an open wound on your ankle or if you are allergic to tobacco. You may notice reactions to the nicotinic acid in the tobacco, such as watery eyes or dryness in your throat.

Running

You probably will not be able to run on a sprained ankle, but do get active as soon as possible. Movement promotes healing, and you want your ankle to heal quickly because the longer it takes, the more the ligament will deteriorate.

Appropriate Cross-Training

You can do swimming, aquarunning, or anything else that does not cause pain.

Possible Causes

Ankle sprains can be caused by either of the following:

- Weak ankles
- Running on uneven surfaces

Prevention

To prevent sprains, do the following:

- If you are prone to ankle sprains, avoid running on rugged trails or other uneven surfaces.

- Strengthen your ankles by running on grassy surfaces, where your feet and ankles have to work a little harder than on firm roads or the track.

Calf Strain

Calf strain is inflammation in the muscles of the calf.

Symptoms

Symptoms of calf strain include the following:

- Pain and tenderness
- Tightness
- Possible swelling

Treatment

Treat calf strains as follows:

- Use RICE.
- Take anti-inflammatory medications as directed on the containers' labels.
- Stretch the calf frequently throughout the day.
- Wrap a 4-inch Ace bandage tightly around the calf, but not so tightly as to cut off circulation, and wear the bandage throughout the day, removing it before bedtime.
- Wear shoes with a heel to lessen tension on the muscles. Your running shoes may feel most comfortable, however.

Running

Run only if you can do so without pain.

Appropriate Cross-Training

You can do swimming, deep-water running, or cycling or use an elliptical trainer—whatever does not cause pain.

Possible Causes

Calf strain can be caused by either of the following:

- A sudden and dramatic increase in mileage or intensity of running
- Lots of running on hills or uneven surfaces

```
        Barnes & Noble Booksellers #2123
              2439 Sycamore Road
               Dekalb, IL 60115
                 815-787-3234

STR:2123 REG:003 TRN:8553  CSHR:Demtra D

Complete Book of Running
  9780671017033        T1
  (1 @ 16.99)                         16.99

Subtotal                              16.99
Sales Tax T1 (8.000%)                  1.36
TOTAL                                 18.35
VISA DEBIT                            18.35
  Card#:  XXXXXXXXXXXXX2262

A MEMBER WOULD HAVE SAVED              1.70


             Thanks for shopping at
               Barnes & Noble

101.25C              07/04/2011  10:23A


              CUSTOMER COPY
```

Barnes & Noble retail store (except for purchases made by check less than 7 days prior to the date of return) or (ii) 14 days of delivery date for Barnes & Noble.com purchases (except for purchases made via PayPal). A store credit for the purchase price will be issued for (i) purchases made by check less than 7 days prior to the date of return, (ii) when a gift receipt is presented within 60 days of purchase, (iii) textbooks returned with a receipt within 14 days of purchase, or (iv) original purchase was made through Barnes & Noble.com via PayPal. Opened music/DVDs/audio may not be returned, but can be exchanged only for the same title if defective.

<u>After 14 days or without a sales receipt,</u> returns or exchanges will not be permitted.

Magazines, newspapers, and used books are not returnable. *Product not carried by Barnes & Noble or Barnes & Noble.com will not be accepted for return.*

Policy on receipt may appear in two sections.

Return Policy

<u>With a sales receipt,</u> a full refund in the original form of payment will be issued from any Barnes & Noble store for returns of new and unread books (except textbooks) and unopened music/DVDs/audio made within (i) 14 days of purchase from a Barnes & Noble retail store (except for purchases made by check less than 7 days prior to the date of return) or (ii) 14 days of delivery date for Barnes & Noble.com purchases (except for purchases made via PayPal). A store credit for the purchase price will be issued for (i) purchases made by check less than 7 days prior to the date of return, (ii) when a gift receipt is presented within 60 days of purchase, (iii) textbooks returned with a receipt within 14 days of purchase, or (iv) original purchase was made through Barnes & Noble.com via PayPal. Opened music/DVDs/audio may not be returned, but can be exchanged only for the same title if defective.

B&N RECOMMENDS

We think you'll like these great titles:

Marathoning for Mortals: A Regular...
by John Bingham

The Non-Runner's Marathon Trainer
by David A. Whitsett

The Beginning Runner's Handbook: The...
by

Running Forward - Looking Back
by Lynn T. Seely

The Courage to Start: A Guide to Running...
by John "The Penguin" Bingham

Prevention

To prevent calf strain, do the following:

- Stretch your calves regularly.
- Follow appropriate guidelines for increasing mileage and intensity of training.
- Don't forget to warm up at the beginning of every run.
- If you experience recurring calf problems, try running shoes that are thick in the heel and have a sturdy heel counter.

Hamstring Pull

A hamstring pull is inflammation or tearing of the hamstring muscles—in the back of the thigh—which usually occurs with the sudden movements of speed training.

Symptoms

Symptoms of a hamstring pull include the following:

- Pain in the hamstrings that is sharper and more localized than general muscle soreness
- Black and blue discoloration in the area; this indicates a tear to the muscle, so you should see a sports physician immediately

Treatment

Treat a hamstring pull as follows:

- Use RICE.
- Take anti-inflammatory medications as directed on the containers' labels.
- Gently stretch the hamstrings several times a day.
- Wrap your thigh with a 6-inch Ace bandage to provide added relief.

Running

You can continue to run if your injury doesn't cause pain, but run easy (no speed training) so as not to turn a minor muscle pull into a major tear.

Appropriate Cross-Training

You can do swimming (use your arms only), deep-water running, cycling, or rowing or use an elliptical trainer—whatever does not cause pain.

Possible Causes

Hamstring pulls can be caused by either of the following:

- Sprinting or speed training, when the muscles work more explosively
- A tight spot that develops into a pull during a long run when your muscles have become overly fatigued

Prevention

To prevent hamstring pulls, do the following:

- Regularly stretch and strengthen the hamstrings.
- Follow the guidelines for increasing mileage and intensity of running safely.
- Be sure to warm up at the beginning of every run.
- If on a long run you feel your hamstrings tighten, stop and stretch them.

Iliotibial Band Syndrome

The iliotibial band (ITB) is a strip of connective tissue that runs from the hip along the outside of the thigh muscle and attaches to the outside of the tibia (shin bone) just below the knee. During running, the tendon moves back and forth over the bony protuberance at the side of your knee. If the ITB is tight (which can occur with overpronation, during downhill running, or simply from tightness of the band itself), the friction caused by this rubbing produces inflammation and pain.

A tight ITB can also result in pain and inflammation at the hip—bursitis—where the band crosses a bursa sac. You might even notice a "snapping" of the tendon on the outside of your hip while you are running. Treatment and prevention are the same for the hip as for the knee.

Symptoms

Symptoms of ITB syndrome are as follows:

- Dull or sharp pain along the outside of the knee that occurs after 1 or 2 miles running (earlier in more severe cases) but goes away when you stop running
- As the injury progresses, more severe pain during running that may affect your gait

Treatment

Treat ITB syndrome as follows:

- Use RICE.
- Take anti-inflammatory medications as described on the containers' labels.
- Stretch the hamstrings, quadriceps, and ITB—in that order—frequently throughout the day.

Running

You may be able to continue to run with ITB syndrome, depending on how quickly pain develops, but stay away from hills and uneven surfaces. As soon as your knee starts to hurt during a run, stop.

Appropriate Cross-Training

You can do walking, cycling, swimming, or deep-water running—any activity that does not irritate the injured area.

Possible Causes

ITB syndrome may be caused by any of the following:

- High weekly mileage
- Sudden and dramatic increases in training
- Lots of downhill running
- Running on cambered roads (which slope from the center down to the sides) always on the same side of the road; this can cause ITB syndrome in the outside leg (running on the left side of the road, facing traffic, the outside leg would be your left leg)
- Leg length discrepancy

SHORT LEG, LONG LEG

When one leg is shorter than the other, it can cause all kinds of trouble for runners, from foot injuries on up to lower back pain. A difference of even a quarter of an inch can be hazardous, especially if you run more than 20 to 30 miles a week. A leg length discrepancy forces your body to tilt a little during running. This might not be noticeable to you or your running partners, but your legs and feet will know because they will have to bear uneven stress.

A leg length discrepancy can be a true difference in the length of your bones or it may result from a muscular imbalance or scoliosis. For example, if the right side of your back is tighter than the other, your right leg will appear shorter.

How do you know if one leg is actually longer than the other? Ultimately, you should see a podiatrist or orthopedist and have your legs measured (this is fairly complex and he or she should take several measurements to ensure accuracy), but you can do a couple of checks at home. Stand erect in your underwear in front of a mirror. Place your fingers on the bony protuberances on each side of your pelvis and look to see if your hands are even. Also, check the wear on the bottom of your running shoes. If one leg is longer than the other, the shoe on that leg will wear out more quickly.

If the cause is a muscular imbalance, your physician will treat the imbalance. For true leg length discrepancies, a series of heel lifts will be prescribed for the shorter leg. In severe cases, the shoe itself will be built up.

- High-arched feet
- Bowlegs
- Underpronation

Prevention

To prevent ITB syndrome, do the following:

- Avoid overdoing downhill running
- When you are on cambered roads, change the side of the street that you run on.
- If you are an underpronator, check your shoes—they should be cushioned and have a curved last to allow foot motion.
- If ITB syndrome recurs, regularly stretch your ITB even when you are not injured.

Morton's Neuroma

The metatarsals are the five bones in the ball of the foot that lie directly behind the bones of your toes. When one of the nerves between the metatarsals (usually the third and fourth) becomes pinched and develops an enlargement, the condition is called Morton's neuroma.

Symptoms

The symptoms of Morton's neuroma are as follows:

- Pain in the ball of your foot that gets worse with running
- Any discoloration is a sign of blood, and you should see a podiatrist or sports medicine physician

Treatment

Treat Morton's neuroma as follows:

- Use RICE.
- Take anti-inflammatory medications as directed on the containers' labels.
- Wear wider running shoes.
- Wear wider street shoes.
- Try placing a metatarsal pad (available in pharmacies) in your shoe under the arch and behind the ball of your foot. This will spread the metatarsals and relieve pinching. If the pad causes discomfort after a couple hours, however, remove it.
- Walking barefoot may provide the most comfort because it allows the bones of the foot to spread.
- If the problem persists, surgery may be required.

Running

You can continue to run if you can do so without pain.

Appropriate Cross-Training

You can do swimming or deep-water running—any activity that does not cause pain.

Possible Causes

Morton's neuroma can be caused by the following:

- Wearing street shoes that are very narrow in the forefoot (often the case in women's shoes), which pushes the bones closer together and may cause pinching and friction around nerves. In general, women have narrow heels relative to the girth of their forefeet.
- Wearing running shoes that are too tight in the forefoot, which may happen if you buy running shoes that are snug around the heel.

Prevention

To prevent Morton's neuroma, wear shoes—for running, work, and evening—that have enough room in the forefoot so that your feet are not pinched.

Plantar Fasciitis

The plantar fascia is a thick band of connective tissue that begins at the base of your toes, runs along the bottom of your foot, and attaches on the bottom of the heel bone. Stress to the plantar fascia causes tears and inflammation of the tissue in the area of the heel. Left untreated, this problem can plague you for up to a year.

Symptoms

You'll recognize plantar fasciitis by pain on the bottom of the heel that increases when you rise up on your toes. It usually feels worst in the morning when the plantar fascia is tightest and stiffest, and it will hurt more at the beginning of a run than after you've warmed up.

Treatment

Treat plantar fasciitis as follows:

- Try icing the plantar fascia by rolling your foot over a cylindrical piece of ice (freeze water in a paper cup), but doing this may not be effective, because the fascia has a layer of fat over it.

- Take anti-inflammatory medications as directed on the containers' labels.
- Stretch your calves and Achilles tendons frequently throughout the day.
- Massage the bottom of your foot, avoiding the tender area.
- Wear street shoes with heels to lessen the tension on the plantar fascia.

Running

If it hurts to run, don't do it. Resume running when you can do so without pain.

Appropriate Cross-Training

You can do swimming, deep-water running, or cycling—anything that doesn't cause pain.

Possible Causes

Plantar fasciitis can be caused by any of the following:

- A tight Achilles tendon
- Tight calves
- Improper or worn-out shoes
- Underpronation
- Overpronation

Prevention

To prevent plantar fasciitis, do the following:

- Regularly stretch your calves and Achilles tendon.
- Make sure you have the right shoe for your foot type and running style, and if the shoes you've been wearing are particularly stiff, try a more flexible pair. A podiatrist may recommend orthotics (devices that are molded to your foot and that you place in your shoe to help direct foot motion).
- Strengthen the muscles of your foot by repeatedly picking up a small object or a towel with your toes.
- Try stretching the fascia by rolling your foot over a golf ball or by pulling your toes up and back toward your ankles.

What are orthotics and how will I know if I need them?

Orthotics is the common term for orthoses or orthotic devices. They are made from rigid plastic that has been shaped using a mold of your foot and are inserted into your shoes to help correct improper foot motion and prevent injury. Your podiatrist or orthopedist may prescribe them if you overpronate or underpronate to a severe degree.

Check that whoever constructs your orthoses is very experienced. Also, you should wear them in all your shoes, not just your running shoes. Orthotics take some getting used to, so don't expect them to be comfortable at first.

Runner's Knee

Runner's knee is the most common injury among runners, both male and female. The patella, or kneecap, fits in a groove at the end of the femur (thighbone). During walking and running, the patella is supposed to move smoothly up and down in the center of that groove. If instead it moves off center and to the side (called improper tracking), it will rub against the femur, which causes pain and inflammation.

Allowed to progress, runner's knee develops into chondromalacia, which specifically involves a wearing away of the cartilage under the kneecap. Chondromalacia cannot be diagnosed without actually seeing the cartilage through magnetic resonance imaging (MRI) or surgery.

Symptoms

The symptoms of runner's knee are as follows:

- Pain around and under the kneecap that becomes worse with running
- Stiffness in the knee
- Swelling around the knee indicates a severe injury, so see a sports physician immediately

Treatment

Treat runner's knee as follows:

- Press your fingers around your knee, and if you find a tender area, ice it. If you don't, ice won't help.

- Take anti-inflammatory medications as directed on the containers' labels.
- Stretch hamstrings and quadriceps (quads) frequently.
- Do strengthening exercises for the hamstrings and quads.
- Try wearing a rubber sleeve with a hole for the kneecap (available from pharmacies); this helps keep the patella in place during walking and running.

Running

If you can run without pain, you can continue to do so, but avoid running downhill. If it hurts to run, cross-train instead.

Appropriate Cross-Training

You can do swimming, deep-water running, rowing, cycling if it does not cause pain (make sure the seat height is adjusted properly, do not clip your foot in, and spin at a low resistance) or use an elliptical trainer—any activity that you can do without pain.

Possible Causes

Runner's knee can be caused by any of the following:

- High weekly mileage or sudden and dramatic increases in mileage or running intensity
- Overpronation
- Weak quads or a strength imbalance between the hamstrings and quads
- Malalignment of the patella and the femur, which prevents the kneecap from sitting properly in the groove of the femur

Prevention

To prevent runner's knee, do the following:

- Wear shoes that control foot motion if you are an overpronator (see chapter 14). A podiatrist may recommend orthotics.
- Regularly stretch and strengthen your quadriceps and hamstring muscles.
- Follow appropriate guidelines for increasing mileage and intensity of running.

Shinsplints

The term *shinsplints* refers to several different minor injuries that cause dull pain in the front of the lower leg. Though a variety of theories have been put forth as to the exact cause of shinsplints—inflammation of the muscles of the shin, an inflammation of the periosteum (a thin sheath of tissue that wraps around the tibia), or muscle tears—there's no consensus among the experts as to the exact definition of shinsplints.

Symptoms

The symptoms of shinsplints include the following:

- Throbbing pain usually on the inner side of the shin about midway down the lower leg
- Tenderness when you touch your shin

Treatment

Treat shinsplints as follows:

- Use RICE.
- Take anti-inflammatory medications as directed on the containers' labels.
- Stretch your calves frequently throughout the day.
- Stretch your shins several times a day.

Running

If you can run without pain, avoid uneven surfaces and hills until the injury has healed completely. If it hurts to run, take a few days off and then try again.

Appropriate Cross-Training

You can do swimming, cycling, deep-water running, or rowing or use an elliptical trainer—whatever does not cause pain.

Possible Causes

Shinsplints can be caused by the following:

- Overtraining—too many miles, too much speed work, or a sudden and dramatic increase in mileage or intensity of running

- Wearing improper or worn-out shoes
- Tight calves

Prevention

To prevent shinsplints, do the following:

- Wear appropriate running shoes.
- Stretch your calves regularly.
- Follow guidelines for increasing mileage and intensity of running safely.

Stress Fractures

A stress fracture is a tiny crack in the surface of the bone caused by the repeated impact of running. Stress fractures most often occur in the metatarsals (the bones in the feet directly behind the toes) and the tibia or shin bone, but they can also occur in the pelvis or groin.

Symptoms

As the stress fracture develops, you may experience muscle soreness and stiffness over a general area of the shin or top of the foot, but with the fracture comes a sharp pain that you can pinpoint. This is what distinguishes a stress fracture from shinsplints or other injuries. If you suspect a stress fracture, see a sports physician to have a bone scan taken to confirm the diagnosis.

Treatment

Treat stress fractures as follows:

- Use RICE.
- Take anti-inflammatory medications as directed on the containers' labels.

Running

Stop running for 3 to 6 weeks until you can run without pain.

Appropriate Cross-Training

You can do cycling (don't clip your feet to the pedals), swimming, deep-water running, or rowing or use an elliptical trainer—any activity that does not cause pain.

Possible Causes

Stress fractures can be caused by the following:

- A sudden and dramatic increase in mileage or intensity of running
- Erratic menstrual periods or amenorrhea, which may produce weaker bones because of a lack of estrogen, making bones more susceptible to fractures
- Underpronation
- High-arched feet (poor shock absorption)

Prevention

To prevent stress fractures, do the following:

- If you are an underpronator, wear cushioned shoes that promote foot motion and improve your ability to absorb the shock of running.
- Consult your gynecologist if you have irregular periods; be vigilant about getting 1,200 milligrams of calcium daily. (See chapter 11 for more information about menstrual dysfunction.)
- Follow guidelines for increasing mileage and running intensity safely.

27

Stitches and Other Running Glitches

We are so fond of one another, because our ailments are the same.

—JONATHAN SWIFT

MOST OF THE TIME, RUNNING GOES PRETTY smoothly. You cruise along at a comfortable pace and before you know it, you've finished your 5-mile run and are ready for a shower and a plate of pancakes. Every now and then, though, a little glitch pops up, some inconvenience—such as a side stitch, a blister, a bit of chafing—that makes your run less than perfect. Following are several common complaints, from allergies to incontinence. They're not life-threatening (with the exception of heatstroke), and most are easily treated and prevented.

Allergies

Sniffing, wheezing, watery eyes—allergies can deliver a whole package of annoyances to your run. From March to May, you have to contend with tree pollen; May to July, grass; August and September, ragweed. It can be enough to turn you into a winter runner. Fortunately, there is relief.

The Cure

You'll find an array of antihistamines that will relieve symptoms, but most cause drowsiness. Some prescription medications do not; see your doctor about them.

The Prevention

Pollen counts are highest during the morning and then again later in the day, so try to plan your runs for noontime during allergy season. Don't run tree-lined streets or trails during the spring; stick to open spaces. Come summer, stay away from lawns and fields and head for the woods. Air pollutants can also cause allergic reactions, so run roads that are not heavily trafficked.

Asthma

Exercise-induced asthma usually strikes after several minutes of running. It can cause chest tightness, shortness of breath, and wheezing and becomes more of a problem in cold, dry weather; during allergy season when pollen counts are high; when running at altitude; and in the presence of air pollution.

The Cure

An asthma attack may subside after several minutes of running, owing to the phenomenon of the "refractory period"—after an initial attack of exercise-induced asthma, symptoms subside for 60 to 90 minutes, during which you can run comfortably. This is why experts recommend that before a race or an important run, you warm up with some fast running to bring on an asthma attack, so that you can then race during the refractory period.

The medications most often prescribed by doctors are a group of drugs called beta-agonists. These include albuterol, bitolterol mesylate, metaproterenol sulfate, pirbuterol acetate, and terbutaline sulfate (all generic names). You should use them 15 minutes before running.

The Prevention

When the weather's cold and dry, wear a face mask during running. This will create warm, humid air around your mouth, which is much less likely to induce asthma. Since pollen and air pollutants can stimulate an attack, try to run midday, when the pollen counts are lowest, and avoid running on roads heavy with traffic.

Athlete's Foot

Itching, burning, scaliness, and redness between the toes and on the soles of your feet are the symptoms of athlete's foot, a fungal infection that's usually picked up in moist locker rooms.

The Cure

Apply a fungicide, such as Desenex or Tinactin, two or three times a day and continue using it for about 2 weeks after the irritation has cleared up, because the fungus hangs on even after symptoms are gone. Relieve itching by soaking your feet in a mixture of baking soda and water or Domeboro solution.

The Prevention

Keep your feet clean and dry and change sweaty socks right after you run. If you work out in a gym and use the locker room to shower and change, consider wearing a pair of flip-flops around the room.

Black Toenails

Black toenails occur when blood forms under nails from repeated rubbing or bumping of the toes against the top of your shoe during running. The condition can be mild to very painful.

The Cure

To relieve the pain, you need to release the pressure caused by the buildup of blood. Disinfect a sharp, thinly pointed object—a paper clip or an X-Acto knife—by heating it in a flame or dipping it in alcohol, then use it to make a hole in the nail. Then stick your foot in a pan of warm water and let the blood drain. Put a little antifungal cream over the nail and cover it with a bandage. In a couple of days, the nail will likely loosen and fall off, or you can pull it off so that it doesn't tear and cut your toe when it does become loose.

The Prevention

Wear shoes that have enough room for your toes. There should be a thumb width of space between the end of your longest toe and the top of the shoe, and the shoe should not fit too snugly over the top of your foot.

Blisters

We all get blisters at one time or another. They are caused by constant friction against an area of the skin. Fluid accumulates between the layers of the skin to form a sac.

The Cure

Leave the blister alone for 24 hours. Most blisters heal on their own. If yours doesn't, sterilize a needle in a flame or alcohol, prick a couple of holes in the blister, and gently squeeze out the fluid. Don't remove the skin; you'll expose the very tender and sensitive layer of skin beneath. Apply Preparation H—sounds gross but it speeds healing—and cover the blister with a gauze pad. Before you put on shoes, cut a doughnut shape out of moleskin to put around the blister and then cover the whole thing with another piece of moleskin.

The Prevention

Wear proper-fitting shoes. Break in new shoes gradually and wear socks made from breathable fabrics that wick moisture away from your skin and help keep your feet dry. Before running, try applying petroleum jelly to areas prone to blisters.

Bunions

Bunions are a common problem among women who wear dress shoes that squeeze the top of the foot into a very narrow space. The big toe becomes turned in toward the little toes and a bony protuberance, called a bunion, develops at the base of the big toe on the outside. The bunion can become painful during running if your shoes put too much pressure on the area.

The Cure

Bunions are something you'll have to live with unless you choose to get surgery, which is rarely necessary. To relieve discomfort, place a bunion shield (available at drugstores) over the area. You can also put a toe spacer made from sponge rubber between your first and second toe. They come in sizes: begin with a small one and gradually increase the size as each one becomes comfortable. If your running shoes put too much pressure on the bunion, make a small incision in the upper where contact occurs.

The Prevention

Wear shoes for work, running, and dress that have adequate room for your feet.

Chafing

When you're sweaty, a rough spot on your clothing, such as a seam, can irritate your skin and may even cause bleeding. Sports bras and running tops can cause chafing. Also, women with well-endowed thighs may experience friction and irritation during running.

The Cure and the Prevention

For chafing, the cure lies in the prevention. Wear clothing made from breathable fabrics, as moisture increases friction and irritation. Before you buy a sports bra or singlet, check for rough seams that might irritate the skin. If you experience chafing along the insides of your thighs, run in long Lycra shorts. Also, Junonia, a mail-order supplier of women's activewear, sells double-layer shorts specifically to prevent chafing during exercise (see chapter 15). Try applying petroleum jelly or olive oil to areas that are prone to irritation.

Dehydration

Dehydration can cause dizziness, weakness, nausea, and in severe cases, chills, cramps, and mental confusion.

The Cure

Stop running immediately; find a cool, shady place; and drink fluids. Water or sports beverages are best because they empty faster from your stomach to the rest of your body. Also, cold beverages are more quickly absorbed than warm ones are.

The Prevention

Drink plenty of fluids throughout the day every day, before running and during long runs, especially in hot weather. (For more information on hydration, see chapter 8.)

Diarrhea

It's no fun when the runs send you running into the bushes, especially during a race. Also called "runner's trots," diarrhea can be brought on by intense physical activity, such as running.

The Prevention

Keep track of what you eat and drink before running and racing; this way, you'll learn which foods and beverages cause trouble. Common culprits include high-fiber foods, caffeinated beverages, and dairy products, for those who are lactose intolerant. How do you know if you are lactose intolerant? After consuming dairy products, you'll produce a lot of gas. Chewing gum, which contains sorbitol, can also cause gastrointestinal problems in certain people. Dehydration can cause diarrhea—another reason to drink plenty of fluids. You'll also be less likely to get into trouble during a run if you have regular bowel movements.

Heat Exhaustion and Heatstroke

Heat exhaustion and heatstroke are similar but not identical. Heat exhaustion is an overheating of the body caused by dehydration. Symptoms include thirst, headache, dizziness, nausea, and in severe cases, a rapid heartbeat and disorientation. Heatstroke specifically refers to the failure of your body's thermoregulatory system. What distinguishes heatstroke from heat exhaustion is that with the former, the runner will stop sweating, will have difficulty walking, and will become disoriented—so much so that she won't be able to take care of herself. Therefore, you should be able to recognize signs of heatstroke so that you can help other runners.

The Cure

If you are experiencing signs of any kind of heat trouble, stop running, find a cool and shady place, and drink water or a sports beverage. If you don't feel better in half an hour, go to the hospital.

Heat stroke can be fatal; mental disorientation means that the runner is in serious condition. Place ice packs around the neck and groin and under the armpits, splash water on the skin, and elevate the legs. Assuming the runner is conscious, get her to drink fluids even if she feels nauseated and doesn't want them. Call for medical assistance.

The Prevention

Dress appropriately for hot-weather running in light breathable fabrics and stay well-hydrated, which helps keep you cool and your thermoregulatory system functioning properly. If you have ever experienced heatstroke, you are more likely to get it again, and you should take extra precautions to protect yourself from the heat. Run in the morning or early evening when temperatures are coolest and carry fluids with you or choose a route that has water stops along the way. It's also a good idea to run with a friend.

Nausea

When you push yourself beyond your limit—such as the effort you might put out to run your very fastest 5-K—you can feel nauseated and even pass out. Experts don't know why this happens.

The Cure and the Prevention

Many runners take a natural anti-inflammatory compound called bromelain (found in the stems of pineapple). It's available in health-food stores as Bromelain 2000. Ted L. Edwards, Jr., M.D., a gastroenterologist and sports medicine specialist who has worked with runners and cyclists in Austin, Texas, for 25 years, recommends his athletes take two 250-milligram capsules before and after a race. "And it seems to be working," says Edwards.

Dr. Edwards also advises that you don't eat or drink anything but water in the 2 hours prior to a hard workout or competition. When it comes to drinking a sports beverage, such as Gatorade or Exceed, wait until *after* you've warmed up, when your body has switched to its energy-metabolism mode. During energy metabolism, you won't experience an up-and-down insulin response to these carbohydrate drinks, which can also trigger nausea during hard exercise. Finally, avoid taking ibuprofen or aspirin before an intense effort.

Side Stitches

You're running merrily along and then—ouch!—you feel a sharp, stabbing pain just below your rib cage on the right side. Side stitches are caused by cramping of the diaphragm but may also be brought on by food in the stomach or intestinal gas. They are the bane of all runners.

The Cure

There are several cures:

- If the stitch is on your right, exhale *forcefully* every time your left foot hits the ground, until the pain goes away; if the stitch is on your left, exhale when your right foot hits.
- Run with your hands on top of your head and your elbows pulled back and breathe deeply from your abdomen.
- Push your fist into your chest under your rib cage; bend over to about 90 degrees and run in this position for about 10 steps.
- Stop running and bend sideways to the left if the stitch is on the right or to the right if the stitch is on the left.
- If nothing works, walk until the pain goes away.

The Prevention

Run with good posture and using the 3:2 rhythmic breathing pattern described on page 39 in chapter 5. Don't eat too close to running.

Urinary Incontinence

Urinary incontinence is a problem that many women develop after having children.

The Cure and the Prevention

Do Kegel exercises—lots of them—regularly. For a description of the proper technique, see page 162 in chapter 12.

Yeast Infections

Some women have found they became more prone to yeast infections after taking up running. The reason is moisture buildup from sweating.

The Cure

Use an over-the-counter cream, such as Gyne-Lotrimin or Monistat 7. Continue to apply the cream for 1 day after symptoms have gone. Yeast infections usually take 3 to 5 days to clear up.

The Prevention

Wear shorts made from breathable fabrics and change your clothing as soon as you can after running and racing.

Letting Go

BY MARLENE CIMONS

PERHAPS THERE IS A TIME TO LET GO.

I have been running for nearly 20 years. I started in 1980, when I was in my midthirties—a late bloomer, I liked to joke—and stayed with it. Like many women, running helped me discover who I was. My body began to change, and so did my mind; I became calmer, grounded, if you will. I also began to set goals—and meet them. I began to realize my potential, however limited.

I was 35 years old before I ran my first 10-K race, barely etching out 54 minutes. I was 36 when I ran my first marathon, breaking 4 hours with a 3:55. Like many new runners, I wanted to get better, faster.

It began to happen. I went on long runs and did regular track workouts. I started climbing that decade-long road of improvement, watching my times drop, establishing new goals. I came tantalizingly close to the barriers I had set for myself: I hovered near 3:40 in the marathon, 75 minutes in the 10-mile, and 45 minutes for 10-K. I got very close, but I never quite made it to breaking any of them.

I was getting older, and my life was changing in other important ways. At the age of 42, I became a mother for the first time—a single mother—when my 3-month-old daughter arrived from India. Still, I didn't give up. I bought a baby jogger and used it religiously. I trained for and ran a few more marathons after she came. By then, though, I could no longer break 4 hours.

I kept telling myself, though, that if I put my mind—and my body—to it, I could still do it. Then, my goal was only to break 4 hours and qualify for Boston. But, even though the goals became smaller, they became more elusive. The things I could do easily a decade earlier were now out of reach.

Other things became more important.

Six years after my daughter came, my son followed, a 3-year-old from Russia. I managed to keep running, but track workouts and superlong runs—which had been the mainstay of my serious training—became a memory.

My moment of truth came a few years ago when I decided to run a marathon on "constitutional" memory only, instead of serious training—it wasn't laziness as much as a lack of time, rather than lack of will, to do the work. It was memory, all right. For a little more than 5 hours—jogging and walking—I remembered how hard and painful a marathon could be.

At that point, I told myself, *It's enough just to be able to run.*

We all know how difficult it is—with work and family responsibilities—to keep on training at the same level. My children are growing up quickly, becoming more independent and social beings with lives and activities of their own, yet they remain dependent on me. In my running infancy, I would run a leisurely 2 to 3 hours on a spring or fall Saturday morning, even when I wasn't planning to run a marathon. These days, an hour's run seems a luxury. I have become the quintessential soccer mom.

Also, all those years of pounding have taken a physical toll. My heart and lungs and bones may be strong, but my joints hurt. After 90 minutes of running—on those mornings when I should be so fortunate!—my body begins to ache in places I never even knew existed.

My muscles are tight. My lower back hurts most mornings when I wake up. Ten marathons, hundreds of races, and literally thousands of miles—not to mention the usual aging process—have eroded what little speed and fluidity I might once have had. I have moved (perhaps not so gracefully) from a respectful 7:30- to an 8-minute pace at my best to a lumbering 10-minute pace on even my better days.

But it's okay.

I am coming to peace with all this, knowing in my heart that it is just as thrilling to watch my daughter sink a three-pointer or make that tie-breaking goal, or listen to my son tap out "Für Elise" (the staple of every piano recital) than to qualify for Boston. I am happy that they are thriving. For my running, I am grateful if I can stay injury free and be out there, able to run every day that I can, at whatever pace.

Marlene Cimons lives with her two children in Bethesda, Maryland, and writes on health issues for the *Los Angeles Times*.

PART IX

Running for a Lifetime

28 Running and Family

The challenge and the energy running requires may be a selfish pursuit, but it actually motivates me to be stronger in my relationships. Being an athlete helps me to know I will give that extra effort when it comes to caring for another's needs.

—JOAN BENOIT SAMUELSON,
author of *Joan Samuelson's Running for Women*

AS WOMEN, WE ARE TRADITIONALLY THE nurturers of relationships, the keepers of family. The impact of all our activities inside and outside the home vibrates along the bonds we share with our partners and our children. Our running is no exception. Fortunately, most of us find the effect enhances our relationships with our partners and our children. Just as our running strengthens our bodies, it can benefit the health and well-being of our families as well.

381

Partners have found each other because of running, drawn together by shared passion, the synergy of like minds, but more significantly by the honesty that running forces. When we run, we don't have the usual accoutrements of dating to enhance our images: no perfect hair or painted face; no sparkling jewels or stunning fashions; no wine or perfume or candlelight. Our meeting place is the road. We sweat, we breathe hard, sometimes we grimace—our bodies, our faces, our athleticism, our attitudes exposed.

Running gives us the courage to be ourselves. We feel strong when we run, less vulnerable, more willing to speak our minds. Running provides the perfect environment in which to grow trust, and from trust, strong relationships develop. Perhaps this is why many couples who run together stay together.

Running can provide a meeting place for parents who struggle to find time together in the steady stream of family, work, and housekeeping responsibilities. Running becomes the rock at the center of all things rushing. It provides a new vantage point from which to observe and discuss the happenings of our lives.

Aside from all the meaningful significance running can add to a relationship, it's just nice having a partner who understands why you are getting up at 5:00 in the morning on weekdays to get your run in before the activities of the day carry you away from any possibility of running. It's nice to have a partner who won't frown when you leave a party early on a Friday evening so you can get a good night's sleep before a Saturday-morning race, someone who doesn't think you're crazy to train for a marathon and who might even join you for a couple of those long Sunday-morning runs.

When Your Partner Doesn't Run

Of course, not all of us are so fortunate. Some of us have partners who not only don't run but don't understand why we do. They may be jealous of our passion for running or resentful of the time it takes from the relationship or the family.

Invite Your Partner's Support

Many women solve the problem of lack of support by involving their partners in their running. "My husband was rather unsupportive of my running," says Michele Peterson of Goffstown, New Hampshire, "but I found a way to get him involved. When I was training for

HIS AND HERS

"My husband is a golfer, so I encourage him to attend coaching and training sessions to improve his game as well as become involved in local tournaments. We keep a calendar of our upcoming events and training schedules, and we have dinner later in the evening after I've had the opportunity to complete my evening run and he's had the opportunity to golf nine holes. By encouraging and supporting his sport, I found he was more supportive of mine."

—BEV DEGEORGE, RUNNER

the Bay State Marathon, which is held in October, I had many hot and humid long runs to do on the weekend, and I asked him to bring me drinks on the course. He'd park his car at our designated meeting places and drink his coffee and read the Sunday paper, waiting for me to come exchange my empty water bottle for a full one. Just seeing our white car gave me energy. He was always there, ready for the exchange, and that meant a lot to me. Although my husband can't relate to the drive that makes me run through heat, humidity, and physical fatigue, I know that deep down, he has come to believe in me and respect my stick-to-itiveness."

Others have coaxed their spouses to races with promises of post-race beer and food. For most people, watching an event gives them an appreciation of the effort, enjoyment, and satisfaction that come with running and racing, and many spectators (including partners) themselves become runners.

Find Acceptance

In the end, it doesn't matter really whether your partner runs. What's important is that there is mutual support for each other's passions. Reaching this mutual support requires communication—talking about why running is important and how it relieves stress, gives you energy, keeps you healthy, and makes you feel good about yourself. Likewise, find out about your partner's interests. The goal isn't conversion but acceptance and love despite differences.

Something for Ourselves

Though it can be fun and meaningful to run with our partners, running is something we first do for ourselves. We choose it from our desire for fitness or competition or pure physical enjoyment; we do it because it enhances our individual well-being. So many of us are constantly doing for others—our partners, our children, our parents, our siblings. "Running is the one thing I do for me," many women say.

Maryann McCambridge started running in 1968 when she was 31 and a mother of six. "I wanted a big family, but I was overwhelmed by the responsibility," she says. "I thought, *I should have at least 20 minutes to myself.* One day, I heard a doctor on the radio recommend running. He pointed out that you didn't need a partner or any equipment—that you could just head right out the door. I thought, *That's for me.*" Maryann has been running ever since—with a few months' break to have her seventh child. "Running makes me appreciate life to the fullest," says Maryann. "I'm in tip-top shape, I'm never sick, and I'm a happy person."

To say that we run for ourselves doesn't mean we are selfish. The good that comes of it benefits everyone we touch. You know that old saying, You need to love yourself before you can truly love anyone else. When you take care of yourself, you are better able to care for others. When you feel good, your joy and energy are felt by everyone around you. "When Mom is happy, everybody is happy. When Mom is sad, everyone is sad," says Maryann. "The responsibility is great."

The gift you give yourself by running multiplies into many gifts that you give back to your partner and children: energy, happiness, patience, health, and self-worth.

Passing the Baton

One of the gifts you give through running is the example of good health and fitness and the importance of taking care of your body. You can inspire your children to take up an active lifestyle, and whether they choose running, swimming, cycling, or team sports, what matters is that they participate regularly in an activity that's good for their health and enhances their total well-being.

Maryann McCambridge has inspired her children through her running. "We are a sports family," she says. Four of her seven children are or have been runners. "I never pushed my children into running or any other sport, but I think they saw by example that being active is healthy and good for you.

"Running teaches me discipline and shows me reward for my dis-

RUNNING WITH BABY

Finding time to run can be difficult even when you're single. When you're in a relationship, it gets even harder; there are your partner's needs to consider. Then comes baby. You can leave your partner at home alone, but not the little one.

Most likely, you and your partner can trade off taking care of your baby, to give the other some free time. If not, perhaps you can trade baby-sitting with a friend or neighbor or organize a group of running mothers who take turns sitting the children while the others go for a run (see chapter 7 for other creative solutions to fitting running into family life). If there's simply no one to leave your baby with while you run, just take her with you.

Get a running stroller. They are perfectly safe when it's just the two of you, but not in races, where they can be hazardous to other runners, you, and your baby. Here are a few tips on buying and using a running stroller:

- The larger the wheelbase, the easier the stroller is to run with but the more difficult it is to transport.
- Adjustable height is important if both you and your partner will be running with the stroller.
- Make sure there's a hand brake to help you slow down the stroller when you need to.
- Storage compartments are convenient for taking along diapers, bottles, and other accessories.
- When running, always use the wrist tether so that you and the stroller stay connected.
- Be careful about parking the stroller on an incline or hanging gear on the handlebars—running strollers can tip backward rather easily.
- You can get a very good stroller at a reasonable price by buying a used one.

cipline. I love running and what it does for me," adds Maryann. "Children pick up on this attitude."

Maryann's son Jack took up running in high school and he and his mom often trained together for road races, including their first marathon in Philadelphia, where Maryann qualified for Boston. Jack's wife, Elaine, and now their children are runners, too. Every year, the McCambridges—Maryann; her children, Jack, Elaine, Matthew, Alisa, and Suzanne; and her grandson, Jason—participate in Miles for Matt, a 24-hour track relay event that raises money for cancer research.

Sometimes it's our children who inspire us to run. Bernie Pongranz started running shortly after her daughter Ann became involved in cross-country. "Ann wanted to run, but there wasn't a girls' team at her school, so she organized one," says Bernie. "She'd often go running at night by herself and my husband would follow her in the car to make sure she was safe. Then he took up running so he could run with her. I'd go to her races and my husband's races, and one day, I just decided to take up running myself."

That was 19 years ago, when Bernie was 40. Since then, she's run many races, including several marathons. In 1996, she and her son's daughter won the grandmother-granddaughter division at the Advil Mini Marathon.

Bernie's daughter, Ann, clearly was so strong-willed that she overcame all obstacles to girls' participation in running, including the absence of a girls' team at her school. Many other girls and women, however, have been held back from sports participation because of lack of encouragement and opportunity. Though the social climate has changed since the 1970s and girls are encouraged and invited to play sports of all kinds, attitudes linger. It seems we *expect* boys to play sports, whereas we *accept* that girls play.

As mothers, we can have the greatest effect in changing those attitudes. One of the gifts we give to our daughters through our running is to show them that an active lifestyle is just as natural and essential to women as it is to men; that women not only are the caretakers of others but that we place a high priority on our own well-being, too; that we do what we need to for our own good health and happiness. With such an example, your children will naturally assume these same attitudes and live by them.

Children's Fitness

You hear yourself so often telling your children to stop running that it seems unlikely you'll ever have to concern yourself with encouraging them to be more active. Children have always loved to play; however, these days, there are more and more opportunities for children to entertain themselves while sitting—in front of television screens or computer monitors. More time inside staring into a screen means less time outside running around.

Experts speculate that children's fitness has declined since the 1970s, but they can't point to any concrete statistics because means of measuring physical fitness in children have changed. They do know that children weigh more today and have more body fat than ever. In 1995, the National Center for Health Statistics in Hyattsville, Maryland, looked at health information for 3,000 children between the ages of 6 and 17 and found that 11 percent were seriously over-weight, twice the percentage noted among children in the 1960s.

An active lifestyle offers the same benefits to your children as it does you. It controls weight, lowers blood pressure (yes, even 8-year-olds can have high blood pressure), improves motor skills, reduces stress, and helps them feel better about themselves. These effects can last into adulthood, provided an active lifestyle is maintained. Studies show that children of average weight become adults who have an easier time maintaining their weight than do adults who were obese as children.

Providing Motivation

A survey conducted by the Melpomene Institute for Women's Health Research in St. Paul, Minnesota, found that children of physi-cally active women are more likely to lead active lifestyles them-selves. Other studies confirm this finding and emphasize that the atti-tudes a child's family and friends take toward sports and physical activity are some of the most important influences on that child's level of activity.

By running, you show your children the value of physical activity, but by doing sports together as a family, you begin to make it a real part of your children's lifestyles. Play outdoors with your kids—tag, kickball, Frisbee, catch. Go for family hikes, bike rides, camping trips. Involve your children in your running. Invite them to bike or skate along while you run. Take them to your races. Many events now have fun runs of a mile or less to allow children to participate.

Talk to your kids about organized sports—soccer, softball, base-ball, football. Offer them the opportunity to participate but don't push them into anything they don't want to do. Praise your children's efforts at whatever activity they choose, and avoid being critical and disappointed by poor performances. It's regular participation and good effort that should be applauded. You don't want your child to measure his or her self-worth by the number of soccer goals scored each week. An overemphasis on performance and competition takes away the fun. When sports stop being fun, children stop playing.

Children's Running

Your child may decide she'd like to come running with you. Take her along, but just as you started by alternating walking and running, do the same with your daughter or son. Go at a pace set by your child, and pay attention to signs of fatigue—don't continue to the point of exhaustion. Also, kids can become overheated more quickly than adults do, so make sure your child drinks plenty of liquids and is dressed in appropriate clothing if the weather is warm.

How far should your child run? That depends on how far she wants to go and how far she is capable of going. Kids are generally better than adults are at stopping an activity when it becomes unpleasant, but if you notice that your child is laboring or seems uncomfortable, *you* make the suggestion to stop for the day.

Lyle Micheli, M.D., director of the Division of Sports Medicine at Children's Hospital in Boston, recommends that children under the age of 14 run no farther than 3 miles at a time. The reason, he says, is that bones are still growing and the growth cartilage at the ends of the bones is softer than adult cartilage and more vulnerable to injury.

High-schoolers who participate in cross-country can and do run more. How much they run usually depends on what their coach requires. Michael Sargent, M.D., a pediatrician specializing in adolescent and college-age runners and the director of athletic medicine at the University of Vermont, believes that in general high school runners can perform quite well on 30 to 40 miles a week, with no more than three hard runs a week.

Some coaches push their athletes to do even more, 50 to 60 miles a week, and though high schoolers may do fine on higher mileage, Sargent cautions that such a high intensity of running at such a young age might result in burnout. "The goal should be to make running a lifetime sport," he says.

MORE ON KIDS' RUNNING

The Road Runners Club of America (RRCA) offers two booklets on children and running: *Children's Running—A Guide for Teachers and Coaches* and *Children's Running—A Guide for Parents and Kids.* They are available for a minimal fee by writing the RRCA at 1150 S. Washington Street, suite 250, Alexandria, VA 22314 or by calling (703) 836-0558.

At what age is it okay for my child to run a marathon?

"I believe you should have two to three years' experience as a 10-K runner before thinking about the marathon," says pediatrician Michael Sargent, M.D., director of athletic medicine at the University of Vermont. "Sure, some high-school and college students run marathons, and they do all right, but the marathon requires maturity—in both body and mind. It's an event that involves a lot of physical and psychological stress. I would discourage runners from attempting the marathon until after their college career."

Running, Adolescence, and Girls

The teenage years can shine with activity and achievement, but for many, this transition to adulthood has its moments of turbulence. Bodies change, hormones rise, and the sexual gap widens. For girls especially, these years can pose significant challenges to self-esteem.

Carol Gilligan, a Harvard University professor who has spent years researching girls' psychological development and passage into adolescence, points out that teens become more relationship oriented and more concerned with being accepted and pleasing others, sometimes compromising their own needs to do so.

It's a time when girls become easily influenced by society's standards of ideal beauty and pressures to be thin. Body-image problems and distortions can develop and may lead to disordered eating, amenorrhea, and possibly anorexia or bulimia. For some girls, running becomes part of their means to drive themselves toward this ideal beauty and thinness. Others may seek acceptance and approval through running performance, and eating disorders and thinness become their means to try to achieve faster race times. No one knows the extent of eating disorders among young female athletes. It is important that as a parent, you be aware of these possibilities, not to worry about them but to be able to recognize signs of an unhealthy pattern so that you can address it before it becomes a problem. Signs that your daughter may be overtraining or undereating include fatigue, irritability, disturbed sleeping patterns, and excess weight loss. If she stops menstruating, it could be a sign that she isn't taking in enough calories to meet her energy requirements. If she misses more than three periods in a row, she should see her gynecologist and consider consulting a sports-oriented nutritionist as well.

Amenorrhea, of course, leads to bone loss. Though we think of osteoporosis as a disease of older women, it can begin in teenagers who experience menstrual dysfunction and aren't conscientious about getting enough calcium. Adolescent girls need 1,200 milligrams of calcium a day.

If you suspect your daughter may be heading toward a health problem or that she may have an eating disorder, experts advise that you not question her about her eating or tell her she looks too thin, but rather express concern about her fatigue or perhaps her lackluster running performances and ask how she's feeling. Then talk with an expert—a physician, nutritionist, or psychologist who specializes in eating disorders. These issues are complicated and difficult to confront. (See chapter 10 for more on body image and eating disorders.) Know, too, that running is not the culprit; it just happened to get caught up in the tangle of bigger issues of self-esteem and desire for control.

For most girls, running is the solution because it builds self-esteem and confidence. In 1991, the Melpomene Institute for Women's Health Research in St. Paul, Minnesota, explored the relationship between sports participation and self-esteem by surveying and meeting with girls between the ages of 9 and 17. "The girls who had the highest self-esteem scores were the ones who were physically active at the highest levels," reports Judy Mahle Lutter, M.A. "The girls talked a great deal about ways they gained self-esteem through sports. Many told about times they were challenged or took a risk. Others shared stories about achievement—not just winning, but learning a new skill or even being a member of a team." Running can help make your daughter's teenage years happy ones.

29 Fifty-Plus

With luck, and if I train right, in the year 2027 I will be signing up for the 5-K and 10-K races for women over 90.

—EVE PELL, who competed at the World Association of Veteran Athletes games in 1997 at the age of 60

LOUISE ADAMS WAS 56 WHEN SHE took up running for the first time since high school. She saw an ad in her hometown newspaper in Boulder, Colorado, for the Rocky Mountain Senior Games and decided to enter. Without any training at all, she won her age group in every sprint event, from 50 meters to the 400.

Twenty years later, Louise is still running and racing. She turned 77 in December 1998 and plans to continue to run until she's 80 at least.

She competes on the track in the middle distances (400 meters to 10-K) and runs a number of 5-K and 10-K road races. Her race times for the 5-K and 10-K are in the mid-twenties and mid-fifties, respectively. In March 1997, she set indoor world records for the 75-to-79 age group in the 400 meters, 800 meters, mile, and 3,000 meters.

"I had been divorced when I decided to start running," says Louise. "I was looking for a new direction. If I were married, I wouldn't be doing this. I was John's wife. We did more things that he wanted to do and with his friends."

Louise runs 3 or 4 days a week with the Boulder Road Runners and does lots of walking. She also lifts weights, bikes, and swims.

"I enjoy the camaraderie," says Louise. "The Boulder Road Runners are very supportive, and I have a good friend, Nancy Smalley. She's 5 years younger. We train together and run a lot of the same races. We're quite competitive.

"When I started running, I had no idea it would evolve into this," adds Louise. "If anyone had told me I'd be running around Boulder in Lycra tights and a brassiere, I'd have said they were out of their mind."

It wasn't all that long ago that people might have thought *Louise* was out of her mind, pounding the streets and scrambling over the trails of Boulder, Colorado, at the age of 77. It's women like Louise, though, who have shown us that there are no age limits to physical activity. Now, more women than ever are maintaining their active lifestyles or taking up sports on into their fifties, sixties, seventies, and eighties.

Running Rewards

The benefits that running offers don't really change as we get older, but certain of them become more significant.

A Healthy Heart

Aging tends to stiffen the arteries, and the walls of the heart's pumping chamber (the left ventricle) becomes thicker because of an increase in the size of the muscle cells. With running, you can keep your blood vessels in good condition and your heart strong. As we age, our hearts function a little differently during exercise. Our heart rate doesn't rise as high as it did when we were younger. Instead, the heart dilates more to take in more blood, and then it contracts forcefully to pump that blood through arteries to working muscles. Heart muscle that has become deconditioned from inactivity, however, loses much of its ability to contract forcefully.

Strong Bones

After menopause, we lose bone at a fairly rapid rate for the first 10 years, and then the rate slows. If we didn't build strong bones in our youth, we become very susceptible to osteoporosis (porous, fragile bones that are easily broken) in our later years. A study done by the Melpomene Institute for Women's Research in St. Paul, Minnesota, found that in a group of women between the ages of 46 and 80, those who were physically active had 25.6 percent higher bone density than did those who were not very active.

Running strengthens the bones in your legs, of course, and your hips and spine—the areas where osteoporosis is most likely to strike. To firm up the bones in your upper body, do some regular resistance training. It's also important to get plenty of calcium in your diet (1,500 milligrams daily) because as we age, our intestines become less efficient at absorbing calcium.

Strong Muscles

Muscle mass also declines as we get older, which makes us more prone to injury—running or otherwise—and as we lose muscle, our resting metabolisms slow down, which can lead to weight gain. Running builds strong legs and will help keep you on your feet during those potentially unsteady years of your seventies and eighties, and with a little weight training for the upper body, you can be strong all over. By maintaining strength, you're better able to take care of yourself, which offers certainly a practical physical benefit but also a psychological one. You'll feel more confident and self-assured, and you'll like your body.

An Easier Menopause

There's no guarantee that running will make a difficult menopause a whole lot easier. Nonetheless, regular running helps you maintain your weight, lessens the moodiness and/or depression that you might experience, and helps you sleep better. (For more on running and menopause, see chapter 13.)

Easier Weight Control

Weight gain seems an inevitable consequence of aging as our metabolisms slow. Most of the women runners I've spoken with who've gone through menopause have noticed some weight gain despite maintaining their running programs. Nonetheless, running is the best calorie burner around, and combined with a healthy diet and some regular strength training to keep your muscle mass up, you'll stay slim. Louise Adams reports that she weighs the same as she did in high school. "It's distributed a little differently, though," she says.

A Stronger Immune System

Our immune systems weaken as we age, making us more susceptible to illness. Running is an immunity booster, unless you do too much of it.

Relief from Stress

One of life's most stressful events is the death of a loved one. In our older years, such losses become more frequent. Running helps us through those times and gives us the strength to go forward with good memories and continued hope for the future.

A Sharper Mind

According to the *Harvard Women's Health Watch* (June 1997), "results of tests administered to large numbers of people of different ages indicate that short-term memory begins to decline in one's 50s; general intelligence, in one's 60s; and capacity for abstract thought, in one's 70s." They also point out that this varies greatly among individuals.

Fortunately for us runners, researchers have linked physical activity with a slower decline in memory. There's more good news: in a 1991 study reported in *U.S. News and World Report* (May 1995), a group of women between the ages of 57 and 85 who began exercising regularly in aerobics classes or by walking were able to *gain back* some of the mental speed they had lost.

A Youthful Attitude

Of course, it takes a youthful attitude to keep running as we get older, but running helps perpetuate that attitude. Running gives you energy. You feel alive, strong, confident. You know that you are fit, attractive, and athletic.

Friendships

Through running, we find friendship and support, whether we run with the members of our local running club or a group from our neighborhood. When our children have all grown and gone and we no longer have the office and its social environment, our running friendships fill the empty places and help give meaning to our lives.

Greater Longevity

Given all the benefits we've just discussed, it's not surprising that by continuing to run into our later years, we can increase the quality and the length of our lives. In a study reported in the *Journal of the American Medical Association* (April 23/30, 1997), Lawrence Kushi, Sc.D., and his colleagues at the University of Minnesota School of Public Health looked at a group of 40,417 postmenopausal women, 55 to 69 years old, whose activity levels ranged from low (moderate to vigorous physical activity a few times a month) to medium (vigorous activity once a week or moderate activity one to four times a week) to high (vigorous activity two or more times a week or moderate activity more than four times a week). Moderate activities included golf, bowling, gardening, taking long walks, and light sports. Vigorous activity included running, racquet sports, aerobics, and other strenuous activities. After 7 years, the researchers found that the more active women showed a lower risk of death from all causes, with the most active women having a 30 percent lower risk of death from all causes compared with those who were least active. The researchers noted that risk of death from cardiovascular and respiratory diseases in particular were much lower in the more active groups.

I'm 52 years old and haven't exercised regularly since I was in high school. I'd like to try running. Do I need a physical before I get started?

The American Heart Association recommends that anyone of any age have a complete physical exam before starting an exercise program, reports Walter M. Bortz, M.D., in the *Fifty-Plus Fitness Association Bulletin*. Bortz also recommends a stress test to make sure your heart is in good working order. "It is my feeling that all physically active people should have a stress test every three years," he says. Once you get the okay from your physician, begin by walking and then move into a walk–run program (see page 47 in chapter 5 for a complete schedule).

THE FIFTY-PLUS FITNESS ASSOCIATION

To learn more about fitness and aging and to take an active role in advancing our knowledge about physical fitness among older adults, consider joining the Fifty-Plus Fitness Association. Members of this nonprofit organization are often the subjects of studies on exercise and aging. You'll receive a quarterly bulletin with advice on various topics in the areas of exercise, nutrition, and health as well as opportunities to meet other members for active outings, seminars, and conferences that are held around the country. For more information, write Fifty-Plus at Box D, Stanford, CA 94309; call them at (415) 323-6160; or check out their web site at **www.pamf.org/fiftyplus/fiftyindex.html**.

Running As We Age

The guidelines for running in your later years are the same as for your youth:

- Don't increase your mileage or intensity too quickly (go by the 10 percent rule).
- Add new training elements—such as speed work, hill running, or long runs—gradually, not all at once.
- Always follow a hard day of running with an easy day.
- Always wear good running shoes and replace them before they become too worn (every 500 miles).

How long or fast or often you run depends what you want to do, how much time you have, and what your body can handle. These are the same parameters you would follow if you were 25. Signs that you are doing too much include the typical symptoms of overtraining: fatigue, irritability, disordered sleeping patterns, sluggishness during running, poor race performances, and injury.

Listen to your body. You can tell when you're overdoing it, especially if you've been running for 10 years or more. Cut back on mileage and/or intensity or mix in some cross-training. If, on the other hand, your running simply energizes you and you want to do more, go for it. At 62, Maryann McCambridge runs 40 miles a week and does 75 "men's" push-ups every morning.

Some Things Do Change

When asked whether she found disappointment in her slower race times now that she's 62, Maryann McCambridge shook her head. "No, I'm happy that I have my health and that I can be there on the starting line."

We get wiser with age, and perhaps this helps us accept that we also, unfortunately, get slower as we age. If you want to maintain as much speed as possible, you may find you'll be more successful by doing more quality running and fewer total miles each week. For example, rather than running 6 or 7 days with just one pace workout on the track, you might cut back to 4 or 5 days of running each week that would include a pace workout, a *fartlek* run, and a longer run. On the other days, go easy, rest completely, or do some light cross-training.

Don't forget to stretch and lift weights. We also lose muscle and flexibility as we get older, making stretching and strength training more important than ever for injury prevention and overall total fitness. Not only do stretching and strength training enhance our running but they also prevent the loss of good balance that can come with age.

What About Injuries?

Injuries occur in older runners for the same reason they do in young runners—overuse. Too many miles, increasing mileage or intensity of running too quickly, or too many hard runs can lead to injury. Age doesn't make you prone to injury, overtraining does.

If an injury does occur, recovery time is the same as it was when you were younger. Many of us mistakenly think that as we age, the healing process slows down. Warren Scott, M.D., chief of sports medicine at Kaiser Permanente Medical Center in Santa Clara, California, says many of his older patients recover from injury just as quickly as the younger ones do. He points out that teenagers do heal fastest, but adults of any age recover at about the same rate.

Scott also warns that family members may view any injury you get as a sign of frailty and may discourage you from cross-training during the recovery period or from resuming running at all once you're healed. There is no reason, though, that you can't recover completely and get back out on the roads.

Some runners do complain of more little aches and pains and stiffness as they age. They say they need more time to warm up before running at their usual pace. If that's the case with you, simply do what your body asks. Treat your body with respect, and it will reward you with miles and miles of enjoyable running—even if they may go by a little more slowly than they once did.

Can I continue to run if I have arthritis in my knees?

"I don't discourage anyone with osteoarthritis from any form of pain-free exercise," says Warren Scott, M.D. "Regular movement speeds the rate at which cartilage is replaced by your body, making it stronger." That being said, Scott does find that for some individuals, running is too painful, and he recommends they take up another activity, such as swimming, cycling, deep-water running, or water aerobics.

Doctors now prescribe exercise as part of the treatment for osteoarthritis. In a study reported in the January 1, 1997, issue of the *Journal of the American Medical Association,* Walter H. Ettinger, Jr., M.D., and his colleagues at Wake Forest University in Winston-Salem, North Carolina, examined the effects of resistance training and aerobic exercise on a group of men and women aged 60 and older who suffered from arthritis of the knee. The researchers found that both resistance training and aerobic exercise (40 minutes of walking at a brisk pace, with a 10-minute warmup and 10-minute cool-down) resulted in moderate improvements in pain and knee function. Furthermore, the researchers suspected that a *higher* intensity of activity would have had an even *greater* effect.

A Few Special Considerations

If you are taking any medications, know that many of them produce side effects that can be a bit hazardous during running. Some drugs affect balance and coordination; others can cause blurred vision or dehydration. Many reduce your ability to regulate heat during exercise. If you happen to experience any unusual symptoms, consult your doctor. Also, any time a drug is prescribed, ask what its side effects might be during exercise. In many cases, medications can be adjusted or alternatives prescribed so as not to interfere with your running.

Don't let poor nutrition interfere with your running either. "I have found that many seniors don't eat enough because they think they don't need as much food as they did when they were younger," says Scott. Running burns a lot of calories; if you aren't eating enough, you risk muscle glycogen depletion during your longer and harder runs and races. (See chapter 8 for more information on nutrition.)

Also, as we get older, we become less heat tolerant. This may be less so for runners, however. A study of marathoners done at the University of Queensland in Australia found that those in their fifties were as good at regulating body temperature as were runners in their twenties. Nonetheless, acclimate to hot weather gradually (keep mileage low and don't do any fast running until your body has become accustomed to the heat); drink plenty of fluids; wear light, breathable clothing; and avoid running during the hottest parts of the day.

The precautions we take as older runners are really not much different from those we should follow in our youth. Getting old doesn't mean we become fragile and vulnerable, as our society has thought for so long. As Warren Scott, M.D., puts it, "the frailty associated with old age is due to lack of exercise more than age."

The myth of the frail old lady has been irrevocably dispelled by women like Louise Adams and many others who are running and racing in their fifties, sixties, seventies, eighties, and beyond. All of us running behind them who continue to follow our dreams of a lifetime of running can look forward to many years of good health, strong bodies, sharp minds, and personal fulfillment.

30 A Celebration of Women's Running*

The biggest change is the mass social acceptance. People used to think I was a freak. Now women of all shapes and sizes run all the time, and everyone just ignores them because they're part of the landscape. That's what I love.

—KATHRINE SWITZER, who ran the Boston Marathon in 1967 before women were officially allowed

ON THE MORNING OF JUNE 21, 1998, OVER 18,000 runners lined up at the start of the Suzuki Rock 'N' Roll Marathon in San Diego, California. More than half of them were women. The significance brings pause when you consider that as recently as 1970, women were not officially allowed to run the marathon in the United States. Men, on the other hand, have been running it since the first Boston held in 1897. In fact, the longest official distance women could race in 1970 was 2½ miles. Long distances—particularly the marathon—would ruin our reproductive systems, according to the intelligentsia of the time.

This didn't stop women from racing longer distances anyway (with no harmful consequences to their uteruses). In 1959, Arlene Pieper ran the Pikes Peak Marathon, a grueling 26.2-mile journey up and down one of Colorado's highest mountains, finishing in 9 hours and 16 minutes. Through the 1960s, women raced a variety of distances, including the marathon. However, the American Athletic Union (AAU), which governed track and field and long-distance running at the time, did not recognize women's race times, meaning that when Mary Lepper finished the Culver City Marathon in California in 1963 in 3:37:03, her time was not recorded in the official results. Though she had in fact broken the world record for the women's marathon, bettering the 3:40:22 that Great Britain's Violet Percy ran in 1926, she was never given credit for having done so. Women ran but were not counted. In the eyes of the sport, we were invisible.

We were not entirely without support. In 1958, H. Browning Ross, a former Olympian and the publisher of *Long Distance Log,* a pulp journal for runners, helped form the Road Runners Club of America (RRCA), which became an advocate for women's right to enter races officially. The RRCA also invited women to run in its distance events, which increased women's participation in running and racing during the 1960s, even though our finishing times were still not nationally recognized by running's governing body.

Women also came to distance running through college cross-country, which is how Kathrine Switzer discovered her love of running, first at Lynchburg College in Virginia and then at Syracuse University in New York as a member of the men's cross-country team. It was Syracuse coach Arnie Briggs who helped Switzer gain entry to the 1967 Boston Marathon, in which race director Jock Semple physically tried to remove her from the course. (See the essay "Running to Catch the Hero Inside" on pages 410 through 413 for the complete

*Author's note: My gratitude goes to Pamela Cooper, author of *The American Marathon,* a history published by Syracuse University Press (Syracuse, New York: 1998), for supplying most of the historical facts in this chapter as well as for providing invaluable insights into the development of women's distance running in this country.

story). The series of photos taken of this struggle hit the front page of newspapers around the world, sparking outrage from women and supporters of women's running everywhere and fueling the fight to gain women's acceptance in the sport. The barriers to women's distance racing had cracked and would soon begin to crumble.

At about the same time, the feminist movement had gained considerable momentum. The National Organization for Women (NOW) had been established in 1966, and women were fighting for their rights and proclaiming their strengths like never before.

By 1970, women runners were actively pursuing equal rights at major races across the country. At the 1970 Bay to Breakers 12-K race in San Francisco, roughly a dozen women carried placards that read AAU UNFAIR TO WOMEN and WHO SAYS WOMEN CAN'T RUN? The next year, the AAU raised the race distance limit to 10 miles for all women and also allowed that "selected women" (those who had already run 26.2 miles) could officially race the marathon. Finally, the way had opened for women to become counted as athletes at every distance.

On April 17, 1972, Nina Kuscsik became the first woman to win the Boston Marathon officially. (Kuscsik finished first in 1968 and Sarah Mae Berman won in 1969, 1970, and 1971, but their times were not recorded.) It was also in 1972 that the first running of the Mini Marathon (later known as the L'eggs Mini Marathon, then Advil and now Avon) took place in New York City. This all-women's 10-K grew to 6,000 runners by the late 1970s, drawing not just the fastest runners but women of all abilities because they felt welcomed by this event and comfortable running among women. The Mini, with its festive atmosphere—music, balloons, refreshments afterward—became a model not only for other women's events but for mixed races as well, which embraced the concept of celebration.

Women's running continued to grow through the 1970s and 1980s as races attracted sponsorship. Avon in particular was instrumental in advancing women's running with an international race series that eventually helped lead to the acceptance of the women's marathon in the Olympics. In 1984 in Los Angeles, Joan Benoit Samuelson ran into the coliseum amid the deafening cheers of the crowd and on to the finish line to become the first woman to win an Olympic gold medal in the marathon. Women had indelibly made their mark in distance running. We can thank every woman who would not be denied her right to race, every woman who ran farther than she was supposed to, every woman who fought the bureaucracy for all women's rights to be counted. They opened the way for all of us to run and race and be recognized regardless of ability.

Today, we run not just as training to race but for health and fitness reasons. We participate in races not only to compete but to have fun, to socialize, and sometimes to support a cause, such as breast cancer research.

The 1990s have seen staggering growth in women's running. Perhaps because we were starved for so long from physical and competitive expression through sports, we now gobble it up hungrily. Women's races have exploded in recent years. The Race for the Cure series of mostly women's 5-Ks took place in nearly 90 cities in 1998. The Idaho Women's Fitness Celebration counted more than 19,000 women at its sixth running in September 1998. And consider the marathon, our greatest symbol of women's strength and endurance in running. In 1976, there were only about 800 competitive women marathoners in the world. Only 20 years later, in 1996, 110,880 women completed the marathon in the United States alone. Women's struggle for equality is an international one, however, and although we in the United States now enjoy our place on the roads, we also celebrate the emergence of African runners from the oppression of their culture. Ethiopian Fatuma Roba's victories at the 1997 and 1998 Boston Marathons and Kenyan Tegla Loroupe's world record at the Rotterdam Marathon in The Netherlands in April 1998 signal a new future for the young women of Africa. These women are the heroines and pioneers for a whole new generation.

Significant Moments in the History of Women's Running

Before 1500 B.C.

In ancient Egypt and Sparta, women are encouraged to participate in sports in the belief that it improves reproductive capabilities.

776 B.C.

In Greece, women are not allowed to participate in or even watch any Olympic event. "The punishment for any woman found in Olympia during the games is to be hurled off a cliff." (Jaffe, Rebecca, M.D.: "History of Women in Sports," in Agostini, Rosemary [ed]: *Medical and Orthopedic Issues of Active and Athletic Women,* Philadelphia: Hanley & Belfus, 1994.)

Mid to Late 1800s

- Society considers women frail and unsuited for physical labor or sport. In reality, many women work very hard in factories and fields and in the pioneer movement westward.
- The feminine "ideal" is a woman who is soft and delicate. Her place is in the home, taking care of her husband and children. "Lack of muscles is seen as a virtue, meaning that the husband could afford to hire servants." (Lutter, Judy Mahle: "Sociologic Considerations on Women and Sports," in Agostini, Rosemary [ed]: *Medical and Orthopedic Issues of Active and Athletic Women,* Philadelphia: Hanley & Belfus, 1994.)
- Society emphasizes the importance of the female reproductive system. Too much intellectual or physical activity is said to be harmful to reproduction.
- Physicians and social theorists develop beliefs based on Darwin's concept of "survival of the fittest," which call for restricting women from too much mental or physical effort. "The laws of nature were advanced as reason to closely regulate the mental and physical efforts of women. Perceived as a discrete energy field, the body was believed to contain a specific amount of energy. If excess energy was used in one direction, less would be available for other needs. . . . A woman, it seemed, could not do two things at the same time. Because she was required to spend her energy on the needs of reproduction, any extra effort used in intellectual endeavor or in vigorous physical activity resulted in weakness, disease, infertility, or damage to future generations." (Vertinsky, Patricia: "Women, Sport, and Exercise in the 19th Century," in Costa, D. Margaret, and Guthrie, Sharon R. [eds]: *Women and Sport,* Champaign, Illinois: Human Kinetics, 1994).

1891

The first recorded woman's running event takes place near Dublin, Ireland. "It was approximately 100 yards and was won by Eva Francisco in 13 seconds" (Colliton, Julie Wentworth, M.D.: "Running," in Costa, D. Margaret, and Guthrie, Sharon R. [eds.]: *Women and Sport,* Champaign, Illinois: Human Kinetics, 1994).

1896

At the first modern Olympic games held in Athens, a woman named Melpomene runs the marathon unofficially. She spends 3 weeks training in secret and then runs the distance in 4 1/2 hours—1 1/2 hours slower than the winner but ahead of other male contestants.

Early 1920s

The Industrial Leagues are formed; companies sponsor teams to compete in various sports. In 1923, the Prudential Insurance Company becomes one of the first to field a women's track team.

1918

Marie Ledru completes the French Marathon.

1921

Alice Milliat of France becomes the leader of the Fédération Sportive Féminine Internationale, which organizes the Women's Olympics in response to the International Olympic Committee's (IOC) rejection of petitions to include more events for women, including track and field, in the Olympic games. Milliat is also extremely influential in bringing about nine international conferences on women's sports held in cities all over Europe.

1922

The first Women's Olympic Games (Olympiques Féminins) are held in Paris. They take place every 4 years until 1934 in London, where teams from 19 countries compete.

1924

Violet Percy of Great Britain runs a marathon in 3 hours 40 minutes 22 seconds.

1928

The success of the Women's Olympics and the strength of Milliat's federation is an embarrassment to the International Amateur Athletic Federation (IAAF), which convinces the IOC to allow track and field at the Amsterdam Games. The events are the 100 meters, 800 meters, 4 × 100-meter relay, high jump, and discus throw.

At the end of the 800-meter race, it was reported that several of the runners staggered across the finish line. Some were said to have collapsed, and the *New York Times* blamed women's physical inadequacy. International pressure forces the IOC to reverse their decision and strike women's track and field from the games.

1930

Gustavus Kirby, president of the AAU and the American representative to the IAAF, threatens a boycott of men's track and field at the 1932 Olympics if women are not accepted. The IOC again reverses its decision but does not allow women to compete in races longer than 200 meters, and this ban is not lifted until the 1960 games.

1932

At the Los Angeles Olympics, Tidye Pickett of Chicago and Louise Stokes of Malden, Massachusetts, become the first black women to be selected to a U.S. Olympic team. "When they arrived in Los Angeles with the women's track squad as part of the relay team for the Games, however, they were denied the opportunity to compete" (Welch, Paula, and Costa, D. Margaret: "A Century of Olympic Competition," in Costa, D. Margaret, and Guthrie, Sharon R. [eds] *Women and Sport,* Champaign, Illinois: Human Kinetics, 1994).

1948

Ignoring assertions that she is too old to compete at a world-class level, Francina (Fanny) Blankers-Koen of Amsterdam, The Netherlands, age 30, a housewife and mother of two, wins a record four Olympic gold medals in track and field (100 meters, 200 meters, 80 meters, and 4 × 100-meter relay). She is nicknamed the "Flying Dutch Housewife." The following headline appears in the *Daily Graphic,* a London newspaper: FASTEST WOMAN IN THE WORLD IS AN EXPERT COOK.

1958

The RRCA is formed. Part of its mission is to get the AAU to officially approve women's long-distance running.

1960

At the Rome Olympics, Wilma Rudolph wins gold medals in the 100 meters, 200 meters, and the 4 × 100-meter relay. On returning to the United States, she is given the Sullivan Award as the year's outstanding female athlete. Rudolph was born in Clarksville, Tennessee, the twentieth of 22 children of a railroad porter and cleaning woman. She overcame polio in her youth to become an athlete and gain a scholarship to Tennessee State University, where she excelled at track prior to competing in the Olympics.

Thanksgiving Day, 1960

Julia Chase, an 18-year-old first-year student at Smith College and the New England AAU 880-yard women's champion, is denied entry to the 4.75-mile Manchester Road Race. The next year, she is allowed to participate, though not officially, and is not permitted through the finishing chutes.

1965

The first women's cross-country race to be officially recognized in the United States takes place in Seattle. The distance is 1.5 miles, and Marie Mulder wins.

1966

Roberta Gibb Bingay jumps into the Boston Marathon with no runner's number and completes the distance in 3 hours 20 minutes.

1967

Kathrine Switzer gains official entry to the Boston Marathon, which is still not open to women. When race director Jock Semple sees that a woman is running his race, he tries to remove her physically but is prevented from doing so. Switzer goes on to finish the marathon in a time of 4 hours 20 minutes. (For more on her story, see "Running to Catch the Hero Inside" on pages 410 to 413)

1972

Title IX of the Education Act of 1972 is passed:

No person . . . shall, on the basis of sex, be excluded from participation in, be denied the benefits of, or be subjected to discrimination under any educational programs or activities receiving federal financial assistance.

1972

At the Munich Olympics, women compete in the 1,500 meters for the first time. The gold medal goes to Soviet Lyudmila Bragina, who runs 4:01.

1973

Susan Hollander of Hamden, Connecticut, sues the local school board for the right to run on the boys' cross-country team, since there is no girls' team. The judge rules against her, saying, "Athletic competition builds character in our boys. We do not need that kind of character in our girls" (Guttman, Allen: *Women's Sports: A History,* New York: Columbia University Press, 1991).

1974

The first International Women's Marathon, organized by physician and women's running advocate Ernst van Aaken, is held in Waldniel, West Germany, on September 22. There are 45 entrants, 9 from the United States.

1978

- Avon sponsors and organizes (under the direction of Kathrine Switzer) an international circuit of women's races, which culminates in the International Women's Marathon championship race.
- On October 22, Grete Waitz of Norway wins her first of nine New York City Marathon titles in a world record time of 2:32:30.

1982

The IAAF finally recognizes women's world records in 5,000- and 10,000-meter races.

1984

At the Los Angeles Olympics, women are finally allowed to compete in the marathon. Joan Benoit (later Samuelson) wins the gold. The women's 3,000 is also added for the first time and is won by Romanian Maricica Puica in a time of 8:35.

A LEGENDARY RUNNER

Ovid, in *Metamorphoses,* tells a story of Atalanta, who, abandoned in infancy, is raised by a she-bear. She becomes a woman of exceptional physical prowess and can match any man in hunting, wrestling, and running, the latter of which she uses as a means to escape matrimony—for a while, anyway. Not too keen on the idea of marriage, Atalanta declares that she will marry the first man who can outrun her. Several suitors try, but she defeats them all. One, Melanion, has a plan. He acquires three golden apples from Aphrodite, which he carries with him in his race with Atalanta. Whenever she begins to get too far ahead, he tosses one of the apples in her path, for which she pauses. Eventually, Melanion outruns her and takes her for his wife.

1985

Ingrid Kristiansen breaks the world record for the marathon with a 2:21:06 victory at London. This mark will stand for 13 years.

1987

Priscilla Welch, age 42, wins the New York City Marathon.

1988

At the Seoul Olympics, the women's 10,000-meter race is added to the games and Soviet Olga Bondarenko wins the gold in 31:05.

1989

Liz McColgan of Great Britain runs 30:39 for the 10-K to set a new world record.

1992

- Derartu Tulu of Ethiopia wins the 10,000-meter at the Barcelona Olympics, to become the first African woman ever to win an Olympic gold medal.
- Lynn Jennings wins her third straight World Cross-Country Championships.

1996

The women's 5,000 meters replaces the 3,000 at the Olympics in Atlanta, and Wang Junxia of China wins the gold in 14:59. Previously, men had been allowed to run the 5,000, whereas women ran the 3,000.

1997

Lydia Cheromei of Kenya sets a new world record for the 5-K with a time of 14:58.

1998

- Elana Meyer of South Africa sets a new world record for the half-marathon with a time of 1:07:29.
- Kenyan Tegla Loroupe sets a new world record for the marathon on April 19 at the Rotterdam Marathon in The Netherlands, finishing in 2:20:47.

Running to Catch the
Hero Inside

BY KATHRINE SWITZER

SOMETIMES I SAY I RUN BECAUSE IT MAKES ME FEEL POWERFUL, accomplished, and confident. Other times, I run because running gives me vision, creativity, and religion. It's also true that I run because it helps me keep my weight down, keeps me regular, prevents headaches, and puts workday frazzles in perspective. Mostly, though, I run because it makes me feel like a hero.

I think I would always have run and been active in the women's running movement, but a unique history compelled me to make running, in one way or the other, my life's work. Because my life's work also makes me feel like a hero, that history is worth retelling.

In 1967, I was a 20-year-old student at Syracuse University in New York, training with the men's cross-country team. The university had no intercollegiate women's sports. I felt privileged to be an equal among these men and to call them my friends.

That included my 50-year-old coach, Arnie Briggs. Inspired by his Boston stories, I ran 31 miles with him one day in practice and asked him to take me to Boston. Despite the publicity that followed Roberta Gibb's unofficial first run in a quality time of 3 hours 20 minutes the year before, Arnie, like many men, needed convincing. Boston was my mecca. I craved running with the 600 other pilgrims who went annually. I finally persuaded Arnie, and he insisted that I register officially. We found no rules forbidding women.

I signed my name with my initials: K. V. Switzer. It is now the stuff of legends how the Boston official Jock Semple thought I was a man and issued me race numbers along with those for my Syracuse teammates, Arnie and my boyfriend, Tom Miller, a 235-pound hammer thrower. Tom was sure he could run it if I could. It was a miserable, sleeting, 33-degree day, and I dressed in baggy gray sweats. My prerace jitters dissipated as more and more men approached me with encouragement. Many asked how to get their wives to run. The gun went off. My dream was beginning.

At 4 miles, it turned into a nightmare. The press truck passed us and I could hear a barrage of cameras snapping. The race director, Will Cloney, stepped into my path to shake a menacing finger at me. I sidestepped him.

Then I heard quick scrabbling steps behind me and turned as a ferocious Semple grabbed me by the shirt and shoulders, spun me around, and screamed, "Get the hell out of my race and give me those numbers!" For a second, I was paralyzed with fear, embarrassed beyond words.

Arnie tried to pull Jock away, saying, "She's okay; I've trained her," but Jock was like a terrier, clenching my shirt. "Stay out of this, Arnie!"

There was a flash in my peripheral vision, then a crunch. Big Tom hit Jock with a flying shoulder block and sent him through the air. There was another thump when he landed. Now I was truly frightened. A wide-eyed Arnie shouted, "Run like hell!" and away we ran, cursing and crying, the press truck accelerating in hot pursuit, spilling cameramen.

It's appalling and funny in the retelling. Jock raced to the finish to have me expelled from the Amateur Athletic Union, an institution never known for its flexibility. The press truck hovered until they realized I was serious about finishing. I had 22 miles ahead and was sure the cops would drag me off (fear creates paranoia), but I was going to finish. If I didn't, people would say that women couldn't do it. Proving women's capability wasn't my original motive, but priorities change.

In those 22 miles, I grew from girl to woman. I realized that I was lucky to have parents and someone like Arnie who had encouraged my daring. I knew other women would run if they had the opportunities. By the time I finished, 4 hours 20 minutes later, I was determined to create opportunities for them. I was also determined to be a better athlete.

The photos of the Semple clash flashed around the world. Other women began to take Boston as their proving ground and spiritual center. Night after night, training 100 miles a week in the dark after work, I'd think of Nina Kuscsik and Sara Mae Berman doing the same. We ran times the world noticed. We organized clubs and events. We strategized together. Today, when times are tough with jobs and kids, it still inspires me.

In 1972, Boston accepted the legislative changes we worked for and admitted us officially. Jock and Will became ebullient supporters. Jock loved being teased as the man who blazed the trail for women's running . . . in spite of himself.

I was able to make training a priority and finished second in 2:51 in 1975, my seventh Boston. Although it was the third best time in the United States and sixth best in the world that year, my overwhelming feeling was that thousands of women could run better if they had the opportunity. Other strong-willed runners felt the same. We made inclusion of the marathon into the Olympic games our goal.

The International Olympic Committee (IOC) still believed that women were too weak for distance running. They confirmed this myth by having no programs to disprove it, so event organization became my focus.

I came up with a plan for a grand prix of women's distance races, culminating in an annual international marathon—in effect, a world championship. Avon Cosmetics hired me and within 3 years, we had events in 21 countries. A public-relations program turned into a social revolution when thousands of women responded.

The national federations were stunned. I'll never forget seeing women in Brazil and Thailand turning up with no shoes . . . not running shoes—no shoes at all. These Avon races gave them self-esteem and gave me the proudest moments of my life.

They also provided statistics the IOC couldn't ignore. The medical evidence demolished the final myth, showing women have inherent capability in endurance events. In 1981, the IOC voted to include the women's marathon event.

The revolution was won at the moment in 1984 when Joan Benoit ran out of the tunnel and into the Olympic stadium in Los Angeles in front of a television audience of 2.2 billion. The finish was beamed into tradition-bound households from Saudi Arabia to America. Every culture knows that 26 miles 385 yards (42.2 kilometers) is a long race. To see a woman run it with such courage and brilliance showed the world that women, too, can be heroes.

I was working in the TV booth then, trying to keep calm while my mind was reeling back to Bostons I'd seen Joan run—and that so many of us had run—laying the groundwork for this moment.

Since then, I've worked in lots of TV booths, covering 20 Boston and 14 New York City Marathons, as well as hundreds of other races. The women in those races today—Tegla Loroupe, Uta Pippig, Elana Meyer—

all are heroes and inspire me, just as their predecessors—Lorraine Moller, Grete Waitz, Ingrid Kristiansen—did.

Equally inspiring, however, are the unknown girls and women I'm working with in places like Malaysia, China, and the Philippines. They have so little, and it's a thrill to give them a start. As I write this, I'm back as program director of Avon Running Global Women's Circuit. After a 12-year hiatus, Avon has returned to the sponsorship that transformed the sport for women and helped create equality in it. Now our ambition is to take the acceptance we strove so hard to achieve to the next level: to accessibility. We want to give every woman an opportunity to use running as a means to fitness and health and, if she wants, competitive development.

The great thing is, she'll say she's running for her weight or her health or whatever, but the real reason she runs is for the same reason I do. She runs because she feels like a hero.

Kathrine Switzer is the author of *Running and Walking for Women Over 40: The Road to Sanity and Vanity* (New York: St. Martin's Press, 1998). Parts of this article appeared previously in the *New York Times*.

Appendix

Pace Yourself

The following chart was developed by Jack Daniels, Ph.D., an exercise physiologist and the head track and cross-country coach at the State University of New York at Cortland in New York.

You can use this chart in two ways. First, by finding your current race time in one column, you can look across to see what your predicted finishing race time would be at another distance. For example, if you can run a 5-K in about 25 minutes, you should be able to finish a marathon in just under 4 hours.

Second, you can use this chart to figure out how fast to do your different training runs. Let's say your most recent race time for a 5-K is about 24 minutes; you should do your easy runs or long runs at a little under a 10-minute-per-mile pace. If you were doing a tempo workout, you would run the tempo portion at roughly an 8:10-minute-per-mile pace. Pace workouts (also called intervals) are run at your 5-K race pace, which for a 24-minute 5-K is about a 7:45-minute-per-mile pace.

PACE PER MILE

5-K	10-K	Half-Marathon	Marathon	Easy Long Runs	Tempo Run	Pace Workout
32:27	67:29	2:29:09	5:05:09	12:55	10:48	10:28
30:40	63:46	2:21:04	4:49:17	12:16	10:18	9:53
29:05	60:26	2:13:49	4:34:59	11:41	9:47	9:23
27:39	57:26	2:07:16	4:22:03	11:09	9:20	8:55
26:22	54:44	2:01:19	4:10:19	10:40	8:55	8:30
25:12	52:17	1:55:55	3:59:35	10:14	8:33	8:08
24:08	50:03	1:50:59	3:49:35	9:50	8:12	7:47
23:09	48:01	1:46:27	3:40:43	9:28	7:52	7:28
22:15	46:09	1:42:17	3:32:23	9:07	7:33	7:10
21:25	44:25	1:38:27	3:24:39	8:48	7:17	6:55
20:39	42:50	1:34:53	3:17:29	8:31	7:03	6:40
19:57	41:21	1:31:35	3:10:49	8:14	6:50	6:26
19:17	39:59	1:28:31	3:04:36	7:59	6:38	6:13
18:40	38:42	1:25:40	2:58:47	7:45	6:26	6:01
18:05	37:31	1:23:00	2:53:20	7:31	6:15	5:50
17:33	36:24	1:20:30	2:48:14	7:19	6:04	5:40

For More Information

There are many resources for information on running, racing, health, and nutrition, but the following are some of my favorites.

Magazines and Newsletters

Runner's World magazine, available at newsstands everywhere
web site: **www.runnersworld.com**

Running Research News (monthly newsletter on training and nutrition)
P.O. Box 27041
Lansing, MI 48909
phone: (517) 371-4897
web site: **www.gisd.com/rrn/**

On the Roads (the official monthly publication of the Road Running Information Center of USA Track and Field)
5522 Camino Cerralvo
Santa Barbara, CA 93111
phone: (805) 683-5868

National Masters News (monthly publication dedicated to the master—over-40—runner)
P.O. Box 16597
North Hollywood, CA 91615
phone: (818) 760-8983

Books

HEALTH AND EXERCISE

The Bodywise Woman, 2nd ed., by Judy Mahle Lutter and Lynn Jaffe (Champaign, Illinois: Human Kinetics, 1996)
The Exercise–Health Connection, by David C. Nieman, Dr. P.H. (Champaign, Illinois: Human Kinetics, 1998)
Exercising Through Your Pregnancy, by James F. Clapp III, M.D. (Champaign, Illinois: Human Kinetics, 1998)

SPORTS NUTRITION

Nancy Clark's Sports Nutrition Guidebook, 2nd ed., by Nancy Clark, M.S., R.D. (Champaign, Illinois: Human Kinetics, 1997)

INSPIRATION
The Quotable Runner, by Mark Will-Weber (New York: Breakaway Books, 1995)

The Elements of Effort, by John Jerome (New York: Breakaway Books, 1997)

THE MIND AND PERFORMANCE
Thinking Body, Dancing Mind, by Chungliang Al Huang and Jerry Lynch (New York: Bantam, 1992)

INJURIES
Healthy Runner's Handbook, by Lyle J. Micheli and Mark Jenkins (Champaign, Illinois: Human Kinetics, 1996)

HISTORY
Boston: A Century of Running, by Hal Higdon (Emmaus, Pennsylvania: Rodale Press, 1995)

The American Marathon, by Pamela Cooper (Syracuse, New York: Syracuse University Press, 1998)

Women's Sports: A History, by Allen Guttmann (New York: Columbia University Press, 1991)

Organizations

American Running and Fitness Association
Provides information on training, health, injury prevention, and more

4405 East West Highway, suite 405

Bethesda, MD 20814

phone: 800-776-2732

web site: **www.arfa.org**

Fifty-Plus Fitness Association
An organization dedicated to research on aging and exercise and providing information to active older adults

Box D

Stanford, CA 94309

phone: (415) 323-6160

web site: **www.pamf.org/fiftyplus/fiftyindex.html**

Melpomene Institute for Women's Research
The only nonprofit research organization dedicated to women's health and physical activity
1010 University Avenue
St. Paul, MN 55104
phone: 612-642-1951
web site: **www.melpomene.org**

Road Runners Club of America
The national association of not-for-profit running clubs; offers publications on women's running, safety, children's running, how to start a running club and more
1150 S. Washington Street, suite 250
Arlington, VA 22314
phone: (703) 836-0558
web site: **www.rrca.org**

Index